T0325353

ing Slip

Page 1 of 1

Purchase Order Number	
53639579	

Invoice #	Shipment #	Date
2247051	S433329001	04/12/2016

& NOBLE DISTRIBUTION
ES AND NOBLE WAY STE B
TOWNSHIP, NJ 08831-3417

Send Product Returns to:
WILEY RETURNS
380 FREIGHT STREET
CAMP HILL, PA 17011

	Qty	List Price	Disc.	Net Price	Ext Net Price
	1	129.95	34.00%	85.76	85.76
ed:	1				85.76

erms: COLLECT

# of Cartons: 1
Total Weight: 1.54

| 36824 | 005 | OW5 | 473886 | **002** | ATT 2857 | |

Location	Qty	Item	Description
350 – 036 – 10	1	9781118931653	ENVIRONMENTAL EXPERIENCE

Type OW5   Qty 1   Plan# 36824   Parcel# 152509815

Group# 473886

Seq# 2857   **002**

WILEY

BILL TO

BARNES & NOBLE DISTRIBUTION
PO BOX 1843
WESTBURY, NY 11590-9010

For Customer Service Call: (800) 225-5945

ISBN	Description
9781118931653	ENVIRONMENTAL EXPERIEN

Total Quantit

Carrier: UPS COLLECT GROUND
PRO#:

Frei

Environmental Experience and Plasticity of the Developing Brain

To my Mentors, Teachers, and Friends, Prof. Lamberto Maffei and Prof. Floriano Papi, as a sign of respect and gratitude.

Environmental Experience and Plasticity of the Developing Brain

EDITED BY

Alessandro Sale

WILEY Blackwell

Published by John Wiley & Sons, Inc., Hoboken, New Jersey
Published simultaneously in Canada

For general information on our other products and services or for technical support, please contact our Customer Care Department within the United States at (800) 762-2974, outside the United States at (317) 572-3993 or fax (317) 572-4002.

Wiley also publishes its books in a variety of electronic formats. Some content that appears in print may not be available in electronic formats. For more information about Wiley products, visit our web site at www.wiley.com.

Library of Congress Cataloging-in-Publication Data applied for:

9781118931653 (cloth)

Printed and bound in Malaysia by Vivar Printing Sdn Bhd

1   2016

Contents

List of contributors

Enrico Alleva
Section of Behavioral Neurosciences, Department of Cell Biology and Neurosciences, Istituto Superiore di Sanità, Rome, Italy

Gordon A. Barr
Department of Anesthesiology and Critical Care Medicine, The Children's Hospital of Philadelphia, Philadelphia, Pennsylvania, USA; Perelman School of Medicine, University of Pennsylvania, Philadelphia, Pennsylvania, USA

Nicoletta Berardi
Department of Neuroscience, Psychology, Drug Research and Child Health NEUROFARBA, University of Florence, Florence, Italy

Giovanni Cioni
Department of Clinical and Experimental Medicine, Pisa University, Pisa, Italy; Department of Developmental Neuroscience, Stella Maris Scientific Institute, Pisa, Italy

Francesca Cirulli
Section of Behavioral Neurosciences, Department of Cell Biology and Neurosciences, Istituto Superiore di Sanità, Rome, Italy

Sean P. Coyne
Department of Comparative Human Development, The University of Chicago, Chicago, Illinois, USA

Jenalee R. Doom
Institute of Child Development, University of Minnesota, Minneapolis, Minnesota, USA

Megan R. Gunnar
Institute of Child Development, University of Minnesota, Minneapolis, Minnesota, USA

Andrea Guzzetta
Department of Clinical and Experimental Medicine, Pisa University, Pisa, Italy; Department of Developmental Neuroscience, Stella Maris Scientific Institute, Pisa, Italy; SMILE Lab, Stella Maris Scientific Institute, Pisa, Italy

Anthony J. Hannan
Florey Institute of Neuroscience and Mental Health, University of Melbourne, Parkville, Australia; Department of Anatomy and Neuroscience, University of Melbourne, Parkville, Australia

Mari A. Kondo
Department of Psychiatry and Behavioral Sciences, Johns Hopkins University School of Medicine, Baltimore, Maryland, USA

Michael J. Lewis
Department of Psychology, Hunter College, City University of New York, Manhattan, New York, USA; Institute of Human Nutrition, Columbia College of Physicians and Surgeons, Columbia University, New York, New York, USA

Dario Maestripieri
Department of Comparative Human Development, The University of Chicago, Chicago, Illinois, USA

Lamberto Maffei
Neuroscience Institute, National Research Council (CNR), Pisa, Italy

Rhiannon M. Meredith
Center for Neurogenomics & Cognitive Research (CNCR), VU University Amsterdam, Amsterdam, The Netherlands

Tommaso Pizzorusso
Neuroscience Institute, National Research Council (CNR), Pisa, Italy; Department of Neuroscience, Psychology, Drug Research and Child Health (NEUROFARBA), University of Florence, Florence, Italy

Elena Putignano
Neuroscience Institute, National Research Council (CNR), Pisa, Italy

Tania L. Roth
Department of Psychological and Brain Sciences, University of Delaware, Newark, Delaware, USA

Alessandro Sale
Neuroscience Institute, National Research Council (CNR), Pisa, Italy

Regina M. Sullivan
Emotional Brain Institute, Nathan Kline Institute, Orangeburg, New York, USA; Child and Adolescent Psychiatry, New York University Langone Medical Center, New York, USA

Moshe Szyf
Department of Pharmacology and Therapeutics, McGill University, Montreal, Quebec, Canada

Paola Tognini
Neuroscience Institute, National Research Council (CNR), Pisa, Italy

CHAPTER 1

Environmental enrichment and brain development

Alessandro Sale[1], Nicoletta Berardi[2], and Lamberto Maffei[1]

[1] Neuroscience Institute, National Research Council (CNR), Pisa, Italy

[2] Department of Neuroscience, Psychology, Drug Research and Child Health NEUROFARBA, University of Florence, Florence, Italy

Introduction: critical periods and experience-dependent plasticity in brain circuits

The term "plasticity" refers to the ability of the nervous system to reorganize its connections functionally and structurally in response to changes in environmental experience. This property underlies the adaptive development and remodeling of neuronal circuitry that makes brain development, behavioral flexibility, and long-term memory possible.

Plasticity is particularly high during developmental time windows called critical periods (CPs), when experience is crucial in promoting and regulating neural maturation and, consequently, the behavioral traits of the newborn, in every vertebrate species tested so far, from birds to rodents to primates (Berardi et al., 2000). Essentially, a CP is a phase of exceptionally high sensitivity to experience displayed by developing neural circuits. During CPs, experience exerts a key role in building the precise assembly of connections that endows each individual with his/her unique characteristics. Different species show different CPs for the same function, in good accordance with a different time course of development and life span. On the other hand, distinct functions show different CPs in the same species, correlating with different time courses of development in different brain areas.

Essential information on developmental brain plasticity and CPs has been provided by studies focusing on the primary visual cortex (V1), which has been for decades the election model for studying experience-dependent plasticity in the brain. The pioneering experiments performed by Hubel and Wiesel showed how dramatically can early sensory deprivation affect the anatomy and physiology of the visual cortex (Figure 1.1). Many neurons in the visual cortex are binocular, that is, receive input from both eyes, and exhibit different degrees of dominance from either eye, a property called ocular dominance. Hubel and

Environmental Experience and Plasticity of the Developing Brain, First Edition.
Edited by Alessandro Sale.
© 2016 John Wiley & Sons, Inc. Published 2016 by John Wiley & Sons, Inc.

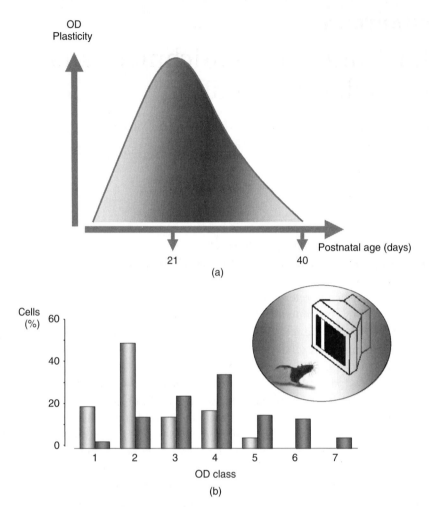

Figure 1.1 Critical period (CP) for ocular dominance plasticity in the rat visual cortex. (a) Schematic representation of the time course of CP for ocular dominance plasticity in the rat, which peaks around postnatal day (P) 21 and is definitively closed by the age of P45. (b) Single unit recordings from the primary visual cortex allow classification of neurons with respect to their ocular preferences: in a typical recording from a nondeprived animal (light cyan columns), cells in class 1 are activated exclusively by the contralateral eye, cells in class 7 are activated exclusively by the ipsilateral eye, neurons in classes 2–3 and 5–6 are activated to varying degrees by both eyes, and neurons in class 4 respond equally to both eyes. Following closure of the contralateral eye from 1 week during the CP, cells become much more responsive toward the ipsilateral open eye, at the expense of the deprived eye (dark cyan columns). (See insert for color representation of this figure.)

Wiesel reported that, early in development, reducing the visual input to one eye by means of lid suture, a treatment classically referred to as monocular deprivation (MD), disrupts ocular dominance of V1 cells, with a loss of neurons driven by the deprived eye and a strong increment in the number of cells driven by the open eye, and reduces the number of binocular neurons (Wiesel and Hubel, 1963). The imbalance of activity between the two eyes results in remarkable anatomical changes in V1, with a shrinkage of the deprived eye ocular dominance columns, those layer IV regions that receive thalamic inputs driven by the closed eye, and in the expansion of the open eye's columns (Hubel et al., 1977; Shatz and Stryker, 1978; LeVay et al., 1980; Antonini and Stryker, 1993), accompanied by a remodeling of cortical horizontal connections (Trachtenberg and Stryker, 2001). At the behavioral level, if the condition of MD is protracted for a long period during development, it eventually leads to lower than normal visual acuity and contrast sensitivity values for the deprived eye (amblyopia), together with a deterioration of binocular vision. Strikingly, the same manipulation of visual experience appeared to be ineffective in the adult (LeVay et al., 1980), leading to the characterization of the first and most widely studied example of CP (Berardi et al., 2000; Berardi et al., 2003; Knudsen, 2004; Hensch, 2005a, 2005b; Levelt and Hubener, 2012).

Another well-studied CP is that regulating age-dependent changes in fear memory acquisition, which in rodents emerges at the end of the second postnatal week of life (Akers et al., 2012). Interestingly, the potential for fear extinction does also follow a CP, displaying a permanent fear erasure in preadolescent mice but leading to incomplete erasure and thus persisting or returning fear responses in juveniles about 10 days older.

In humans, CPs have been documented for several brain modalities (Figure 1.2). Examples of CPs in the sensory domain are those for the maturation of visual acuity and stereopsis, the acquisition of language-specific abilities in phonemic perception, and the acquisition of gustatory and olfactory preferences (Lewis and Maurer, 2005; Werker and Tees, 2005; Ventura and Worobey, 2013). A particularly relevant case of olfactory learning regulated by a CP is that underlying maternal attachment, clearly present in newborn babies and well described at the neurobiological level in rodents (see also the chapter by Sullivan and colleagues in this book [Chapter 6]). CPs in humans have been also found for second language acquisition, both speech and sign language, or for proficient performance in musical instrument playing (Bengtsson et al., 2005; Kuhl, 2010).

As in the case of MD, the importance of a proper experience during the CP is made particularly clear by the detrimental effects caused by its absence or deterioration, like in the classic example of the negative effects in the social/affective domain produced by rearing under conditions in which the mother is absent or early removed and sufficient maternal care levels are not available (Sullivan et al., 2006). Developmental plasticity, indeed, is by itself neither good nor bad, it simply takes its course, allowing the system to proceed toward an adaptive developmental trajectory when the stimuli are adequate and available, or instead resulting in severe and even permanent deficits under harsh environmental conditions. Thus, while the existence of a mechanism by which high levels of plasticity during the CP are followed by an abrupt reduction of circuit modifiability after its closure is likely to provide adaptive advantages

Plasticity

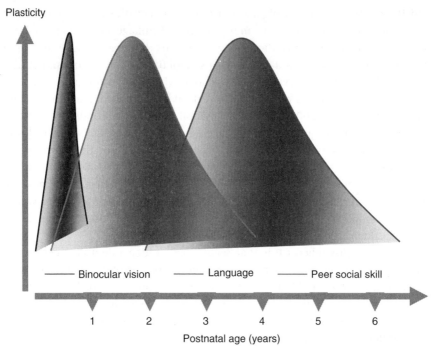

———— Binocular vision   ———— Language   ———— Peer social skill

1   2   3   4   5   6

Postnatal age (years)

Figure 1.2 Critical periods across brain functions in humans. The picture represents a schematic of the critical period time course for acquisition of binocular vision, language learning, and adequate peer social skills in children. Different functions display different time courses, both in terms of total duration of the heightened sensitivity window and concerning the age of onset and closure of the potential for plasticity. In the three curves, levels of plasticity have been normalized to the peak. (See insert for color representation of this figure.)

in terms of the possibility to fix the acquired neural assemblies without the need of continuous maintenance, it may also expose the nervous system to severe dysfunctions when development is perturbed.

Importantly, the potential for recovery after reestablishment of proper environmental conditions can also be regulated by CPs, with studies in postinstitutionalized children demonstrating that the most severe and persisting effects of raising children in impoverished environments lacking sufficient social stimuli are more likely to be documented when adoption occurs beyond 4–6 months of age (for a comprehensive survey of the literature on the effects of institutional deprivation, see the chapter by Doom and Gunar in this book [Chapter 9]).

Not surprisingly, much effort in Neuroscience research is currently devoted to understanding the molecular mechanisms underlying the closure or the sudden reduction of plasticity at the end of the CPs. Among the most promising candidates are factors exerting a key role as plasticity brakes, such as critical components of the extracellular matrix, that is, the chondroitin sulphate proteoglycans that surround neuronal cell bodies in structures called perineuronal nets, myelin-related Nogo receptors, proteins belonging to the newly discovered class called Lynx family, epigenetic regulators of the functional state of chromatin such as histone deacetylase inhibitors, and the maturation of intracortical GABAergic interneurons (Bavelier et al., 2010; Nabel and Morishita, 2013).

Optimization of environmental stimulation: environmental enrichment

In parallel to the Hubel and Wiesel seminal work based on a sensory depriva-tion approach, fundamental contributions to the knowledge of how experience affects brain development have been provided by the group of Rosenzweig and colleagues, using the so-called environmental enrichment (EE) paradigm. Origi-nally defined as "a combination of complex inanimate and social stimulation" (Rosenzweig et al., 1978), EE is performed in wide cages where the animals are reared in large social groups and in the presence of a variety of objects, like tunnels, nesting material, stairs, and plastic recoveries, that are changed by the experimenter at least once a week in order to stimulate the explorative behav-ior, curiosity, and attentional processes of the animals. An essential component of EE is voluntary physical exercise, the opportunity to attain high levels of motor activity on dedicated devices, such as running wheels. The EE definition and description is based on the comparison with alternative rearing conditions, such as the standard condition, in which the animals are reared in small social groups and in very simple cages where no particular objects other than nesting mate-rial, food, and water are present, and the very simple impoverished condition, in which social interactions are impossible because the animals are reared alone in individual cages. Compared with these more simplified environments, EE gives the animals the opportunity for structured social interaction, multisensory stimulation, and increased levels of physical activity.

Since its original introduction in the early 1960s, extensive work has been done investigating the impact of EE on the morphology, chemistry, and physiol-ogy of the brain, for the vast majority focusing on adult subjects (Rosenzweig and Bennett, 1996; van Praag et al., 2000; Diamond, 2001; Sale et al., 2009). The ben-eficial results associated with EE are as various as the fantasy of the researchers in documenting them: enriched animals display a marked improvement in complex cognitive functions and reduced stress reactivity, are characterized by increased levels of hippocampal long-term potentiation (LTP) and have robust increments in cortical thickness and weight, together with modifications of neuronal mor-phology in terms of increased dendritic arborization, number of dendritic spines, synaptic density, and postsynaptic thickening, occurring in several brain regions (Baroncelli et al., 2010).

Even if EE may appear as a way of rearing the animals in a semi-naturalistic setting more similar to the wild life, the beneficial effects observed in enriched

animals cannot be simply interpreted as a functional restoration to a more physiological condition from deficits caused by living in the typical deprived setting
imposed on laboratory animals. Indeed, the most commonly used strains of rats
and mice are highly inbred animals, maintained for hundreds of generations in
artificial enclosures, thus subjected to a strong genetic drift responsible for main
differences in their gene pool with respect to the natural populations (see Sale
et al., 2014). Thus, which kind of environmental stimuli can be considered physiological or "naturalistic" is not immediately clear for these strains. Moreover,
differently from the condition characterized by multiple contingencies and risks
associated with living in the wild, enriched animals are totally free to choose
when and how much to explore the surroundings and thus to experience the
enriched stimuli, living in a danger-free environment much more similar, in
human terms, to a well-equipped playroom than a jungle.

Environmental enrichment and visual system development

Despite the interest raised by the possibility to induce beneficial effects on brain
and behavior by means of environmental manipulations, most studies addressing
the impact of EE remained focused on adults, leaving almost unexplored the
question of whether an enhanced environmental stimulation can also affect
brain development, modulating the processes that govern maturation of neural
circuits in the central nervous system. This fundamental issue is at the core of
the classic debate about the role of nature and nurture, or, in more biological
terms, genes and environment, in the construction of brain architecture and its
functional output, the behavior. While the widely accepted consensus is that
genes and environment work in concert in shaping neural circuits and behavior,
the contribution of specific genetic programs to brain development has been
characterized much earlier in the debate, with studies concerning the impact of
environment remaining for a long time at a merely descriptive level of analysis.

Since early EE provides increased sensory stimulation during CPs, when
anatomical and functional rearrangements of the cerebral cortex proceed at
their maximum level, it might be expected that procedures aimed at increasing
the intensity and optimizing the quality of experience might elicit robust
brain changes through experience-dependent plasticity processes. Accordingly,
preweaning EE has been sporadically shown to result in more complex dendritic
branching in cortical pyramidal cells, particularly in the parieto-occipital cortex
(Venable et al., 1989), to promote an earlier neuronal cytodifferentiation in
the rat motor cortex, correlating with better performance in a number of
motor adaptive responses (Pascual and Figueroa, 1996), and to significantly
increase ippocampal and cortical expression levels of the neural cell adhesion
molecule (NCAM), synaptophysin, and brain-derived neurotrophic factor
(BDNF) (Koo et al., 2003).

What remained almost unknown for long time was the actual extent of the impact of the environment on brain development at the very functional level, such as in terms of maturation of fine neuronal properties. With the aim to fill this gap, some years ago our group started a series of studies focusing on visual system maturation in environmentally enriched rodents. In this new approach, the rigorous and highly quantitative methodology typical of visual system research has been combined with the theoretical framework of the EE paradigm, resulting in quite a powerful new tool that allowed us to open a window on the dynamic building of the brain according to different levels of environmental stimulation (Sale et al., 2009) (Figure 1.3).

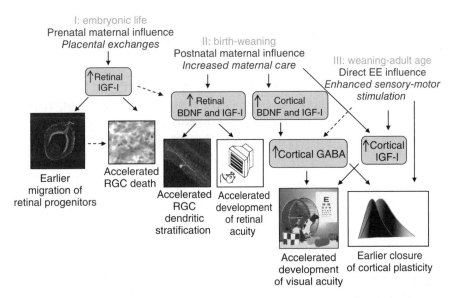

Figure 1.3 Environmental enrichment and visual system development acceleration: a three phases model. The figure depicts an interpretative framework of the data regarding EE effects on the developing visual system. Three consecutive temporal phases are differently controlled by the richness of the environment: (I) a prenatal phase in which the mother mediates the influence of the environment through placental exchanges with the fetus, leading to an accelerated anatomical retinal development that is mostly due to increased levels of IGF-1; (II) an early postnatal phase in which enhanced maternal care received by EE pups stimulates the expression of experience-dependent factors in the visual system, resulting in an early increase of BDNF and IGF-1 in the retina and the visual cortex; this guides the accelerated maturation of retinal ganglion cells (RGCs) observed in EE pups and, through an increased GABAergic inhibitory transmission, triggers a faster visual cortex development; and (III) a third and final phase in which the autonomous interaction of the developing pup with the enriched environment further increases cortical IGF-1, which promotes the maturation of the GABAergic system, also leading to an acceleration in visual acuity maturation. Continuous lines represent well-documented interactions between boxes; dashed lines indicate likely interactions in the context of visual cortex development requiring further experimental characterization. (See insert for color representation of this figure.)

A first result was the demonstration of a marked acceleration in the visual system development in mice and rats exposed to EE since birth (Cancedda et al., 2004; Landi et al., 2007b). This effect was particularly evident for the maturation of visual acuity, a highly sensitive parameter of visual development. Moreover, early exposure to EE was also able to induce an earlier closure of the time window during which it is possible, during the first postnatal weeks of life, to induce LTP in visual cortical slices through theta-frequency stimulation from the white matter (Cancedda et al., 2004). Looking for possible molecular mediators underlying the EE-induced acceleration of visual system development, the neurotrophin BDNF and its action as regulator of the maturation of the GABAergic system emerged as key factors. Indeed, BDNF increased at the end of the first postnatal week of life in the visual cortex of enriched pups, and this increase was paralleled by an enhanced expression of the two GABA biosynthetic enzymes, GAD65 and 67.

The impact of EE on visual system development appeared to be very similar to what was previously established for an artificial BDNF overexpression obtained by genetic engineering (see Sale et al., 2009 for review), which was shown to drive an earlier development of intracortical GABAergic inhibition, followed by faster visual acuity maturation, likely due to the refinement of visual receptive fields under the direct control of inhibitory interneurons (Huang et al., 1999). In both enriched and BDNF overexpressing mice, the acceleration of visual system development elicited by BDNF and the intracortical GABAergic system do not require vision at all, considering that it is evident before eye opening and even before photoreceptor formation. This striking conclusion was also confirmed by results obtained in enriched rats raised in darkness during development (Bartoletti et al., 2004), a procedure that usually prolongs the duration of the CP and impairs visual acuity maturation (Timney et al., 1978; Fagiolini et al., 1994). Indeed, the detrimental effects of dark rearing were completely counteracted by either EE (Bartoletti et al., 2004) or BDNF overexpression (Gianfranceschi et al., 2003). This strongly demonstrates that the maturation of a sensory system can be forced to proceed even in the absence of specific sensory experience impinging on it, provided that adequate levels of some critical molecular factors are available to the developing neural circuits.

A second major finding was the demonstration of a key role in visual development exerted by the insulin-like growth factor-1 (IGF-1), a molecule that promotes the survival and proliferation of neural cells, thus exerting a wide variety of actions both during development and in adulthood (O'Kusky and Ye, 2012). IGF-1 expression is increased during the second postnatal week in the visual cortex of rats raised in EE compared to standard-reared animals, and exogenous IGF-1 supply mimics, whereas its blocking prevents, EE effects on visual acuity maturation (Ciucci et al., 2007). Interestingly, IGF-1 eventually converges on the same biochemical pathway as BDNF, that is, the inhibitory GABAergic system, leading to an increased GAD65 expression in V1 (Ciucci et al., 2007). The essential role of IGF-1 as a key mediator of the EE control on experience-dependent development has been recently reinforced by Wang and colleagues (Wang et al., 2013). They found that a mismatch between two visual developmental processes, ocular dominance development and binocular matching of orientation selectivity development, can be caused by overexpression of BDNF, which acts on ocular dominance development and cortical plasticity decline but is unable to drive binocular matching of orientation selectivity, with negative results for the quality of binocular vision; EE exposure and IGF-1 are able to correct this mismatch, ensuring an harmonic development of all properties of visual cortical neurons.

While the classic sensory deprivation approach based on dark rearing or eye-lid suture led to postulate that the prime site for experience-dependent plasticity is the cerebral cortex, the impact of EE on visual system development turned out not to be restricted to the visual cortex. The retina, a peripheral part of the central nervous system traditionally considered little plastic in response to changes of sensory inputs (Baro et al., 1990; Fagiolini et al., 1994; Fine et al., 2003), indeed appeared much responsive to EE: retinal acuity, which is the spatial discrimination limit of the retinal output, was accelerated in enriched rats to the same extent as the visual cortex (Landi et al., 2007b), an effect accompanied, at the morphological level, by an earlier segregation of retinal ganglion cell dendrites into ON and OFF sublaminae (Landi et al., 2007a). The similarity of the response displayed by the visual cortex extended to the molecular level of analysis, with increased retinal IGF-1 and BDNF in the retinal ganglion cell layer of developing rats raised under enriched conditions (Landi et al., 2007a; Landi et al., 2007b).

Based on the convincing finding that the environment can be exploited as a driving force to increase the expression of neuronal protective factors, a recent work investigated the impact of EE on a mouse model of Retinitis Pigmentosa, a family of inherited disorders in which a mutation in a retinal-specific gene causes the primary degeneration of rods, followed by the secondary death of cones, leading to near blindness. The results show that early EE delays the loss of rod photoreceptors and the secondary death of cones, thus preventing vision for a much longer time than control animals maintained in conventional standard-rearing conditions (Barone et al., 2012).

Maternal touch

What might cause such very early changes in the developing brain of an enriched pup? Answering this question is not trivial, considering that the offspring mostly spend the whole time in the nest during the first days of postnatal life, with very few chances to explore the surroundings and receive an enhanced sensory stimulation. During the initial phase of postnatal development, maternal influence is certainly the most important source of sensory experience for the developing subject (Hofer, 1984; Ronca et al., 1993; Liu et al., 2000), directly regulating physical growth and promoting the neural maturation of brain structures through highly adaptive behaviors such as licking, grooming, and feeding (Fleming et al., 1999; Meaney and Szyf, 2005; Champagne et al., 2008).

We postulated that maternal behavior could be the solution to the mystery of visual system acceleration in very young pups born in enriched conditions, with the possibility of maternal behavior differences between enriched and nonenriched dams. Our theory stood up to the facts quite well. Enriched pups were demonstrated to receive higher levels of maternal stimulation compared to standard-reared animals (Sale et al., 2004), experiencing an almost continuous physical contact provided by the mother or other adult females, and receiving increased levels of licking during the first 10 days of life. Moreover, when we willingly replaced enriched mothers mimicking maternal behavior with an artificial tactile stimulation (massage), we were able to reproduce the EE-dependent acceleration of visual development, an effect mediated by increased IGF-1 levels in the primary visual cortex (Guzzetta et al., 2009).

Mimicking early enrichment with maternal stimulation offered a fascinating chance for clinical application. In parallel to the effects obtained in massaged rats, together with Prof. Cioni's group at the Stella Maris Hospital (Calambrone, Pisa), we reported that enriching the environment in terms of body massage ("massage therapy") accelerates brain development in healthy preterm infants (gestational age between 30 and 33 weeks) (see the chapter by Guzzetta and Cioni in this book [Chapter 10]). Massaged infants displayed increased levels of plasma IGF-1 and exhibited a faster developmental reduction in the latency of flash visual evoked potentials and an increase in behavioral visual acuity, which persisted above 2 months past the end of the treatment (Guzzetta et al., 2009, 2011).

Despite this first attempt to investigate the effects elicited by enriched living conditions in children, very little is known on the impact of early EE in humans. Previous studies showed that early educational and health enrichment at ages 3–5 years is associated with long-term increases in psychophysiological orienting and arousal at age 11 (Raine et al., 2001), and that early nutritional, educational, and motor enrichment is prophylactic for antisocial and criminal behavior at age 17–23 years (Raine et al., 2003). In our opinion, this is a research field that deserves much more attention, bearing a great potential for translation of the results obtained in well-designed experiments to educational programs and national health services.

As previously noted (Sale et al., 2014), the remarkable ability of an early exposure to EE conditions to accelerate brain development should not be viewed as necessarily always beneficial. As a delicate equilibrium among an orchestra's elements, speeding up the circuit maturation in a system, or feeding an excessive stimulation upon it, might cause that system to either fail an exact temporal matching with the maturation of other developing circuits or to suffer from overstimulation detrimental effects. Again, the same treatment might result in excessively narrow CPs, possibly reducing the chance for a proper interaction with the environment (Wang et al., 2013). Fortunately, it appears that the EE protocols employed in current laboratory practice not only do not force the animals in terms of the amount of received stimulation but in very young individuals are mostly mediated by maternal behavior, an absolutely natural source of experience that is very unlikely to be associated with stressful conditions.

Prenatal effects

Having focused on maternal influence as a key mediator of early EE effects on brain development, we went back to retinal development to also show that a substantial fraction of the acceleration previously reported in this structure as a result of early EE exposure was actually due to prenatal maternal effects. Enriching female rats for the entire length of gestation resulted in faster dynamics of neural progenitor migration and spontaneous apoptosis in the retinal ganglion cell layer, an effect mediated also in this case by IGF-1 (Sale et al., 2007a). To explain how changes in the environment experienced by the mother are finally translated in variations of the developmental trajectories in the offspring, we put forward a model in which sustained physical exercise during pregnancy increases IGF-1 in the mother, promoting placental transfer of nutrients to the fetus; this in turn leads to increased amounts of IGF-1 autonomously produced by the fetus, resulting in an earlier development, detectable at the retinal level (Figure 1.4).

Apart from the visual domain, other systems appear to be influenced by prenatal enrichment. The hippocampus of rat pups born from physically trained mothers displays an increased expression of BDNF and proliferation of progenitor cells in the granule layer (Parnpiansil et al., 2003; Bick-Sander et al., 2006). The beneficial effects of prenatal enrichment are long-lasting, resulting in enhanced cognitive abilities at very early and older postnatal ages (Parnpiansil et al., 2003; Lee et al., 2006), providing enduring protection from neurodegeneration in old age through a reduction of beta-amyloid plaque burden (Herring et al., 2012) and leading to increased synaptic elaboration and complexity in the hippocampus. Moreover, maternal complex housing during pregnancy as a form of prenatal enrichment has been recently shown to alter brain organization and to offer neuroprotection against major consequences of perinatal brain injury (Gibb et al., 2014).

Strikingly, maternal exercise during pregnancy also exerts beneficial effects on human fetal development (Prather et al., 2012), with the recommendation made by the American College Congress of Obstetricians and Gynecologists in 2002 in which at least 30 minutes of moderate exercise during pregnancy on most days of the week is considered as a safe way to promote benefits for the mother, fetus, and future newborn (American College of Obstetricians and Gynecologists, 2002).

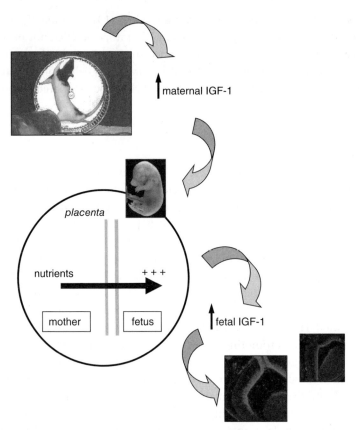

Figure 1.4 Prenatal enrichment modulates retinal development in the fetus. The figure shows a possible explicative model for the effects elicited by maternal enrichment during pregnancy on retinal development. Increased levels of physical exercise in gestating dams lead to higher amounts of circulating IGF-1 in the maternal blood stream, stimulating the supply of nutrients transferred to the fetus through the placental barrier. The enhancement in glucose and placental lactogens received by the fetus stimulates the autonomous production of IGF-1 in his tissues, with an increased expression detectable in the ganglion cell layer of the retina. IGF-1, in turn, stimulates the maturation of retinal circuitries. The photographs depict two examples of one enriched (left) and one nonenriched (right) retinal sections immunostained for double cortin, which labels migrating cells and is a good marker of the temporal and spatial distribution of neural progenitors during the early developmental stages of the rat retina. Reprinted from Sale et al., 2012. (See insert for color representation of this figure.)

Thus while for many years the best-documented maternal effects were those elicited by prenatal stress protocols, which has long been linked to growth retardation and structural malformations in the offspring (Mulder et al., 2002; Seckl, 2004; Graignic-Philippe et al., 2014), the results obtained with prenatal EE underscore the impact of positive changes in the quality and intensity of maternal stimulation during pregnancy as powerful modulators of several growth factors known to be critical for central nervous system development.

Beyond the visual system

An intrinsic strength of the EE paradigm is its remarkable ability to impact on the whole brain and not to specifically act on a single developing system. The beneficial effects of EE, indeed, are not exclusive of the visual system. The auditory cortex, for instance, displays major changes when EE is applied at juvenile developmental stages, with increased strength of auditory responses and improved sound sensitivity and tone frequency/directional selectivity (Engineer et al., 2004; Zhang et al., 2009). Moreover, exposure to enriched environments at very early postnatal ages has been associated with an early maturation of major components of the brain extracellular matrix, the chondroitin sulfate proteoglycans (CSPGs), in the striatum, leading to increased cognitive and motor abilities (Simonetti et al., 2009). As reported for the visual system, an accelerated maturation of GABAergic and glutamatergic synapses has been documented also in the hippocampus of enriched mice, together with a faster transition from excitatory to inhibitory GABA action (He et al., 2010).

A recent study suggests that exposure to EE is also able to modulate the programming of energy balance and food intake. Mice enriched from birth, but not mice exposed to EE when adult, show decreased levels of leptin, despite similar adipose mass and normal food intake. This effect is based on an enhanced leptin signaling and higher excitatory input on anorexigenic neurons in the arcuate nucleus of the hypothalamus found in young EE mice (Mainardi et al., 2010a; Mainardi et al., 2013).

The beneficial effects of EE are not limited to subtle functional changes evoked by the environment in the absence of pre-existing pathologies but extend to include the case of genetically programmed states of brain disability. One paradigmatic example is that of Down syndrome, the most common genetic cause of mental retardation caused by triplication of chromosome 21. People with Down syndrome have a severe cognitive impairment (Nadel, 2003; Pennington et al., 2003) and a number of attention and visual deficits (Brown et al., 2003; Clark and Wilson, 2003; John et al., 2004). The most widely studied animal model of Down syndrome is the Ts65Dn mouse, which carries triplication of a segment of Chr16 syntenic with human Chr21 (Gardiner et al., 2003; Seregaza et al., 2006). Ts65Dn mice recapitulate the main hallmarks of the Down syndrome phenotype, with severe defects in learning abilities and attention and visual functions (e.g., Holtzman et al., 1996; Escorihuela et al., 1998; Scott-McKean et al., 2010). An essential mechanism underlying these defects has been shown to be excessive brain inhibition, leading to a failure of long-term synaptic (LTP) plasticity in the hippocampus (Siarey et al., 1999; Kleschevnikov et al., 2004; Fernandez et al., 2007; Best et al., 2012). The central role of overinhibition in the Down syndrome pathogenesis is confirmed by the demonstration that administration of various classes of antagonists of GABA receptors reverses major cognitive disabilities and LTP deficits in Ts65Dn mice (Rissman and Mobley, 2011). Recently, we tested the EE potential for therapeutic application in the Ts65Dn model of Down syndrome. Our findings show that EE promotes recovery from cognitive impairment and synaptic plasticity failure and induces a full rescue of visual acuity, ocular dominance, and visual neuronal response latencies in Ts65Dn mice compared to their littermates reared in standard conditions, an effect accompanied by normalization of GABA release in hippocampal and visual cortex synaptosomes (Begenisic et al., 2011). Interestingly, it has been reported that transgenic mice with overdosage of Dyrk1A, a key Down syndrome candidate gene, display recovery from their deficits in adult hippocampal neurogenesis after exposure to EE, an effect due to normalization of DYRK1A kinase overdosage (Pons-Espinal et al., 2013). The beneficial effects of EE are not limited to adulthood: indeed, we recently found that exposure to early EE in developing Ts65Dn mice is able to prevent most of their characteristic deficits in terms of declarative memory abilities, hippocampal synaptic plasticity, and visual system maturation (Begenisic et al., 2015).

Other well-established cases of mouse models of syndromes linked to gene mutation having their phenotype ameliorated following exposure to an enriched environment are heterozygous Mecp2 null mice, a model of Rett syndrome, and Fmr1-knockout mice, a model of Fragile X syndrome (Restivo et al., 2005; Lonetti et al., 2010).

Strikingly, there have been recent attempts to directly translate these successful results from the animal models to humans, specifically in the fields of autism and Down syndrome treatment. A randomized controlled trial enrolled 2- to 12-year-old children with autism and assigned them to either a control group or to a sensorimotor enrichment procedure mostly consisting of daily olfactory-tactile stimulation. The results, very encouraging, demonstrated a marked clinical improvement for the enrichment group in terms of the severity of autism as assessed with the Childood Autism Rating Scale, together with a clear improvement in cognition (Woo and Leon, 2013). Moreover, the same procedure of early multisensory massage intervention previously used in preterm babies has been shown to be very effective in also promoting visual acuity and stereopsis maturation in children with Down syndrome (Purpura et al., 2014), who are often at high risk for environmental impoverishment due to prolonged hospitalization and frequent deterioration in parent-infant bonding.

Is it possible to rejuvenate the brain? Impact of EE on adult visual system plasticity

The study of visual system plasticity under environmental conditions of scaled complexities has provided significant advances not only in the field of brain development but also in our knowledge concerning the molecular processes underlying the closure of the CP and the ensuing dramatic decline in the potential for neuronal plasticity.

With the closure of the CP in the primary visual cortex, the possibility to induce functional and structural changes in this structure in response to a modulation of sensory experience abruptly wanes. This leads to permanent brakes to the cerebral potential for recovery from possible defective processes that may have occurred during development, preventing or robustly limiting functional rehabilitation. Certainly one of the most ambitious goals in basic and clinical neuroscience research is to develop suitable procedures able to overcome the major obstacles that reduce plasticity levels in the adult brain (Bavelier et al., 2010). Also in this case, the visual system emerges as one of the favorite testing grounds.

It has to be underlined that the decay of plasticity in the adult visual system may be not as absolute as previously thought, but it seems actually dependent on the specific neural processes under investigation. A striking example of use-dependent plasticity persisting for the entire life span has been described by Bear and colleagues (Frenkel et al., 2006), who showed that repeated exposure to grating stimuli of a single orientation results in a long-lasting increase of VEP amplitudes in response to the test stimulus. Another previously described example is the shift in orientation or spatial frequency selectivity displayed by cat primary visual cortical neurons after a period of adaptation consisting in the presentation of a stimulus at nonpreferred orientations or spatial frequencies (Ghisovan et al., 2008; Marshansky et al., 2011).

Despite these examples of plasticity not restricted to a CP, the possibility to obtain functional recovery from alterations of visual experience starting at early postnatal ages is extremely limited. One paradigmatic example of a permanent loss of visual abilities that is still orphan of treatment is amblyopia (lazy eye), a severe condition with an estimated prevalence of 1–5% in the total world population (Holmes and Clarke, 2006). Amblyopia is caused by an early imbalance between the two eyes, typically caused by unequal refractive power in the two eyes (anisometropia), abnormal alignment of ocular axes (strabismus), or visual clouding (Mittelman, 2003). If not precociously recognized and reversed, these defects eventually lead amblyopic subjects to develop a dramatic degradation of visual acuity and contrast sensitivity in the affected eye, experiencing multiple perceptual deficits that include stereopsis defects (Holmes and Clarke, 2006; Kiorpes, 2006; Levi, 2006).

In rats and mice, amblyopia can be very efficiently induced by means of a long-term occlusion of vision through one eye, using an enduring MD procedure that starts early in development and is protracted until adulthood (Figure 1.5). Using this useful model of experimental amblyopia, we showed that exposure to an enriched environment setting is one of the most effective procedures to reverse visual deficits in adult rodents, challenging the CP dogma. Indeed we reported that adult amblyopic rats transferred to an EE enclosure for 3 weeks undergo a full recovery of visual acuity and binocularity, with beneficial

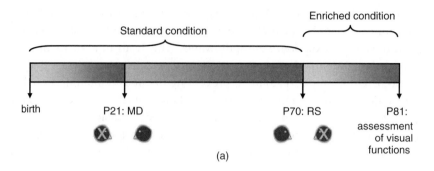

(a)

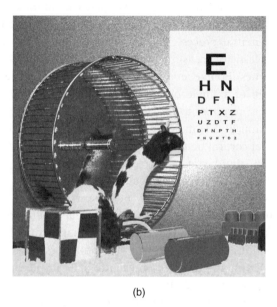

(b)

Figure 1.5 Exposure to enriched conditions promotes recovery of visual functions in adult amblyopic rats. (a) Experimental amblyopia is easily induced in juvenile rats by imposing an artificial closure of one eye through lid suture (monocular deprivation [MD]), started at the peak of the critical period (postnatal day 21) and maintained until the animals reach the adult age (around P70). Then, reverse suture (RS) is performed, consisting in the reopening of the long-term deprived eye and simultaneous closure of the fellow eye, in order to force the animals to use their lazy eye. After RS, the animals are divided in two groups, one left undisturbed under standard-rearing conditions, the other one being transferred to an enriched environment setting. (b) Rearing adult amblyopic rats in an enriched environment for 3 weeks leads to a complete recovery of visual functions, in terms of visual acuity, binocularity, and stereopsis. (See insert for color representation of this figure.)

effects detectable at both the electrophysiological and the behavioral level, and outlasting the end of the treatment for at least 10 days (Sale et al., 2007b). The recovery of plasticity in enriched rats is accompanied by a three-fold reduction in GABA release detected in the visual cortex contralateral to the previously deprived eye, without any significant change in the release of glutamate, and it is totally prevented by intracortical infusion of the GABAergic agonist diazepam. These observations led to the now widely accepted notion that the compelling ability of EE to promote adult brain plasticity is tightly linked to its impact on the brain excitation/inhibition balance, with a marked decrease in GABAergic transmission (Baroncelli et al., 2011). The possibility to reinstate juvenile-like levels of plasticity in the adult brain by manipulating the excitation/inhibition balance has been subsequently confirmed in more artificial conditions, with the demonstration that a pharmacological reduction of inhibition levels obtained through intracortical infusion of either MPA (an inhibitor of GABA synthesis) or picrotoxin (a GABAA antagonist) or through systemic administration of fluoxetine reactivates plasticity in response to MD in adult rats (Maya Vetencourt et al., 2008; Harauzov et al., 2010).

One case of particularly relevant clinical interest in the amblyopia field is that of those patients who lose the more functional eye due to an accident or ocular illnesses, thus becoming severely visually impaired. We recently addressed the possibility to rescue visual acuity in long-term deprived adult rats exposed to EE immediately after silencing of retino-thalamic projections of the fellow (nonamblyopic) eye due to optic nerve dissection (Tognini et al., 2012). Exposure to EE induced a full recovery of visual acuity in monocular rats, leading to lower numbers of GAD67+ cells and increased BDNF in the visual cortex.

The positive results obtained in enriched amblyopic animals strongly encourage researchers to find possible ways of application to clinics of the promising and noninvasive approach of EE. An intermediate and reasonable step might be that of investigating the impact of various independent EE components (e.g., social, sensory, motor). The general aim here is to design possible therapeutic approaches based on the most promising and effective variables.

Following this idea, we separately assessed the effects of either enhanced physical exercise, increased levels of social interaction, or sustained visual stimulation for their potential in promoting recovery from amblyopia in adult rats (Baroncelli et al., 2012). Our results show a full recovery of ocular dominance and visual acuity in exercised animals and in rats exposed to a protocol of visual enrichment. To further characterize the contribution of visual stimuli, we reused a protocol of classic EE (social, cognitive, motor and sensory stimuli together), but we placed enriched amblyopic animals under complete dark-rearing conditions, showing that they failed to recover their visual functions; visual recovery was also impossible even under normal light conditions, when the long-term deprived eye was maintained closed to prevent visual pattern perception; thus, EE must be coupled with proper visual stimulation in order to exert its beneficial effects. In agreement with this result, binocular lid suture has been shown to be unable to stimulate visual recovery from a preceding amblyogenic period of MD in kittens (Duffy et al., 2014).

In contrast to motor and visual enrichment, enhancing social stimulation alone was not able to induce restoration of normal visual acuity and ocular dominance. Recovery from amblyopia was faithfully associated with a reduction of GABAergic intracortical inhibition, as revealed by decreased GABA release in synaptosome analysis. Thus, potentiation of single environmental components is able to reproduce the effect of visual function recovery from amblyopia previously reported in classically enriched animals (Baroncelli et al., 2012), possibly encouraging the implementation of new environmental strategies devoted to promote stimulation of the amblyopic eye in adult patients as a way to increase their chance of visual functional improvements.

A second way toward future applications of EE strategies to clinics is to find paradigms of increased sensory and/or motor activity that, resembling part or the whole ensemble of the EE beneficial effects, appear more promising in terms of the ensuing results on brain and behavior. In the visual system model, increasing evidence shows that experimental procedures akin to EE, such as playing videogames or practicing visual perceptual learning (PL), are quite effective in promoting recovery from amblyopia in adulthood (Levi and Li, 2009; Astle et al., 2011; Li et al., 2011; Green and Bavelier, 2012), likely acting by either modulating levels of molecular brakes or by promoting the expression of endogenous permissive factors such as neuromodulators.

PL is currently considered one of the most promising active strategies for treating amblyopia in adulthood (see Levi, 2012; Bonaccorsi et al., 2014). PL consists in the improvement in performance on a variety of simple sensory tasks, following practice and, in the visual system, involves identifying small differences in simple visual attributes, such as position, orientation, texture, or shape. Despite its suitability for inducing vision recovery in human subjects, the cellular and molecular mechanisms underlying PL effects are still scarcely known. Recently, we set up a new model of visual PL in rodents that led us to the possibility to test the impact of this procedure on visual cortical plasticity at the cellular and molecular level, a kind of analysis normally prevented when working on human subjects (Sale et al., 2011). To elicit visual PL, we first trained a group of adult animals to practice in a forced-choice visual discrimination task that requires them to distinguish between two vertical gratings differing only for their spatial frequency; then, we made the two stimuli progressively more similar to each other, until the animal performance reached a steady plateau (Figure 1.6(a)). This task requires activation of V1 circuitries, as indicated by the strong selectivity of PL for the orientation of gratings employed during training (Sale et al., 2011) (Figure 1.6(b)). Control animals only learned the association task, that is, they were only required to discriminate between a grating and a homogeneous gray panel, matching the overall swim time and number of training days in the water maze with those of PL rats (Figure 1.6(a)). Within 1 hour from the last discrimination trial, LTP from layer II-III of V1 slices appeared occluded in PL animals compared to controls, both when testing its inducibility in vertical connections (stimulating electrode placed in layer IV) and when

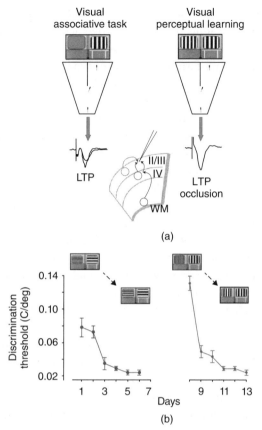

Figure 1.6 Visual perceptual learning induces long-term potentiation in the primary visual cortex. (a) A modified version of the visual water box task (Prusky et al., 2000; Cancedda et al., 2004) was used to induce visual perceptual learning in a group of adult rats that were first trained to distinguish a low 0.117 cycles per degree (c/deg) spatial frequency (SF) grating (reference grating) from a 0.712 c/deg SF grating (test grating) (right panel) and then learned to distinguish the two gratings when they became more and more similar to each other. A group of control animals was trained to distinguish the reference grating from a homogeneous gray (left panel). After training, LTP from layer II–III of V1 slices was occluded in PL animals compared to controls, at the level of both vertical (blue arrow) and horizontal (red arrow) connections. Sample traces from PL and control slices 5 minutes before (thin line) and 25 minutes after (thick line) induction of LTP are shown. (b) Visual perceptual learning is specific for stimulus orientation. The graphs show daily discrimination threshold values obtained in PL animals trained in discriminating first horizontal gratings and then tested with vertical. After the orientation change, the animals displayed a marked impairment in their discrimination abilities. Reprinted from Sale et al., 2012. (See insert for color representation of this figure.)

stimulating at the level of horizontal connections (stimulating electrode placed in layer II/III) (Figure 1.6(a)). Moreover, a significant shift toward increased amplitude of fEPSPs was found in the input/output curves of trained animals compared to controls (Sale et al., 2011). Thus, the data fulfill two of the most commonly accepted criteria used to relate LTP with learning, that is, occlusion and mimicry, demonstrating that the improvements displayed by PL rats in discriminating visual gratings of progressively closer spatial frequencies can be explained in terms of long-term increments of synaptic efficacy in V1, the same cortical area at work during perception. This is consistent with the critical role of LTP in mediating learning processes previously reported in other brain areas such as the amygdala, the hippocampus, and the motor cortex (Rogan et al., 1997; Rioult-Pedotti et al., 2000; Whitlock et al., 2006). An impact on V1 LTP appears to be a common prerogative of visual PL and EE. Indeed, enriched rats also show an enhancement of thalamocortical LTP triggered by theta-burst stimulation (TBS) of the dorsal lateral geniculate nucleus of the thalamus (Mainardi et al., 2010b), leading to an enhancement in VEP responses to visual stimulation across a wide range of contrasts.

Since potentiation of synaptic transmission might help the recovery process of visual responses for the long-term deprived eye, practice with visual PL through the amblyopic eye is expected to favor a functional rescue in amblyopic animals. In agreement with this hypothesis, a marked recovery of visual functions was evident in amblyopic rats subjected to visual PL, while no recovery occurred in two control groups in which the treatment did not induce LTP in V1, that is, in rats that only learned the associative visual task and in animals that were trained only until the first step of the discrimination procedure between the test and the reference grating, without proceeding further with a progression of finer discrimination trials (Baroncelli et al., 2012). Recovery of visual abilities in PL animals was accompanied by a robust decrease of the inhibition-excitation balance.

Concluding remarks

The data reviewed in this chapter demonstrate that exposure to EE conditions is a powerful tool to modulate the development of the central nervous system and to boost plasticity in the adult brain. The secret of the EE approach resides in its ability to impact, under physiological developmental conditions, on molecules critically involved in brain maturation and plasticity, such as growth and neurotrophic factors or GABA-ergic inhibition levels, or to successfully implement, in the presence of concurrent developmental pathologies, a kind of endogenous pharmacotherapy (Sale et al., 2014), that is, the stimulation of the spontaneous reparative potential held by the brain even without the concomitant administration of external artificial substances. Finding suitable strategies for translating EE in human terms in order to apply its framework to the treatment of several neurodevelopmental disorders and adult neurological diseases emerges as an urgent need for clinical practice and a major challenge for future neuroscience research.

References

Akers KG, Arruda–Carvalho M, Josselyn SA, Frankland PW. (2012). Ontogeny of contextual fear memory formation, specificity, and persistence in mice. *Learn Mem* 19:598–604.

American College of Obstetricians and Gynecologists. (2002). ACOG committee opinion. Exercise during pregnancy and the postpartum period. Number 267, January 2002. American College of Obstetricians and Gynecologists. *Int J Gynaecol Obstet* 77:79–81.

Antonini A, Stryker MP. (1993). Rapid remodeling of axonal arbors in the visual cortex. *Science* 260:1819–1821.

Astle AT, Webb BS, McGraw PV. (2011). Can perceptual learning be used to treat amblyopia beyond the critical period of visual development? *Ophthalmic Physiol Opt* 31:564–573.

Baro JA, Lehmkuhle S, Kratz KE. (1990). Electroretinograms and visual evoked potentials in long–term monocularly deprived cats. *Invest Ophthalmol Vis Sci* 31:1405–1409.

Baroncelli L, Braschi C, Spolidoro M, Begenisic T, Sale A, Maffei L. (2010). Nurturing brain plasticity: impact of environmental enrichment. *Cell Death Differ* 17:1092–1103.

Baroncelli L, Braschi C, Spolidoro M, Begenisic T, Maffei L, Sale A. (2011). Brain plasticity and disease: a matter of inhibition. *Neural Plast* 2011:286073.

Baroncelli L, Bonaccorsi J, Milanese M, Bonifacino T, Giribaldi F, Manno I, Cenni MC, Berardi N, Bonanno G, Maffei L, Sale A. (2012). Enriched experience and recovery from amblyopia in adult rats: impact of motor, social and sensory components. *Neuropharmacology* 62:2388–2397.

Barone I, Novelli E, Piano I, Gargini C, Strettoi E. (2012). Environmental enrichment extends photoreceptor survival and visual function in a mouse model of retinitis pigmentosa. *PLoS One* 7:e50726.

Bartoletti A, Medini P, Berardi N, Maffei L. (2004). Environmental enrichment prevents effects of dark–rearing in the rat visual cortex. *Nat Neurosci* 7:215–216.

Bavelier D, Levi DM, Li RW, Dan Y, Hensch TK. (2010). Removing brakes on adult brain plasticity: from molecular to behavioral interventions. *J Neurosci* 30:14964–14971.

Begenisic T, Spolidoro M, Braschi C, Baroncelli L, Milanese M, Pietra G, Fabbri ME, Bonanno G, Cioni G, Maffei L, Sale A. (2011). Environmental enrichment decreases GABAergic inhibition and improves cognitive abilities, synaptic plasticity, and visual functions in a mouse model of Down syndrome. *Front Cell Neurosci* 5:29.

Begenisic T, Sansevero G, Baroncelli L, Cioni G, Sale A. (2015). Early environmental therapy rescues brain development in a mouse model of Down syndrome. *Neurobiol Dis* 82:409–419.

Bengtsson SL, Nagy Z, Skare S, Forsman L, Forssberg H, Ullen F. (2005). Extensive piano practicing has regionally specific effects on white matter development. *Nat Neurosci* 8:1148–1150.

Berardi N, Pizzorusso T, Maffei L. (2000). Critical periods during sensory development. *Curr Opin Neurobiol* 10:138–145.

Berardi N, Pizzorusso T, Ratto GM, Maffei L. (2003). Molecular basis of plasticity in the visual cortex. *Trends Neurosci* 26:369–378.

Best TK, Cramer NP, Chakrabarti L, Haydar TF, Galdzicki Z. (2012). Dysfunctional hippocampal inhibition in the Ts65Dn mouse model of Down syndrome. *Exp Neurol* 233:749–757.

Bick–Sander A, Steiner B, Wolf SA, Babu H, Kempermann G. (2006). Running in pregnancy transiently increases postnatal hippocampal neurogenesis in the offspring. *Proc Natl Acad Sci USA* 103:3852–3857.

Bonaccorsi J, Berardi N, Sale A. (2014). Treatment of amblyopia in the adult: insights from a new rodent model of visual perceptual learning. *Front Neural Circuits* 8:82.

Brown JH, Johnson MH, Paterson SJ, Gilmore R, Longhi E, Karmiloff–Smith A. (2003). Spatial representation and attention in toddlers with Williams syndrome and Down syndrome. *Neuropsychologia* 41:1037–1046.

Cancedda L, Putignano E, Sale A, Viegi A, Berardi N, Maffei L. (2004). Acceleration of visual system development by environmental enrichment. *J Neurosci* 24:4840–4848.

Champagne DL, Bagot RC, van Hasselt F, Ramakers G, Meaney MJ, de Kloet ER, Joels M, Krugers H. (2008). Maternal care and hippocampal plasticity: evidence for experience–dependent structural plasticity, altered synaptic functioning, and differential responsiveness to glucocorticoids and stress. *J Neurosci* 28:6037–6045.

Ciucci F, Putignano E, Baroncelli L, Landi S, Berardi N, Maffei L. (2007). Insulin–like growth factor 1. (IGF–1) mediates the effects of enriched environment (EE) on visual cortical development. *PLoS ONE* 2:e475.

Clark D, Wilson GN. (2003). Behavioral assessment of children with Down syndrome using the Reiss psychopathology scale. *Am J Med Genet A* 118A:210–216.

Diamond MC. (2001). Response of the brain to enrichment. *An Acad Bras Cienc* 73:211–220.

Duffy KR, Bukhamseen DH, Smithen MJ, Mitchell DE. (2014). Binocular eyelid closure promotes anatomical but not behavioral recovery from monocular deprivation. *Vision Res* 114:151–160.

Engineer ND, Percaccio CR, Pandya PK, Moucha R, Rathbun DL, Kilgard MP. (2004). Environmental enrichment improves response strength, threshold, selectivity, and latency of auditory cortex neurons. *J Neurophysiol* 92:73–82.

Escorihuela RM, Vallina IF, Martinez–Cue C, Baamonde C, Dierssen M, Tobena A, Florez J, Fernandez–Teruel A. (1998). Impaired short– and long–term memory in Ts65Dn mice, a model for Down syndrome. *Neurosci Lett* 247:171–174.

Fagiolini M, Pizzorusso T, Berardi N, Domenici L, Maffei L. (1994). Functional postnatal development of the rat primary visual cortex and the role of visual experience: dark rearing and monocular deprivation. *Vision Res* 34:709–720.

Fernandez F, Morishita W, Zuniga E, Nguyen J, Blank M, Malenka RC, Garner CC. (2007). Pharmacotherapy for cognitive impairment in a mouse model of Down syndrome. *Nat Neurosci* 10:411–413.

Fine I, Wade AR, Brewer AA, May MG, Goodman DF, Boynton GM, Wandell BA, MacLeod DI. (2003). Long–term deprivation affects visual perception and cortex. *Nat Neurosci* 6: 915–916.

Fleming AS, O'Day DH, Kraemer GW. (1999). Neurobiology of mother–infant interactions: experience and central nervous system plasticity across development and generations. *Neurosci Biobehav Rev* 23:673–685.

Frenkel MY, Sawtell NB, Diogo AC, Yoon B, Neve RL, Bear MF. (2006). Instructive effect of visual experience in mouse visual cortex. *Neuron* 51:339–349.

Gardiner K, Fortna A, Bechtel L, Davisson MT. (2003). Mouse models of Down syndrome: how useful can they be? Comparison of the gene content of human chromosome 21 with orthologous mouse genomic regions. *Gene* 318:137–147.

Ghisovan N, Nemri A, Shumikhina S, Molotchnikoff S. (2008). Visual cells remember earlier applied target: plasticity of orientation selectivity. *PLoS One* 3:e3689.

Gianfranceschi L, Siciliano R, Walls J, Morales B, Kirkwood A, Huang ZJ, Tonegawa S, Maffei L. (2003). Visual cortex is rescued from the effects of dark rearing by overexpression of BDNF. *Proc Natl Acad Sci USA* 100:12486–12491.

Gibb RL, Gonzalez CL, Kolb B. (2014). Prenatal enrichment and recovery from perinatal cortical damage: effects of maternal complex housing. *Front Behav Neurosci* 8:223.

Graignic–Philippe R, Dayan J, Chokron S, Jacquet AY, Tordjman S. (2014). Effects of prenatal stress on fetal and child development: a critical literature review. *Neurosci Biobehav Rev* 43:137–162.

Green CS, Bavelier D. (2012). Learning, attentional control, and action video games. *Curr Biol* 22:R197–206.

Guzzetta A, Baldini S, Bancale A, Baroncelli L, Ciucci F, Ghirri P, Putignano E, Sale A, Viegi A, Berardi N, Boldrini A, Cioni G, Maffei L. (2009). Massage accelerates brain development and the maturation of visual function. *J Neurosci* 29:6042–6051.

Guzzetta A, D'Acunto MG, Carotenuto M, Berardi N, Bancale A, Biagioni E, Boldrini A, Ghirri P, Maffei L, Cioni G. (2011). The effects of preterm infant massage on brain electrical activity. *Dev Med Child Neurol 53 Suppl* 4:46–51.

Harauzov A, Spolidoro M, DiCristo G, De Pasquale R, Cancedda L, Pizzorusso T, Viegi A, Berardi N, Maffei L. (2010). Reducing intracortical inhibition in the adult visual cortex promotes ocular dominance plasticity. *J Neurosci* 30:361–371.

He S, Ma J, Liu N, Yu X. (2010). Early enriched environment promotes neonatal GABAergic neurotransmission and accelerates synapse maturation. *J Neurosci* 30:7910–7916.

Hensch TK. (2005a). Critical period mechanisms in developing visual cortex. *Curr Top Dev Biol* 69:215–237.

Hensch TK. (2005b). Critical period plasticity in local cortical circuits. *Nat Rev Neurosci* 6: 877–888.

Herring A, Donath A, Yarmolenko M, Uslar E, Conzen C, Kanakis D, Bosma C, Worm K, Paulus W, Keyvani K. (2012). Exercise during pregnancy mitigates Alzheimer–like pathology in mouse offspring. *Faseb J* 26:117–128.

Hofer MA. (1984). Relationships as regulators: a psychobiologic perspective on bereavement. *Psychosom Med* 46:183–197.

Holmes JM, Clarke MP. (2006). Amblyopia. *Lancet* 367:1343–1351.

Holtzman DM, Santucci D, Kilbridge J, Chua–Couzens J, Fontana DJ, Daniels SE, Johnson RM, Chen K, Sun Y, Carlson E, Alleva E, Epstein CJ, Mobley WC. (1996). Developmental abnormalities and age–related neurodegeneration in a mouse model of Down syndrome. *Proc Natl Acad Sci USA* 93:13333–13338.

Huang ZJ, Kirkwood A, Pizzorusso T, Porciatti V, Morales B, Bear MF, Maffei L, Tonegawa S. (1999). BDNF regulates the maturation of inhibition and the critical period of plasticity in mouse visual cortex. *Cell* 98:739–755.

Hubel DH, Wiesel TN, LeVay S. (1977). Plasticity of ocular dominance columns in monkey striate cortex. *Philos Trans R Soc Lond B Biol Sci* 278:377–409.

John FM, Bromham NR, Woodhouse JM, Candy TR. (2004). Spatial vision deficits in infants and children with Down syndrome. *Invest Ophthalmol Vis Sci* 45:1566–1572.

Kiorpes L. (2006). Visual processing in amblyopia: animal studies. *Strabismus* 14:3–10.

Kleschevnikov AM, Belichenko PV, Villar AJ, Epstein CJ, Malenka RC, Mobley WC. (2004). Hippocampal long–term potentiation suppressed by increased inhibition in the Ts65Dn mouse, a genetic model of Down syndrome. *J Neurosci* 24:8153–8160.

Knudsen EI. (2004). Sensitive periods in the development of the brain and behavior. *J Cogn Neurosci* 16:1412–1425.

Koo JW, Park CH, Choi SH, Kim NJ, Kim HS, Choe JC, Suh YH. (2003). The postnatal environment can counteract prenatal effects on cognitive ability, cell proliferation, and synaptic protein expression. *Faseb J* 17:1556–1558.

Kuhl PK. (2010). Brain mechanisms in early language acquisition. *Neuron* 67:713–727.

Landi S, Cenni MC, Maffei L, Berardi N. (2007a). Environmental enrichment effects on development of retinal ganglion cell dendritic stratification require retinal BDNF. *PLoS One* 2:e346.

Landi S, Sale A, Berardi N, Viegi A, Maffei L, Cenni MC. (2007b). Retinal functional development is sensitive to environmental enrichment: a role for BDNF. *Faseb J* 21:130–139.

Lee HH, Kim H, Lee JW, Kim YS, Yang HY, Chang HK, Lee TH, Shin MC, Lee MH, Shin MS, Park S, Baek S, Kim CJ. (2006). Maternal swimming during pregnancy enhances short–term memory and neurogenesis in the hippocampus of rat pups. *Brain Dev* 28:147–154.

LeVay S, Wiesel TN, Hubel DH. (1980). The development of ocular dominance columns in normal and visually deprived monkeys. *J Comp Neurol* 191:1–51.

Levelt CN, Hubener M. (2012). Critical–period plasticity in the visual cortex. *Annu Rev Neurosci* 35:309–330.

Levi DM. (2006). Visual processing in amblyopia: human studies. *Strabismus* 14:11–19.

Levi DM. (2012). Prentice award lecture 2011: removing the brakes on plasticity in the amblyopic brain. *Optom Vis Sci* 89:827–838.

Levi DM, Li RW. (2009). Perceptual learning as a potential treatment for amblyopia: a mini–review. *Vision Res* 49:2535–2549.

Lewis TL, Maurer D. (2005). Multiple sensitive periods in human visual development: evidence from visually deprived children. *Dev Psychobiol* 46:163–183.

Li RW, Ngo C, Nguyen J, Levi DM. (2011). Video–game play induces plasticity in the visual system of adults with amblyopia. *PLoS Biol* 9:e1001135.

Liu D, Diorio J, Day JC, Francis DD, Meaney MJ. (2000). Maternal care, hippocampal synaptogenesis and cognitive development in rats. *Nat Neurosci* 3:799–806.

Lonetti G, Angelucci A, Morando L, Boggio EM, Giustetto M, Pizzorusso T. (2010). Early environmental enrichment moderates the behavioral and synaptic phenotype of MeCP2 null mice. *Biol Psychiatry* 67:657–665.

Mainardi M, Scabia G, Vottari T, Santini F, Pinchera A, Maffei L, Pizzorusso T, Maffei M. (2010a). A sensitive period for environmental regulation of eating behavior and leptin sensitivity. *Proc Natl Acad Sci USA* 107:16673–16678.

Mainardi M, Landi S, Gianfranceschi L, Baldini S, De Pasquale R, Berardi N, Maffei L, Caleo M. (2010b). Environmental enrichment potentiates thalamocortical transmission and plasticity in the adult rat visual cortex. *J Neurosci Res* 88:3048–3059.

Mainardi M, Pizzorusso T, Maffei M. (2013). Environment, leptin sensitivity, and hypothalamic plasticity. *Neural Plast* 2013:438072.

Marshansky S, Shumikhina S, Molotchnikoff S. (2011). Repetitive adaptation induces plasticity of spatial frequency tuning in cat primary visual cortex. *Neuroscience* 172:355–365.

Maya Vetencourt JF, Sale A, Viegi A, Baroncelli L, De Pasquale R, O'Leary OF, Castren E, Maffei L. (2008). The antidepressant fluoxetine restores plasticity in the adult visual cortex. *Science* 320:385–388.

Meaney MJ, Szyf M. (2005). Maternal care as a model for experience–dependent chromatin plasticity? *Trends Neurosci* 28:456–463.

Mittelman D. (2003). Amblyopia. *Pediatr Clin North Am* 50:189–196.

Mulder EJ, Robles de Medina PG, Huizink AC, Van den Bergh BR, Buitelaar JK, Visser GH. (2002). Prenatal maternal stress: effects on pregnancy and the (unborn) child. *Early Hum Dev* 70:3–14.

Nabel EM, Morishita H. (2013). Regulating critical period plasticity: insight from the visual system to fear circuitry for therapeutic interventions. *Front Psychiatry* 4:146.

Nadel L. (2003). Down's syndrome: a genetic disorder in biobehavioral perspective. *Genes Brain Behav* 2:156–166.

O'Kusky J, Ye P. (2012). Neurodevelopmental effects of insulin–like growth factor signaling. *Front Neuroendocrinol* 33:230–251.

Parnpiansil P, Jutapakdeegul N, Chentanez T, Kotchabhakdi N. (2003). Exercise during pregnancy increases hippocampal brain–derived neurotrophic factor mRNA expression and spatial learning in neonatal rat pup. *Neurosci Lett* 352:45–48.

Pascual R, Figueroa H. (1996). Effects of preweaning sensorimotor stimulation on behavioral and neuronal development in motor and visual cortex of the rat. *Biol Neonate* 69: 399–404.

Pennington BF, Moon J, Edgin J, Stedron J, Nadel L. (2003). The neuropsychology of Down syndrome: evidence for hippocampal dysfunction. *Child Dev* 74:75–93.

Pons–Espinal M, Martinez de Lagran M, Dierssen M. (2013). Environmental enrichment rescues DYRK1A activity and hippocampal adult neurogenesis in TgDyrk1A. *Neurobiol Dis* 60:18–31.

Prather H, Spitznagle T, Hunt D. (2012). Benefits of exercise during pregnancy. *Pm R* 4:845–850; quiz 850.

Prusky GT, West PW, Douglas RM. (2000). Behavioral assessment of visual acuity in mice and rats. *Vision Res* 40:2201–2209.

Purpura G, Tinelli F, Bargagna S, Bozza M, Bastiani L, Cioni G. (2014). Effect of early multisensory massage intervention on visual functions in infants with Down syndrome. *Early Hum Dev* 90:809–813.

Raine A, Venables PH, Dalais C, Mellingen K, Reynolds C, Mednick SA. (2001). Early educational and health enrichment at age 3–5 years is associated with increased autonomic and central nervous system arousal and orienting at age 11 years: evidence from the Mauritius Child Health Project. *Psychophysiology* 38:254–266.

Raine A, Mellingen K, Liu J, Venables P, Mednick SA. (2003). Effects of environmental enrichment at ages 3–5 years on schizotypal personality and antisocial behavior at ages 17 and 23 years. *Am J Psychiatry* 160:1627–1635.

Restivo L, Ferrari F, Passino E, Sgobio C, Bock J, Oostra BA, Bagni C, Ammassari–Teule M. (2005). Enriched environment promotes behavioral and morphological recovery in a mouse model for the fragile X syndrome. *Proc Natl Acad Sci USA* 102:11557–11562.

Rioult–Pedotti MS, Friedman D, Donoghue JP. (2000). Learning–induced LTP in neocortex. *Science* 290:533–536.

Rissman RA, Mobley WC. (2011). Implications for treatment: GABAA receptors in aging, Down syndrome and Alzheimer's disease. *J Neurochem* 117:613–622.

Rogan MT, Staubli UV, LeDoux JE. (1997). Fear conditioning induces associative long–term potentiation in the amygdala. *Nature* 390:604–607.

Ronca AE, Lamkin CA, Alberts JR. (1993). Maternal contributions to sensory experience in the fetal and newborn rat. (Rattus norvegicus). *J Comp Psychol* 107:61–74.

Rosenzweig MR, Bennett EL. (1996). Psychobiology of plasticity: effects of training and experience on brain and behavior. *Behav Brain Res* 78:57–65.

Rosenzweig MR, Bennett EL, Hebert M, Morimoto H. (1978). Social grouping cannot account for cerebral effects of enriched environments. *Brain Res* 153:563–576.

Sale A, Putignano E, Cancedda L, Landi S, Cirulli F, Berardi N, Maffei L. (2004). Enriched environment and acceleration of visual system development. *Neuropharmacology* 47:649–660.

Sale A, Cenni MC, Ciucci F, Putignano E, Chierzi S, Maffei L. (2007a). Maternal enrichment during pregnancy accelerates retinal development of the fetus. *PLoS ONE* 2:e1160.

Sale A, Maya Vetencourt JF, Medini P, Cenni MC, Baroncelli L, De Pasquale R, Maffei L. (2007b). Environmental enrichment in adulthood promotes amblyopia recovery through a reduction of intracortical inhibition. *Nat Neurosci* 10:679–681.

Sale A, Berardi N, Maffei L. (2009). Enrich the environment to empower the brain. *Trends Neurosci* 32:233–239.

Sale A, De Pasquale R, Bonaccorsi J, Pietra G, Olivieri D, Berardi N, Maffei L. (2011). Visual perceptual learning induces long–term potentiation in the visual cortex. *Neuroscience* 172:219–225.

Sale A, Berardi N, Maffei L. (2012). Environmental influences on visual cortex development and plasticity. In: Visual Cortex, Eds. S. Molotchnikoff and J. Rouat, Intech.

Sale A, Berardi N, Maffei L. (2014). Environment and brain plasticity: towards an endogenous pharmacotherapy. *Physiol Rev* 94:189–234.

Scott–McKean JJ, Chang B, Hurd RE, Nusinowitz S, Schmidt C, Davisson MT, Costa AC. (2010). The mouse model of Down syndrome Ts65Dn presents visual deficits as assessed by pattern visual evoked potentials. *Invest Ophthalmol Vis Sci* 51:3300–3308.

Seckl JR. (2004). Prenatal glucocorticoids and long–term programming. *Eur J Endocrinol 151 Suppl* 3:U49–62.

Seregaza Z, Roubertoux PL, Jamon M, Soumireu–Mourat B. (2006). Mouse models of cognitive disorders in trisomy 21: a review. *Behav Genet* 36:387–404.

Shatz CJ, Stryker MP. (1978). Ocular dominance in layer IV of the cat's visual cortex and the effects of monocular deprivation. *J Physiol* 281:267–283.

Siarey RJ, Carlson EJ, Epstein CJ, Balbo A, Rapoport SI, Galdzicki Z. (1999). Increased synaptic depression in the Ts65Dn mouse, a model for mental retardation in Down syndrome. *Neuropharmacology* 38:1917–1920.

Simonetti T, Lee H, Bourke M, Leamey CA, Sawatari A. (2009). Enrichment from birth accelerates the functional and cellular development of a motor control area in the mouse. *PLoS One* 4:e6780.

Sullivan R, Wilson DA, Feldon J, Yee BK, Meyer U, Richter–Levin G, Avi A, Michael T, Gruss M, Bock J, Helmeke C, Braun K. (2006). The International Society for Developmental Psychobiology annual meeting symposium: impact of early life experiences on brain and behavioral development. *Dev Psychobiol* 48:583–602.

Timney B, Mitchell DE, Giffin F. (1978). The development of vision in cats after extended periods of dark–rearing. *Exp Brain Res* 31:547–560.

Tognini P, Manno I, Bonaccorsi J, Cenni MC, Sale A, Maffei L. (2012). Environmental enrichment promotes plasticity and visual acuity recovery in adult monocular amblyopic rats. *PLoS One* 7:e34815.

Trachtenberg JT, Stryker MP. (2001). Rapid anatomical plasticity of horizontal connections in the developing visual cortex. *J Neurosci* 21:3476–3482.

van Praag H, Kempermann G, Gage FH. (2000). Neural consequences of environmental enrichment. *Nat Rev Neurosci* 1:191–198.

Venable N, Fernandez V, Diaz E, Pinto–Hamuy T. (1989). Effects of preweaning environmental enrichment on basilar dendrites of pyramidal neurons in occipital cortex: a Golgi study. *Brain Res Dev Brain Res* 49:140–144.

Ventura AK, Worobey J. (2013). Early influences on the development of food preferences. *Curr Biol* 23:R401–408.

Wang BS, Feng L, Liu M, Liu X, Cang J. (2013). Environmental enrichment rescues binocular matching of orientation preference in mice that have a precocious critical period. *Neuron* 80:198–209.

Werker JF, Tees RC. (2005). Speech perception as a window for understanding plasticity and commitment in language systems of the brain. *Dev Psychobiol* 46:233–251.

Whitlock JR, Heynen AJ, Shuler MG, Bear MF. (2006). Learning induces long–term potentiation in the hippocampus. *Science* 313:1093–1097.

Wiesel TN, Hubel DH. (1963). Single–cell responses in striate cortex of kittens deprived of vision in one eye. *J Neurophysiol* 26:1003–1017.

Woo CC, Leon M. (2013). Environmental enrichment as an effective treatment for autism: a randomized controlled trial. *Behav Neurosci* 127:487–497.

Zhang H, Cai R, Zhang J, Pan Y, Sun X. (2009). Environmental enrichment enhances directional selectivity of primary auditory cortical neurons in rats. *Neurosci Lett* 463:162–165.

CHAPTER 2

Epigenetic control of visual cortex development and plasticity

Paola Tognini[1], Elena Putignano[1], and Tommaso Pizzorusso[1,2]

[1] *Neuroscience Institute, National Research Council (CNR), Pisa, Italy*
[2] *Department of Neuroscience, Psychology, Drug Research and Child Health (NEUROFARBA), University of Florence, Florence, Italy*

Introduction

Neuroplasticity is a multifaceted and dynamic process involving gene–environment interactions that result in both short- and long-term changes in gene expression, cellular function, circuit formation, neuronal morphology, and thereby in modification of behavior. Elevated plasticity marks the early stages of mammalian neurodevelopment when brain circuits and synaptic connections are malleable and easily shaped by experience and environmental cues. Following terminal differentiation, neurons undergo periods of axonal and dendritic branching that allow for fine-tuning of synaptic contacts and the generation of elaborate circuits, many of which can persist throughout the lifetime of an individual. As the brain matures, such connections become progressively more stable and resistant to environmental stimuli; however, they can remain in part malleable permitting, although at a lesser extent, plasticity phenomena (Citri and Malenka, 2008). The mammalian brain depends on complex and highly regulated mechanisms to appropriately activate or silence gene programs in response to inputs from the environment. At the molecular level, these events are controlled by activity-dependent signalling pathways that mediate gene expression by modifying the activity, localization, and/or expression of transcriptional-regulatory enzymes in combination with alterations in chromatin structure in the nucleus (McClung and Nestler, 2008). Therefore, epigenetic mechanisms play a key role in activating the transcriptional program responsible for the establishment and refinement of synaptic connections and neuronal circuits especially during development but not only. Recent studies indicate that alterations in chromatin state and gene expression are important for mediating various aspects of experience-dependent plasticity, such as

Environmental Experience and Plasticity of the Developing Brain, First Edition.
Edited by Alessandro Sale.

developmental plasticity (i.e., visual cortical plasticity), learning and memory, and drug of abuse responses.

The term "epigenetics" (which literally means "above genetics") was introduced for the first time in the early 1940s by Conrad Waddington as "the branch of biology which studies the casual interactions between genes and their products which brings the phenotype into being" (Waddington, 1968). In the original meaning of this definition, epigenetics referred to all molecular pathways modulating the expression of a genotype into a particular phenotype. Over the following years, with the rapid growth of genetics, the meaning of the word has gradually changed, and today, the most widely accepted definition is: "the study of changes in gene function that are mitotically and/or meiotically heritable and that do not entail a change in DNA sequence" (Wu and Morris, 2001). The three key epigenetic mechanisms include histone modifications leading to nucleosome and chromatin remodeling, DNA methylation, and noncoding RNA mediated posttranscriptional regulation. These mechanisms have mostly been explored in the context of embryonic development and stem cell differentiation. However, it is now clear that experience, be it environmental or sensory stimulation, maternal behavior, psychological or physical stress, learning, or drug exposure, causes an active regulation of the chemical and three-dimensional structure of DNA in the nervous system (Borrelli et al., 2008; Dulac, 2010). Epigenetic changes lead to alterations in gene readout in neurons that trigger dynamic and/or long-lasting changes in neural function. It is emerging that chromatin is not a stable and immutable structure but is dynamic and able to integrate a variety of signals from the cell surface in appropriate transcriptional outputs. To achieve this coordinated transcriptional response, specific molecular mechanisms remodel or tag chromatin and DNA. In the following section we are going to analyze more in detail these epigenetic modifications.

Overview of chromatin modifications

Chromatin, the ensemble of genomic DNA with histones, is the physiological form of our genome and the substrate for processes that regulate cellular gene expression. The fundamental repeating unit of chromatin is the nucleosome, which consists of approximately 147 bp of superhelical DNA wrapped around the radial surface of an octamer of highly conserved core histone proteins (two copies each of H2A, H2B, H3, and H4). Histones, particularly histones H3 and H4, are subject to extensive covalent post-translational modifications, including methylation, acetylation, phosphorylation, ubiquitylation, SUMOylation, glycosylation, biotinylation, ADP ribosylation and proline isomerization, and probably others that have yet to be discovered, each occurring at specific sites and amino-acid residues. Most modifications localize to the amino (N)- and carboxy (C)-terminal histone tails, and a few localize to the histone globular domains (Berger, 2007). Some histone modifications act in cis to alter the local chromatin structure directly, whereas others act in trans to influence the recruitment of chromatin-modifying factors. In trans histone modifications enable specific binding partners to dock, often as part of larger multimolecular complexes that induce further chromatin remodeling (Dulac, 2010).

Acetylation is the best characterized of the post-translational modifications (PTMs) on histones. Acetylation of lysine (Lys) residues occurs on the amino group in their side chain, which effectively neutralizes their positive charge, changing nucleosome structure by weakening the electrostatic interaction between the positively charged histone tails and the negatively charged DNA. The reaction is catalyzed by histone acetyltransferases (HATs), which transfer an acetyl group from acetyl-coenzyme A to the ϵ-NH+ group of a Lys residue within a histone (Lau et al., 2000; Tanner et al., 2000). The process is reversible, and the enzymes that catalyze the reversal of histone acetylation are known as histone deacetylases (HDACs). Acetylation of histones ultimately functions to relax chromatin structure allowing for the recruitment of various effector proteins, transcriptional coactivators (some of which contain specific acetyl–lysine recognition motifs, referred to as bromodomains), and members of the general transcriptional machinery (Goldberg et al., 2007).

Histone methylation is another histone-directed epigenetic tag, discovered 50 years ago (Murray, 1964). Similar to acetylation, methylation of histones occurs on ϵ-NH+ groups of Lys residues, but unlike acetylation, methylation of Lys preserves their positive charge. In addition, Lys can accept up to three methyl groups. Arginine residues within histones can also be mono- or dimethylated on their guanidine nitrogen (Kouzarides, 2007). Methyl marks are written by S-adenosylmethionine (SAM)-dependent methyl-transferases and removed by either the Jumonji family of 2-oxoglutarate-dependent demethylases (Tsukada et al., 2006) or the flavin-dependent enzymes lysine-specific histone demethylase 1 (LSD1; also known as KDM1A) and LSD2 (also known as KDM1B) (Shi et al., 2004).

Phosphorylation of histones H1 and H3 was first observed more than 40 years ago in the context of chromosome condensation during mitosis (Gurley et al., 1974). H3 was the first histone whose phosphorylation was characterized in response to the activation of mitogenic signalling pathways and this PTM is correlated with active gene transcription. Phosphorylation of serine 10 on H3 is mediated for example by ribosomal protein S6 kinase 2 (RSK2) and mitogen- and stress-activated protein kinase 1 (MSK1), which are both downstream of extracellular signal-regulated kinase (ERK) (Mahadevan et al., 1991; Sassone-Corsi et al., 1999; Goto et al., 2002). In order to reverse these phosphorylation events, phosphatases remove phosphate groups from histones, for example PP1 and PP2A (Hsu et al., 2000; Nowak et al., 2003).

Acetylation, methylation and phosphorylation involve small chemical groups, whereas ubiquitylation and SUMOylation add large moieties, two-thirds the size of the histone proteins themselves, which may lead to more profound changes in chromatin structure. Another degree of complexity is that methylation can occur several times (mono-, di- or trimethylation) on one lysine side chain, and each level of modification can have different biological outcomes. Some of the functional outcomes of these modifications are clear. For example, there is abundant evidence that acetylation is activating, whereas SUMOylation seems to be repressing for gene expression, and these two types of modification may mutually interfere. By contrast, methylation and ubiquitylation have variable effects, depending on the precise residues and contexts. For example, methylation of lysine 4 or 36 on H3 is associated with transcriptional initiation/pausing and transcriptional elongation, respectively, whereas methylation of lysine 9 or 27 on H3 is more strongly correlated with transcriptional repression/silencing. Two ubiquitylation sites in the C termini of H2B and H2A correlate with active and repressed transcription, respectively (Berger, 2007). The fact that histone modifications can recruit other proteins by recognition of the modified histone via protein domains is a central idea of the histone code hypothesis (Jenuwein and Allis, 2001). The histone code hypothesis refers to the combination of modifications within and between histones that code for information not present in the DNA sequence and predicts that the modification marks on the histone tails should provide binding sites for proteins with regulatory functions that are able to "read" such marks. How those modifications are established or removed is a key step in epigenetic regulation, and a wealth of work has shown that histone tail modifications are established ("written") or removed ("erased") by the action of chromatin-associated enzymatic complexes. Therefore, proteins able to interact with chromatin marks are called: "reader", "writer" or "eraser" based on their function. More recently, due to the complexity of epigenetic tags combinations and to the sophisticated functional outcomes, the scientific community prefers to refer to that as a chromatin language rather than a simple code (Lee et al., 2010).

In the last few years, an epigenetic modification that has caught the attention of neuroscientists has been DNA methylation. Methylation of DNA consists in the transfer of a methyl group on the carbon at position 5 of the cytosine ring and in mammalian cells is preferentially confined to CpG dinucleotides. This modification is known to have a role in the constitutive silencing of chromatin regions, the inactivation of one of the X chromosomes in females, the imprinting of parental alleles, and the silencing of retroviral genes and other individual genes. Cytosine methylation is catalyzed by a class of enzymes called DNA methyl-transferases (DNMT); DNMT3a and DNMT3b can establish a new methylation pattern to unmodified DNA and are thus known as de novo DNMT. On the other hand, DNMT1 functions during DNA replication to copy the DNA methylation pattern from the parental DNA strand onto the newly synthesized daughter strand. Cytosine methylation is not the only covalent modification that has been characterized in DNA. Recent studies demonstrated that 5 methyl-cytosine (5-mC) can be oxidized by specific enzymes called TET (ten-eleven translocation) to

5-hydroxyl-methyl-cytosine (5-hmC). Hydroxymethylcytosine is emerging as the active demethylation mark that targets a specific 5′-methyl group on cytosine for net removal by a complex base excision repair mechanism (Guo et al., 2011a; Guo et al., 2011b). 5-hmC can be deaminated to 5-hydroxyuracil to create a mismatch in the DNA sequence that is removed by glycosylases enzymes. The a-basic site is repaired by the base excision repair machinery resulting in an un-methylated cytosine. Intriguingly, 5-hmC is enriched in the brain with respect to other tissues and changes in its abundance from early postnatal stage to adulthood (Szulwach et al., 2011), rising the possibility that 5-hmC in neurons can play a transcriptional regulatory role. Furthermore, it has been shown that TET1 oxidase is involved in memory formation and storage, providing evidence that DNA methylation and hydroxylmethylation play a role in CNS plasticity (Kaas et al., 2013; Rudenko et al., 2013). The importance of DNA methylation in assisting essential gene regulatory events that are associated with brain function is revealed by neurological disorders caused by deregulation in DNA methylation processes, such as Rett syndrome and Fragile X syndrome. We show examples of disorders connected to DNA methylation more in detail in the next paragraph.

Epigenetics and brain plasticity

Long-term modifications of chromatin are involved in changes in gene expression that lead to neural plasticity. Long-term potentiation (LTP) and long-term depression (LTD) are well-known models of synaptic plasticity, characterized respectively by an up- and a down-regulation of synaptic efficacy. Certain forms of LTP and LTD are long lasting and depend on changes in gene expression. Based on the critical role that chromatin remodeling plays in creating a transcription permissive or silencing state of the genome (Felsenfeld and Groudine, 2003), growing evidence suggests that histone PTMs may be implicated in these processes. For example, H4 acetylation at specific promoters in Aplysia is altered after LTP and LTD (Guan et al., 2002).

Plasticity-induced epigenetic changes are also observed in mammalian models of synaptic plasticity. Several forms of LTP require the activation of NMDA receptors and engagement of the MEK–ERK/MAPK signalling cascade (Morris et al., 1986; English and Sweatt, 1997). Direct activation of NMDA receptors in the hippocampus leads to an increase in acetylation of histone H3, which can be blocked by inhibition of the MEK–ERK/MAPK cascade. In addition, activation of dopaminergic, cholinergic and glutamatergic signalling pathways in the hippocampus induces ERK-dependent increases in the phosphorylation of histone H3. These results suggest that the induction of mammalian synaptic plasticity leads to ERK-dependent increases in histone acetylation and phosphorylation in the hippocampus (Levenson and Sweatt, 2005).

The transcription factor CREB (AMP cyclic response element [CRE] binding protein) is essential for activity-induced gene expression. At the mechanistic level, CREB-associated transcriptional regulation has been shown to involve the recruitment of multicomponent regulator complexes, as well as the initiation of chromatin-remodeling events. Activated CREB recruits CREB-binding protein (CBP; also known as CREBBP) or its paralogue p300 (also known as EP300), which functions as both a scaffolding protein and a HAT. CBP recruitment, in turn, stimulates histone acetylation and transcriptional-complex formation at the promoters, leading to transcriptional activation of many CREB-target genes. Mutations in the gene encoding CBP are responsible for the mental-retardation syndrome Rubinstein–Taybi, the phenotype of which may result from impairment of either or both of the CREB-dependent and CREB-independent functions of CBP. The essential role of HAT activity in CBP-mediated neuronal plasticity has been genetically demonstrated by the selective long-term memory defects of a transgenic mouse line carrying a dominant-negative CBP that blocks the HAT activity of the endogenous protein (Korzus et al., 2004). In another study, the induction of early phase LTP and LTD – forms of plasticity that do not require transcription – was not affected in CBP+/– animals. However, the induction of late-phase LTP, which requires transcription, was significantly impaired in CBP+/– mice. Treatment of hippocampal slices from CBP+/– animals with an HDAC inhibitor significantly improved late-phase LTP induction, which indicates that inhibition of HDACs had compensated for HAT haploinsufficiency (Alarcon et al., 2004). In other studies using hippocampal slices, induction of LTP through high-frequency stimulation was significantly enhanced by two HDAC inhibitors, trichostatin A (TSA) and sodium butyrate (Levenson et al., 2004). In addition, LTP in the amygdala that was induced by forskolin was also enhanced by the HDAC inhibitor TSA (Yeh et al., 2004). These discoveries indicate that the epigenetic state of the genome affects the induction of long-term forms of mammalian synaptic plasticity.

Recent studies implicated histone PTMs in memory formation and storage. Guan et al. (2009) demonstrated that neuronal-specific overexpression of HDAC2, but not that of HDAC1, decreased dendritic spine density, synapse number, synaptic plasticity and memory formation. Conversely, HDAC2 deficiency resulted in increased synapse number and memory facilitation, similar to chronic treatment with HDAC inhibitors in mice. These results suggest that HDAC2 functions in modulating synaptic plasticity and long-lasting changes of neural circuits, which in turn negatively regulates learning and memory (Guan et al., 2009). HDAC3 has also an impact on learning and memory processes. Focal deletion of HDAC3 in hippocampus increased histone acetylation as well as object location memory, although not object recognition memory, in agreement with the role of hippocampus in these forms of memory (McQuown et al., 2011). Moreover, histone methylation is actively regulated in the hippocampus and facilitates long-term memory formation. Trimethylation of histone H3 at lysine 4 (H3K4), an active mark for transcription, is upregulated in hippocampus 1 h following contextual fear conditioning, while dimethylation of histone H3 at lysine 9 (H3K9), a molecular mark associated with transcriptional silencing, is increased 1 h after fear conditioning and decreased 24 h after context exposure alone and contextual fear conditioning. Furthermore, mice deficient in the H3K4-specific histone methyltransferase, Mll, displayed deficits in contextual fear conditioning relative to wild-type animals (Gupta et al., 2010). This suggests that histone methylation is required for proper long-term consolidation of contextual fear memories.

Histone proteins present variants, nonallelic forms of the conventional histones, and their incorporation in the nucleosome is involved in transcriptional regulation, repair, chromosome assembly and segregation. The histone subunit H2A.Z has been involved in memory consolidation, through nucleosome exchange in the promoter region of specific memory genes (Zovkic et al., 2014). Therefore, histone variants exchange seems to be an additional epigenetic contributor to the complexity of gene expression regulation in brain plasticity.

Drug addiction can be viewed as a form of drug-induced neural plasticity or "maladaptive plasticity", whereby repeated exposure to drugs of abuse leads to long-lasting changes in the brain's natural reward centers and associated memory circuits, which underlie the addiction phenotype. Multiple drugs of abuse induce changes in histone acetylation in the brain, and evidence has begun to accumulate that these modifications underlie some of the functional abnormalities found in addiction models. First, global levels of H3 and H4 acetylation are increased in the Nucleus Accumbens (NAc) after acute or chronic exposure to cocaine (Kumar et al., 2005; Renthal and Nestler, 2008), and gene promoters that show increased H3 or H4 acetylation have been mapped genome-wide (Renthal et al., 2009). Despite these global increases, many genes show decreased histone acetylation after chronic cocaine, raising a key question as to what governs gene-specific acetylation changes in the face of global modifications. Histone methylation is also directly regulated by drugs of abuse: global levels of histone 3 lysine 9 dimethylation (H3K9me2) are reduced in the NAc after chronic cocaine exposure (Maze et al., 2010), and a genome-wide screen revealed alterations in H3K9me2 binding on the promoters of numerous genes in this brain region (Renthal et al., 2009); both increases and decreases were observed, indicating again that epigenetic modifications at individual genes often defy global changes. The global decrease in H3K9me2 in the NAc is probably mediated by cocaine-induced downregulation of two histones methyl transferases, G9a and G9a-like protein (GLP), which catalyse the dimethylation of H3K9me2. These adaptations mediate enhanced responsiveness to cocaine, as selective knockout or pharmacological inhibition of G9a in the NAc promotes cocaine-induced behaviours, whereas G9a overexpression has the opposite effect (Maze et al., 2010).

Given the involvement of epigenetic mechanisms in nervous system function, it is not surprising that a growing number of disorders, in particular mental retardation and autism spectrum syndromes, have been linked to chromatin remodeling defects. The most well-studied "epigenetic disease" associated with altered neurological function, is Rett syndrome, an X-linked postnatal autism spectrum disorder characterized by stereotypical motor, learning, and social abnormalities that generally worsen over time (Moretti and Zoghbi, 2006). Candidate gene analyses identified MeCP2 as the gene responsible for this disorder (Amir et al., 1999). MeCP2 binds both methylated and hydroxylmethylated CpG dinucleotides and it regulates gene expression in a repressive or activated fashion (Mellen et al., 2012). Fragile X syndrome, the most commonly inherited form of mental retardation, is brought about by an abnormal expansion of repeated trinucleotide sequences within one of two Fragile X genes: FMR1 and FMR2 (Ashley et al., 1993). FMR1 and FMR2 contain a polymorphic trinucleotide repeat (CGG and CCG, respectively) in their 5′-untranslated regions that are responsible for the loss of gene expression. Expansion of these repeats results in hypermethylation of these regions and flanking CpG islands, leading to transcriptional silencing of the FMR and surrounding genes (Levenson and Sweatt, 2005). These two examples shed light on the importance of DNA methylation for a correct development of brain functions.

In Rubinstein-Taybi syndrome (RSTS), characterized by mental retardation and developmental abnormalities, the DNA-binding hook is provided by CREB. Phosphorylation of CREB leads to CBP recruitment and activation of target promoters. In RSTS, mutations in the CBP gene result in impairment of its HAT activity. Mice haploinsufficient for CBP display impaired cognitive function, altered neuronal plasticity, and aberrant histone acetylation at target gene promoters. Interestingly, the behavioral symptoms can be ameliorated by administration of HDAC inhibitors (Vo and Goodman, 2001).

A striking example of developmental disruption caused by mutations in a chromatin factor gene is alpha-thalassaemia/mental retardation, X-linked syndrome, the gene for which is a helicase (spinocerebellar ataxia-7) involved in chromatin remodeling, by regulating several HAT complexes. Mutations lead to defects in psychomotor, urogenital and haematopoietic development, with maturational defects in erythroid precursors resembling those of alpha-thalassaemia (Feinberg, 2007). These pathologies are just some examples of disorders involving alteration in epigenetic mechanisms (for a review see Portela and Esteller, 2010). All these observations indicate that dysfunction of the normal epigenetic status of the genome can have marked consequences on synaptic plasticity processes and normal cognitive function, indicating that drugs that target the epigenome might represent viable therapies for treating various diseases that affect cognition.

Epigenetic control on visual system development

The visual system has long been one of the most investigated models for the study of experience-dependent plasticity, because visual experience can be easily manipulated and the subsequent effects can be measured at the anatomical, physiological and molecular level. The maturation of the visual circuitry starts before the eye opening and therefore before the onset of vision, although experience is necessary for a correct development of the visual system, especially during a specific window of time called the critical period (P21-P35 in rodents). During this period of heightened plasticity, experience is able to produce permanent and extensive modifications of cortical organizations. Indeed, in animals reared in total darkness from birth (dark rearing [DR]), visual connections do not consolidate and remains plastic even after the closure of the critical period. Furthermore, neuronal cells displayed immature properties such as reduced orientation selectivity, direction tuning and larger receptive fields, which are typical of cortical neurons at the time of eye opening (Timney et al., 1978; Fagiolini et al., 1994). Monocular deprivation (MD), which consists in the closure of one eye, is the classic paradigm used to study ocular dominance (OD) plasticity: the rapid change in the responses of visual cortical neurons, which results from unbalanced inputs from the two eyes. If MD is performed during the critical period, it causes the synaptic reorganization of primary visual (V1) cortex circuits. The deprived eye shows a loss of visual acuity resulting from a decrease in the visual inputs that causes an irreversible reduction of the ability of that eye to drive neuronal responses in the cortex; therefore neurons in the binocular zone of the contralateral V1, previously dominated by the deprived eye, shift their responsiveness toward the ipsilateral open eye (i.e., ocular dominance shift). Behaviorally, animals monocularly deprived during development lose visual acuity and stereoscopic vision (amblyopia) in the deprived eye and any subsequent experience or visual stimulation cannot completely reverse the effects of early deprivation after the closure of the critical period (Berardi et al., 2003). Visual cortical plasticity declines with age. Nonetheless, in mice prolonged periods of altered sensory experience or primed experience can also lead to synaptic modifications during adulthood (Rittenhouse et al., 1999; Sawtell et al., 2003; Hofer et al., 2006), although to a lesser extent and without the profound effects on neuronal circuits observed in young animals.

As previously underlined, several studies have demonstrated that regulation of gene expression is one of the key mechanisms involved in brain plasticity. Indeed, experience-dependent plasticity in the visual cortex activates specific gene programs aimed to reshape neuronal circuits and synaptic connections as shown by genome wide analysis performed both in MD and DR animals (Majdan and Shatz, 2006; Tropea et al., 2006). This suggests that the consequences of visual manipulations could be mediated in part through modifications in the chromatin landscape aimed to activate or repress the transcription of experience-controlled genes. Therefore, visual experience activates mechanisms regulating gene transcription at different levels: an episode of light stimulation after three days of DR in juvenile mice activates CRE-mediated gene expression and induces the phosphorylation of the transcription factor CREB; moreover, visual experience also induces histone H4 acetylation, histone H3 phosphorylation and acetylation. These posttranslational modifications are mediated by visual stimuli induced activation of ERK-MSK signaling cascade (Putignano et al., 2007). It is well known that plasticity in the visual cortex is very pronounced during the critical period and it declines after its end. Different mechanisms have been proposed to be responsible for the closure of the visual sensitive period, such as changes in extracellular matrix composition and axonal myelinization, which could inhibit structural plasticity (Pizzorusso et al., 2002; McGee et al., 2005; Pizzorusso et al., 2006), and maturation of inhibitory circuits that changes the excitatory/inhibitory balance, making the circuitry less favorable to plasticity (Hensch and Fagiolini, 2005; Gandhi et al., 2008; Yazaki-Sugiyama et al., 2009; Iurilli et al., 2013).

Recently, we showed that signaling cascades regulating histone post-translational modifications and subsequently chromatin landscape and gene expression contributes to the closure of the critical period. CREB phosporyla-tion, CRE-mediated gene expression, and histone acetylation are not induced by visual stimulation in adult mice, suggesting epigenetic mechanisms to play a role in experience-dependent gene transcription in developmental experience-dependent plasticity (Putignano et al., 2007). Visual cortical plasticity studies are interesting from a clinical point of view too, because humans frequently are affected by amblyopia (or lazy eye). Visual manipulation or defective visual experience during the critical period cause profound changes in the organization of visual circuits leading to a substantial decrease in visual acuity and stereoscopic vision. For instance, children with congenital cataracts or strabismus could become amblyopic if not treated before 8 years of age. These treatments are generally ineffective in adult persons due to the decline in activity-dependent plasticity as with rodents. Therefore, to find strategies to enhance experience-dependent plasticity in rodents is of great interest with the prospect to develop new therapies for humans. Interestingly, epigenetic manipulation in mice and rats has been demonstrated to be effective in restoring juvenile-like plasticity in the visual cortex. Increasing histone acetylation through an HDAC inhibitor (TSA) treatment, promotes OD plasticity after MD in adult mice (Putignano et al., 2007). Furthermore, epigenetic drugs increasing histone acetylation reverse visual acuity deficits induced by long-term MD initi-ated during the critical period in rodents. Indeed, visual acuity of the amblyopic eye recovers to the normal value in adult rats treated with HDAC inhibitors (valproic acid or sodium butyrate), tested both electrophysiologically and behaviorally (Silingardi et al., 2010). Therefore, altering chromatin landscape can be considered a way to promote functional recovery from early alteration of sensory inputs in the adult cortex.

As previously mentioned, CREB-dependent gene expression has been shown to be a key mechanism in the regulation of developmental plasticity in the visual system (Pham et al., 1999; Mower et al., 2002; Cancedda et al., 2003) or other brain structures (Lonze and Ginty, 2002). Nonetheless, little is known about which specific CREB-dependent genes are involved in the molecular mechanisms implicated in experience-dependent plasticity. Recently, a microRNA, miR-132, raced up our attention as a candidate CREB-regulated gene involved in visual developmental plasticity. MicroRNAs (miRNAs) are endogenous evolutionarily conserved short noncoding RNAs that interact with specific target mRNAs based on sequence imperfect complementarity in the 3′ untranslated region (UTR) of the target mRNAs, resulting in translational repression or mRNA deadenylation and degradation. MiRNAs are processed from RNA polymerase II (RNAPII)-specific transcripts of independent genes or from introns of protein-coding genes. In the canonical pathway, primary precursor (pri-miRNA) processing occurs in two steps, catalysed by two members of the RNase III family of enzymes, Drosha and Dicer, operating in complexes with dsRNA-binding proteins, for example DGCR8 and transactivation-responsive (TAR) RNA-binding protein (TRBP) in mammals. In the first nuclear step, the Drosha–DGCR8 complex processes the pri-miRNA into an ~70-nucleotide precursor hairpin (pre-miRNA), which is exported to the cytoplasm. Some pre-miRNAs are produced from very short introns (mirtrons) as a result of splicing and debranching, thereby bypassing the Drosha–DGCR8 step. In either case, cleavage by Dicer, assisted by TRBP, in the cytoplasm yields an ~20-bp miRNA/miRNA* duplex. Following processing, one strand of the miRNA/miRNA* duplex (the guide strand) is preferentially incorporated into a miRNA-induced silencing complex (miRISC), whereas the other strand (passenger or miRNA*) is released and degraded. Generally, the retained strand is the one that has the less stably base-paired 5′ end in the miRNA/miRNA* duplex. miRNA* strands are not always by-products of miRNA biogenesis and can also be loaded into miRISC to function as miRNAs. Argonaute (AGO) proteins, which directly interact with miRNAs, and glycine-tryptophan protein of 182 kDa (GW182) proteins, which act as downstream effectors in the repression, are key factors in the assembly and function of miRISCs. As part of miRISC, miRNAs base- pair to target mRNAs and induce their translational repression or deadenylation and degradation (Tognini and Pizzorusso, 2012). It is important to note that miRNAs are emerging as key modulators of post-transcriptional gene regulation in many tissues.

Recent evidence points to a widespread role for neural miRNAs at various stages of synaptic development, including dendritogenesis, synapse formation and synapse maturation. Furthermore, they play a role in brain plasticity, learning and memory and their dysregulation has been described in neurological diseases.

MiR-132 belongs to the miR212/132 family, highly conserved in vertebrates, and its expression is strongly enriched in all brain structures tested (Vo et al., 2005; Klein et al., 2007; Remenyi et al., 2010). The miR-132 genomic locus is characterized by the presence of four CRE consensus sites that regulate both miR-132 and miR-212 transcription (Remenyi et al., 2010), for instance miR-132 expression is strongly induced by the activation of CREB pathway both in vitro

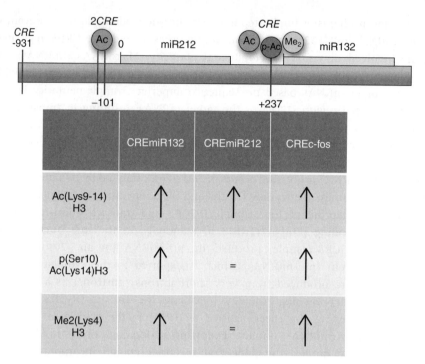

Figure 2.1 Sketch of histone post-translational modifications induced by visual experience on miR212/132 gene. (See insert for color representation of this figure.)

and in vivo (Vo et al., 2005; Hollander et al., 2010). Neuronal cultures treatment with CREB-activating stimuli such as forskolin, depolarizing agents, or neurothrophins (i.e., BDNF) strongly increased miR-132 levels (Vo et al., 2005; Klein et al., 2007; Wayman et al., 2008; Nudelman et al., 2010). Moreover, miR-132 has been involved in regulation of neurite outgrowth and activity-dependent dendritic spine remodeling in neuronal cell cultures (Vo et al., 2005; Wayman et al., 2008; Edbauer et al., 2010).

Experience-dependent miR-132 expression has been demonstrated to play an essential role in visual cortical plasticity (Mellios et al., 2011; Tognini et al., 2011). In the visual cortex miR-132 is strongly induced by visual stimuli during the critical period. Indeed, a short light stimulation after three days of DR is able to increase the level of the mature miR-132 and of the pri-miRNA (pri-miR-132). Strikingly, visual stimulation upregulates histone modifications involved in transcriptional activation on miR-212/132 genomic locus, specifically across the CRE sites necessary for pri-miR-132 expression: Acetyl (Lys9-14), phospho (Ser10) Ac (Lys14) and dimethyl (Lys4) on H3, suggesting that miR-132 expression is epigenetically controlled by light stimuli (Figure 2.1).

Intriguingly, miR-132 is developmentally regulated in the visual cortex, showing a very low expression before eye-opening and a marked increase during the critical period with a peak between P25 and P30. In mice reared in darkness from birth, miR-132 levels remain constantly low at the same range observed before the eye opening, indicating that its expression is strongly driven by visual inputs. Therefore, the miR-132 developmental curve suggests a key role for this microRNA during the sensitive period, a time of intense synaptogenisis, dendritic spines turnover and experience-dependent refinement of neuronal circuits. As expected, in adult mice pri-miR-132 light stimuli-dependent induction is significantly reduced suggesting miR-132 as a player in juvenile plasticity; enhancement of histone acetylation through TSA treatment is able to increase pri-miR-132 induction in the adult visual cortex, confirming that histone posttranslational modifications are involved in experience-dependent miR-132 transcription (Tognini et al., 2011). As explained earlier, MD is the classic paradigm used to study experience-dependent plasticity in the visual cortex. Microarray analysis demonstrated that miR-132 is one of the most highly dowregulated miRNA by MD in juvenile mice (Mellios et al., 2011). Interestingly, a decrease in H3 phosphoacetylation on the miR-212/132 genomic locus was observed during MD too (Tognini et al., 2011), reinforcing the hypothesis that epigenetic mark changes tightly control this microRNA transcription. Interfering with miR-132 downregulation during MD by counteracting its decrease through cortical infusion of a chemically modified miRNA-mimic or further reducing it via miR-132- sequestering –sponge coding virus injection, totally prevents OD plasticity in mice during the critical period. These results were obtained by in vivo electrophysiological recording (Tognini et al., 2011) and two-photon calcium imaging (Mellios et al., 2011) and show that an optimal concentration of miR-132 is necessary for experience-dependent plasticity.

MiR-132 action on cortical neurons involves changes in dendritic spine morphology; indeed miR-132 mimic treatment increases the fraction of mushroom/stubby spines in the visual cortex, representing the mature and stable form of dendritic spines (Tognini et al., 2011). Conversely, miR132 downregulation results in more immature spines (Mellios et al., 2011). Taken together, these two results suggest that the miR-132 decrease induced by MD could be necessary to make dendritic spines less stable, allowing the occurrence of the structural plasticity mechanisms underlying OD plasticity, whereas the strong miR-132 reduction obtained by viral transduction would make spines too unstable to consolidate OD plasticity (Tognini and Pizzorusso, 2012). Therefore, an optimal concentration of miR-132 seems to be necessary for the occurrence of OD plasticity. Interestingly, the necessity to tightly control the amount of miR-132 level to allow plasticity has been proposed for cognitive functions too: a robust overexpression of miR-132 in the hippocampus impaired learning and memory and was correlated with an excessive spine density, whereas a moderate increase of miR-132 enhanced cognitive abilities (Hansen et al., 2013).

Which target proteins mediate the effect of miR-132? In the central nervous system the best candidate proteins are MeCP2 and p250GAP. MeCP2 is a DNA methyl binding protein implicated in transcriptional regulation, and its gene mutations cause Rett syndrome, a form of autism characterized by dendritic spine abnormalities. For instance, it has been shown that MeCP2 ko mice have impairments in visual functions caused by an early upregulation and maturation of parvalbumin cells and hyperconnectivity of perisomatic PV-circuits and a consequent shift in cortical E/I balance favoring inhibition (Durand et al., 2012). P250GAP is a Rho family GTPase activating protein. Previously, it was demonstrated that p250GAP is a bona fide miR-132 target (Vo et al., 2005; Wayman et al., 2008) and it was shown that this protein is enriched in the postsynaptic density (Nakazawa et al., 2003; Okabe et al., 2003). It has been proposed that miR-132 regulates spine formation in hippocampal neurons by downregulating p250GAP and activating the Rac1-PAK actin-remodeling pathway (Impey et al., 2010). Therefore, we can speculate that regulation of p250GAP expression could be a mechanism by which miR132 modulates structural plasticity at the synapse, in particular dynamic changes in spines associated with OD plasticity. However, due to the high number of putative target proteins for each microRNA, deeper studies are necessary to discover the specific miR-132 targets mediating its effect on visual cortical plasticity during development.

Future directions

Although a lot of exciting discoveries have been made during the last decade, we still need to address many questions. The mammalian brain is a very complicated and heterogeneous organ characterized by functionally different areas and a huge variety of cell populations. Glial cells and all the diverse neurons might have different epigenome and transcriptome. So far, the majority of epigenetic studies have used homogenates of the highly heterogeneous cells composing the neural tissue (excitatory and inhibitory neurons, glial cells, etc.) potentially masking the diversity of cell-specific epigenetic marks or gene expression. The solution to this challenge is a single-cell type analysis (i.e., laser capture microdissection, fluorescence-activated cell sorting, etc.) that is not easy to apply and requires careful collection and processing of the sample to avoid induction of expression changes.

Concerning the visual cortex a lot of open issues remain to be addressed: besides acetylation of H3 and H4 and methylation of Lys4 on H3, which other histone PTM are involved in the regulation of ocular dominance plasticity and development of the visual cortex? Are these epigenetic marks highly dynamic or they are long-lasting after the period of deprivation? We might speculate that some specific epigenetic marks acquired during experience early in life could prime gene expression later in adulthood. Moreover, we have just a very little information concerning the genes targeted by histone PTM in ocular dominance plasticity. High throughput techniques (i.e., ChIP – seq) will give precious insights regarding how dynamic is the epigenome. In addition, DNA methylation could further expand our knowledge about chromatin remodeling and transcriptional control in the visual cortex (Tognini et al., 2015).

It is worth to notice that epigenetic drugs have been used in humans to tackle the brake in neuroplasticity induced by the closure of sensitive periods. HDAC inhibitors are not just able to promote plasticity in adult rodents (Putignano et al., 2007; Silingardi et al., 2010; Yang et al., 2012) but even in humans. Valproate facilitates sensory plasticity in adult persons allowing them to identify a pitch (i.e., absolute pitch, the ability to produce or to identify the pitch of a musical sound without any reference point) (Gervain et al., 2013). This pioneering study paves the way to the use of HDAC inhibitors to restore critical-period plasticity in the adult human brain highlighting the power of exploiting the remodeling of the epigenome in the reorganization and rewiring of consolidated neuronal cortical circuits.

Acknowledgments

We thank the Italian Flagship project EPIGEN for financial support of our work.

References

Alarcon JM, Malleret G, Touzani K, Vronskaya S, Ishii S, Kandel ER, Barco A. (2004). Chromatin acetylation, memory, and LTP are impaired in CBP+/− mice: a model for the cognitive deficit in Rubinstein–Taybi syndrome and its amelioration. *Neuron* 42:947–959.

Amir RE, Van den Veyver IB, Wan M, Tran CQ, Francke U, Zoghbi HY. (1999). Rett syndrome is caused by mutations in X-linked MECP2, encoding methyl-CpG-binding protein 2. *Nat Genet* 23:185–188.

Ashley CT, Sutcliffe JS, Kunst CB, Leiner HA, Eichler EE, Nelson DL, Warren ST. (1993). Human and murine FMR-1: alternative splicing and translational initiation downstream of the CGG–repeat. *Nat Genet* 4:244–251.

Berardi N, Pizzorusso T, Ratto GM, Maffei L. (2003). Molecular basis of plasticity in the visual cortex. *Trends Neurosci* 26:369–378.

Berger SL. (2007). The complex language of chromatin regulation during transcription. *Nature* 447:407–412.

Borrelli E, Nestler EJ, Allis CD, Sassone–Corsi P. (2008). Decoding the epigenetic language of neuronal plasticity. *Neuron* 60:961–974.

Cancedda L, Putignano E, Impey S, Maffei L, Ratto GM, Pizzorusso T. (2003). Patterned vision causes CRE-mediated gene expression in the visual cortex through PKA and ERK. *J Neurosci* 23:7012–7020.

Citri A, Malenka RC. (2008). Synaptic plasticity: multiple forms, functions, and mechanisms. *Neuropsychopharmacology* 33:18–41.

Dulac C. (2010). Brain function and chromatin plasticity. *Nature* 465:728–735.

Durand S, Patrizi A, Quast KB, Hachigian L, Pavlyuk R, Saxena A, Carninci P, Hensch TK, Fagiolini M. (2012). NMDA receptor regulation prevents regression of visual cortical function in the absence of Mecp2. *Neuron* 76:1078–1090.

Edbauer D, Neilson JR, Foster KA, Wang CF, Seeburg DP, Batterton MN, Tada T, Dolan BM, Sharp PA, Sheng M. (2010). Regulation of synaptic structure and function by FMRP-associated microRNAs miR–125b and miR–132. *Neuron* 65:373–384.

English JD, Sweatt JD. (1997). A requirement for the mitogen-activated protein kinase cascade in hippocampal long term potentiation. *J Biol Chem* 272:19103–19106.

Fagiolini M, Pizzorusso T, Berardi N, Domenici L, Maffei L. (1994). Functional postnatal development of the rat primary visual cortex and the role of visual experience: dark rearing and monocular deprivation. *Vision Res* 34:709–720.

Feinberg AP. (2007). Phenotypic plasticity and the epigenetics of human disease. *Nature* 447: 433–440.

Felsenfeld G, Groudine M. (2003). Controlling the double helix. *Nature* 421:448–453.

Gandhi SP, Yanagawa Y, Stryker MP. (2008). Delayed plasticity of inhibitory neurons in developing visual cortex. *Proc Natl Acad Sci USA* 105:16797–16802.

Gervain J, Vines BW, Chen LM, Seo RJ, Hensch TK, Werker JF, Young AH. (2013). Valproate reopens critical–period learning of absolute pitch. *Frontiers in Syst Neurosci* 7:102.

Goldberg AD, Allis CD, Bernstein E. (2007). Epigenetics: a landscape takes shape. *Cell* 128:635–638.

Goto H, Yasui Y, Nigg EA, Inagaki M. (2002). Aurora–B phosphorylates Histone H3 at serine28 with regard to the mitotic chromosome condensation. *Genes Cells* 7:11–17.

Guan JS, Haggarty SJ, Giacometti E, Dannenberg JH, Joseph N, Gao J, Nieland TJ, Zhou Y, Wang X, Mazitschek R, et al. (2009). HDAC2 negatively regulates memory formation and synaptic plasticity. *Nature* 459:55–60.

Guan Z, Giustetto M, Lomvardas S, Kim JH, Miniaci MC, Schwartz JH, Thanos D, Kandel ER. (2002). Integration of long-term-memory-related synaptic plasticity involves bidirectional regulation of gene expression and chromatin structure. *Cell* 111:483–493.

Guo JU, Ma DK, Mo H, Ball MP, Jang MH, Bonaguidi MA, Balazer JA, Eaves HL, Xie B, Ford E, et al. (2011a). Neuronal activity modifies the DNA methylation landscape in the adult brain. *Nat Neurosci* 14:1345–1351.

Guo JU, Su Y, Zhong C, Ming GL, Song H. (2011b). Hydroxylation of 5-methylcytosine by TET1 promotes active DNA demethylation in the adult brain. *Cell* 145:423–434.

Gupta S, Kim SY, Artis S, Molfese DL, Schumacher A, Sweatt JD, Paylor RE, Lubin FD. (2010). Histone methylation regulates memory formation. *J Neurosci* 30:3589–3599.

Gurley LR, Walters RA, Tobey RA. (1974). Cell cycle–specific changes in histone phosphorylation associated with cell proliferation and chromosome condensation. *J Cell Biol* 60: 356–364.

Hansen KF, Karelina K, Sakamoto K, Wayman GA, Impey S, Obrietan K. (2013). miRNA–132: a dynamic regulator of cognitive capacity. *Brain StructFunct* 218:817–831.

Hensch TK, Fagiolini M. (2005). Excitatory-inhibitory balance and critical period plasticity in developing visual cortex. *Prog Brain Res* 147:115–124.

Hofer SB, Mrsic–Flogel TD, Bonhoeffer T, Hubener M. (2006). Prior experience enhances plasticity in adult visual cortex. *Nat Neurosci* 9:127–132.

Hollander JA, Im HI, Amelio AL, Kocerha J, Bali P, Lu Q, Willoughby D, Wahlestedt C, Conkright MD, Kenny PJ. (2010). Striatal microRNA controls cocaine intake through CREB signalling. *Nature* 466:197–202.

Hsu JY, Sun ZW, Li X, Reuben M, Tatchell K, Bishop DK, Grushcow JM, Brame CJ, Caldwell JA, Hunt DF, et al. (2000). Mitotic phosphorylation of histone H3 is governed by Ipl1/aurora kinase and Glc7/PP1 phosphatase in budding yeast and nematodes. *Cell* 102: 279–291.

Impey S, Davare M, Lasiek A, Fortin D, Ando H, Varlamova O, Obrietan K, Soderling TR, Goodman RH, Wayman GA. (2010). An activity-induced microRNA controls dendritic spine formation by regulating Rac1–PAK signaling. *Mol Cell Neurosci* 43:146–156.

Iurilli G, Olcese U, Medini P. (2013). Preserved excitatory-inhibitory balance of cortical synaptic inputs following deprived eye stimulation after a saturating period of monocular deprivation in rats. *PloS one* 8, e82044.

Jenuwein T, Allis CD. (2001). Translating the histone code. *Science* 293:1074–1080.

Kaas GA, Zhong C, Eason DE, Ross DL, Vachhani RV, Ming GL, King JR, Song H, Sweatt JD. (2013). TET1 controls CNS 5-methylcytosine hydroxylation, active DNA demethylation, gene transcription, and memory formation. *Neuron* 79:1086–1093.

Klein ME, Lioy DT, Ma L, Impey S, Mandel G, Goodman RH. (2007). Homeostatic regulation of MeCP2 expression by a CREB–induced microRNA. *Nat Neurosci* 10:1513–1514.

Korzus E, Rosenfeld MG, Mayford M. (2004). CBP histone acetyltransferase activity is a critical component of memory consolidation. *Neuron* 42:961–972.

Kouzarides T. (2007). Chromatin modifications and their function. *Cell* 128:693–705.

Kumar A, Choi KH, Renthal W, Tsankova NM, Theobald DE, Truong HT, Russo SJ, Laplant Q, Sasaki TS, Whistler KN, et al. (2005). Chromatin remodeling is a key mechanism underlying cocaine–induced plasticity in striatum. *Neuron* 48:303–314.

Lau OD, Courtney AD, Vassilev A, Marzilli LA, Cotter RJ, Nakatani Y, Cole PA. (2000). p300/CBP-associated factor histone acetyltransferase processing of a peptide substrate. Kinetic analysis of the catalytic mechanism. *J Biol Chem* 275:21953–21959.

Lee JS, Smith E, Shilatifard A. (2010). The language of histone crosstalk. *Cell* 142:682–685.

Levenson JM, O'Riordan KJ, Brown KD, Trinh MA, Molfese DL, Sweatt JD. (2004). Regulation of histone acetylation during memory formation in the hippocampus. *J Biol Chem* 279:40545–40559.

Levenson JM, Sweatt JD. (2005). Epigenetic mechanisms in memory formation. *Nat Rev Neurosci* 6:108–118.

Lonze BE, Ginty DD. (2002). Function and regulation of CREB family transcription factors in the nervous system. *Neuron* 35:605–623.

Mahadevan LC, Willis AC, Barratt MJ. (1991). Rapid histone H3 phosphorylation in response to growth factors, phorbol esters, okadaic acid, and protein synthesis inhibitors. *Cell* 65:775–783.

Majdan M, Shatz CJ. (2006). Effects of visual experience on activity-dependent gene regulation in cortex. *Nat Neurosci* 9:650–659.

Maze I, Covington HE 3rd,, Dietz DM, LaPlant Q, Renthal W, Russo SJ, Mechanic M, Mouzon E, Neve RL, Haggarty SJ, et al. (2010). Essential role of the histone methyltransferase G9a in cocaine–induced plasticity. *Science* 327:213–216.

McClung CA, Nestler EJ. (2008). Neuroplasticity mediated by altered gene expression. *Neuropsychopharmacology* 33:3–17.

McGee AW, Yang Y, Fischer QS, Daw NW, Strittmatter SM. (2005). Experience-driven plasticity of visual cortex limited by myelin and Nogo receptor. *Science* 309:2222–2226.

McQuown SC, Barrett RM, Matheos DP, Post RJ, Rogge GA, Alenghat T, Mullican SE, Jones S, Rusche JR, Lazar MA, et al. (2011). HDAC3 is a critical negative regulator of long-term memory formation. *J Neurosci* 31:764–774.

Mellen M, Ayata P, Dewell S, Kriaucionis S, Heintz N. (2012). MeCP2 binds to 5hmC enriched within active genes and accessible chromatin in the nervous system. *Cell* 151:1417–1430.

Mellios N, Sugihara H, Castro J, Banerjee A, Le C, Kumar A, Crawford B, Strathmann J, Tropea D, Levine SS, et al. (2011). miR-132, an experience–dependent microRNA, is essential for visual cortex plasticity. *Nat Neurosci* 14:1240–1242.

Moretti P, Zoghbi HY. (2006). MeCP2 dysfunction in Rett syndrome and related disorders. *Curr Opin Genet Dev* 16:276–281.

Morris RG, Anderson E, Lynch GS, Baudry M. (1986). Selective impairment of learning and blockade of long-term potentiation by an N-methyl-D-aspartate receptor antagonist, AP5. *Nature* 319:774–776.

Mower AF, Liao DS, Nestler EJ, Neve RL, Ramoa AS. (2002). cAMP/Ca2+ response element-binding protein function is essential for ocular dominance plasticity. *J Neurosci* 22:2237–2245.

Murray K. (1964). The occurrence of epsilon-N-methyl lysine in histones. *Biochemistry* 3:10–15.

Nakazawa T, Watabe AM, Tezuka T, Yoshida Y, Yokoyama K, Umemori H, Inoue A, Okabe S, Manabe T, Yamamoto T. (2003). p250GAP, a novel brain-enriched GTPase–activating protein for Rho family GTPases, is involved in the N-methyl-d-aspartate receptor signaling. *Mol Biol Cell* 14:2921–2934.

Nowak SJ, Pai CY, Corces VG. (2003). Protein phosphatase 2A activity affects histone H3 phosphorylation and transcription in Drosophila melanogaster. *Mol Cell Biol* 23:6129–6138.

Nudelman AS, DiRocco DP, Lambert TJ, Garelick MG, Le J, Nathanson NM, Storm DR. (2010). Neuronal activity rapidly induces transcription of the CREB-regulated microRNA-132, in vivo. *Hippocampus* 20:492–498.

Okabe T, Nakamura T, Nishimura YN, Kohu K, Ohwada S, Morishita Y, Akiyama T. (2003). RICS, a novel GTPase-activating protein for Cdc42 and Rac1, is involved in the beta-catenin-N-cadherin and N-methyl-D-aspartate receptor signaling. *J Biol Chem* 278.9920–9927.

Pham TA, Impey S, Storm DR, Stryker MP. (1999). CRE-mediated gene transcription in neocortical neuronal plasticity during the developmental critical period. *Neuron* 22:63–72.

Pizzorusso T, Medini P, Berardi N, Chierzi S, Fawcett JW, Maffei L. (2002). Reactivation of ocular dominance plasticity in the adult visual cortex. *Science* 298:1248–1251.

Pizzorusso T, Medini P, Landi S, Baldini S, Berardi N, Maffei L. (2006). Structural and functional recovery from early monocular deprivation in adult rats. *Proc Natl Acad Sci USA* 103:8517–8522.

Portela A, Esteller M. (2010). Epigenetic modifications and human disease. *Nat Biotechnol* 28:1057–1068.

Putignano E, Lonetti G, Cancedda L, Ratto G, Costa M, Maffei L, Pizzorusso T. (2007). Developmental downregulation of histone posttranslational modifications regulates visual cortical plasticity. *Neuron* 53:747–759.

Remenyi J, Hunter CJ, Cole C, Ando H, Impey S, Monk CE, Martin KJ, Barton GJ, Hutvagner G, Arthur JS. (2010). Regulation of the miR-212/132 locus by MSK1 and CREB in response to neurotrophins. *Biochem J* 428:281–291.

Renthal W, Nestler EJ. (2008). Epigenetic mechanisms in drug addiction. *Trends Mol Med* 14:341–350.

Renthal W, Kumar A, Xiao G, Wilkinson M, Covington HE 3rd,, Maze I, Sikder D, Robison AJ, LaPlant Q, Dietz DM, et al. (2009). Genome–wide analysis of chromatin regulation by cocaine reveals a role for sirtuins. *Neuron* 62:335–348.

Rittenhouse CD, Shouval HZ, Paradiso MA, Bear MF. (1999). Monocular deprivation induces homosynaptic long-term depression in visual cortex. *Nature* 397:347–350.

Rudenko A, Dawlaty MM, Seo J, Cheng AW, Meng J, Le T, Faull KF, Jaenisch R, Tsai LH. (2013). Tet1 is critical for neuronal activity-regulated gene expression and memory extinction. *Neuron* 79:1109–1122.

Sassone–Corsi P, Mizzen CA, Cheung P, Crosio C, Monaco L, Jacquot S, Hanauer A, Allis CD. (1999). Requirement of Rsk–2 for epidermal growth factor-activated phosphorylation of histone H3. *Science* 285:886–891.

Sawtell NB, Frenkel MY, Philpot BD, Nakazawa K, Tonegawa S, Bear MF. (2003). NMDA receptor-dependent ocular dominance plasticity in adult visual cortex. *Neuron* 38:977–985.

Shi Y, Lan F, Matson C, Mulligan P, Whetstine JR, Cole PA, Casero RA. (2004). Histone demethylation mediated by the nuclear amine oxidase homolog LSD1. *Cell* 119:941–953.

Silingardi D, Scali M, Belluomini G, Pizzorusso T. (2010). Epigenetic treatments of adult rats promote recovery from visual acuity deficits induced by long-term monocular deprivation. *Eur J Neurosci* 31:2185–2192.

Szulwach KE, Li X, Li Y, Song CX, Wu H, Dai Q, Irier H, Upadhyay AK, Gearing M, Levey AI, et al. (2011). 5-hmC-mediated epigenetic dynamics during postnatal neurodevelopment and aging. *Nat Neurosci* 14:1607–1616.

Tanner KG, Langer MR, Denu JM. (2000). Kinetic mechanism of human histone acetyltransferase P/CAF. *Biochemistry* 39:15652.

Timney B, Mitchell DE, Giffin F. (1978). The development of vision in cats after extended periods of dark-rearing. *Exp Brain Res* 31:547–560.

Tognini P, Putignano E, Coatti A, Pizzorusso T. (2011). Experience–dependent expression of miR-132 regulates ocular dominance plasticity. *Nat Neurosci* 14:1237–1239.

Tognini P, Pizzorusso T. (2012). MicroRNA212/132 family: molecular transducer of neuronal function and plasticity. *Int J Biochem Cell Biol* 44:6–10.

Tognini P, Napoli D, Tola J, Silingardi D, Della Ragione F, D'Esposito M, Pizzorusso T. (2015) Experience-dependent DNA methylation regulates plasticity in the developing visual cortex. *Nat Neurosci* 18:956–958.

Tropea D, Kreiman G, Lyckman A, Mukherjee S, Yu H, Horng S, Sur M. (2006). Gene expression changes and molecular pathways mediating activity-dependent plasticity in visual cortex. *Nat Neurosci* 9:660–668.

Tsukada Y, Fang J, Erdjument–Bromage H, Warren ME, Borchers CH, Tempst P, Zhang Y. (2006). Histone demethylation by a family of JmjC domain–containing proteins. *Nature* 439:811–816.

Vo N, Goodman RH. (2001). CREB-binding protein and p300 in transcriptional regulation. *J Biol Chem* 276:13505–13508.

Vo N, Klein ME, Varlamova O, Keller DM, Yamamoto T, Goodman RH, Impey S. (2005). A cAMP-response element binding protein–induced microRNA regulates neuronal morphogenesis. *Proc Natl Acad Sci USA* 102:16426–16431.

Waddington CH. (1968). Towards a theoretical biology. *Nature* 218:525–527.

Wayman GA, Davare M, Ando H, Fortin D, Varlamova O, Cheng HY, Marks D, Obrietan K, Soderling TR, Goodman RH, et al. (2008). An activity-regulated microRNA controls dendritic plasticity by down-regulating p250GAP. *Proc Natl Acad Sci USA* 105:9093–9098.

Wu C, Morris JR. (2001). Genes, genetics, and epigenetics: a correspondence. *Science* 293:1103–1105.

Yang EJ, Lin EW, Hensch TK. (2012). Critical period for acoustic preference in mice. *Proc Natl Acad Sci USA 109 Suppl* 2:17213–17220.

Yazaki–Sugiyama Y, Kang S, Cateau H, Fukai T, Hensch TK. (2009). Bidirectional plasticity in fast-spiking GABA circuits by visual experience. *Nature* 462:218–221.

Yeh SH, Lin CH, Gean PW. (2004). Acetylation of nuclear factor-kappaB in rat amygdala improves long-term but not short–term retention of fear memory. *Mol Pharmacol* 65:1286–1292.

Zovkic IB, Paulukaitis BS, Day JJ, Etikala DM, Sweatt JD. (2014). Histone H2A.Z subunit exchange controls consolidation of recent and remote memory. *Nature* 515:582–586.

CHAPTER 3

Gene–environment interactions in the etiology of psychiatric and neurodevelopmental disorders

Mari A. Kondo[1] and Anthony J. Hannan[2,3]

[1] Department of Psychiatry and Behavioral Sciences, Johns Hopkins University School of Medicine, Baltimore, Maryland, USA
[2] Florey Institute of Neuroscience and Mental Health, University of Melbourne, Parkville, Australia
[3] Department of Anatomy and Neuroscience, University of Melbourne, Parkville, Australia

How animal models help us study human brain disorders

Animal models of human disorders are valuable tools for understanding disease mechanisms as well as trialling potential treatments. Although no model is perfect, they allow us to overcome some of the difficulties of human studies. In many cases the inability to conduct controlled experiments with humans necessitates reliance on reports of behaviors and on epidemiological data in conjunction with complicated statistics to adjust for confounding variables. Furthermore, in the absence of reliable genetic causation or biomarkers, patients are lumped into syndromes based on clinical diagnosis, which increases the likelihood of noisy data and decreases sensitivity. Brain diseases are particularly difficult to study in living humans since, in most cases, the target tissues are inaccessible for biological testing during the patient's lifetime and the reliability of proxy biomarkers, such as blood or olfactory cells, is hotly debated (Horiuchi et al., 2013; Tylee et al., 2013). In addition to imaging technologies and postmortem brain banks that are a window into brain disease, there is a clear need for well-designed and controlled nonhuman studies to help us understand the factors contributing to brain diseases at the molecular, cellular, network and whole organism levels.

Genetic models for complex brain diseases

Complex diseases are thought to arise from the combined effect of multiple susceptibility genes and negative environmental conditions. Even within the

Environmental Experience and Plasticity of the Developing Brain, First Edition.
Edited by Alessandro Sale.
© 2016 John Wiley & Sons, Inc. Published 2016 by John Wiley & Sons, Inc.

same diagnosis, the set of genes and environmental conditions involved will likely differ from person to person. Furthermore accumulating data from humans and animal models suggests the importance of sex-differences and genetic background in susceptibility to stressors, onset, progression and outcome of various brain disorders, as well as the effects of pharmacological or environmental interventions (Martinez-Cue et al., 2002; Pietropaolo et al., 2008; Pang et al., 2009; Franceschelli et al., 2014; Du et al., 2015). Although female mice are often excluded from behavioral studies due to concerns about the effect of estrous cycle phases, this appears to be overstated (Plappert et al., 2005; Meziane et al., 2007). Since we know that factors such as sex and genetic background are important in the biological milieu, these should be actively considered in designing studies to help us to understand mechanisms of brain disorders and responses to environmental factors.

Large genome-wide association studies have started to increase the reliability of loci identified as associated with psychiatric disorders; however, developing good preclinical models for complex psychiatric and neurodevelopmental disorders such as schizophrenia, bipolar disorder, depression, and autism remains a major challenge (Kendler, 2013; Schizophrenia Working Group of the Psychiatric Genomics Consortium, 2014). For this reason, animal models are studied at the level of endophenotypes relevant to disease and are often classified in terms of the validity that they display (usually partitioned as construct, face and predictive validity)(Willner, 1984; Gottesman and Gould, 2003; Burrows et al., 2011). In addition to utilizing mutant mouse models created from candidate gene-based approaches, it may be possible to gain useful biological insights using models for neurodevelopmental or neurodegenerative disorders with psychiatric elements as part of the symptomatology. Huntington's disease and Rett syndrome may be good candidates since patients often show psychiatric symptoms and both have a known, causative single-gene alteration that make it possible to study gene–environment interactions on psychiatric endophenotypes using rodent models of these diseases.

Behavioral outcomes from environmental modulation

Animal models allow us to manipulate and test the effects of environmental factors on the brain, as well as associated behaviors and cognitive processes. An experimental paradigm called environmental enrichment can be employed to examine the effects of interacting with a stimulating and varied environment as a part of everyday life. Here we will discuss environmental manipulations associated with rodent studies. Environmental enrichment involves controlled modification of an animal's environment by housing rodents in spacious, interactive conditions with objects of varying textures, sizes, shapes, and colors that are regularly changed. For postweaning environmental enrichment, mice are generally assigned to mixed genotype, single-sex social housing groups. However, like differences in "standard housing," the details of "environmental enrichment" vary between laboratories and studies, making direct comparisons difficult (Olsson and Dahlborn, 2002; Nithianantharajah and Hannan, 2006; Gonder and Laber, 2007). The objective of the enriched housing condition is to facilitate enhanced sensory, cognitive and motor stimulation in experimental rodents. It is well documented that exposure to environmental enrichment or voluntary physical exercise improves learning and memory, and can decrease anxiety in wild-type animals as well as slow down onset and/or progression in many disease models (Fordyce and Wehner, 1993; Duffy et al., 2001; Fox et al., 2006), reviewed in (van Praag et al., 2000; Nithianantharajah and Hannan, 2006; Laviola et al., 2008; Pang and Hannan, 2013). The benefits of enrichment are most effectively illustrated by the rescue of behavioral abnormalities, such as poor motor coordination and depression-like behavior, as well as BDNF deficits in the hippocampus and striatum, in mouse models of Huntington's disease, which was previously thought to be an archetypal genetically determined disease (van Dellen et al., 2000; Hockly et al., 2002; Spires et al., 2004; Nithianantharajah et al., 2008; Pang et al., 2009). Environmental enrichment can also benefit mouse models of severe, early neurodevelopmental disorders such as Down syndrome (Martinez-Cue et al., 2002; Begenisic et al., 2011), Fragile X syndrome (Restivo et al., 2005), Rett syndrome (Kondo et al., 2008; Nag et al., 2009; Kerr et al., 2010; Lonetti et al., 2010), and amblyopia (Cancedda et al., 2004; Sale et al., 2007; Sale et al., 2009). Environmental enrichment is thought to benefit animals at early stages of disease by rescuing protein deficits and acting as a buffer against detrimental effects on synaptic and neural plasticity, thereby protecting neural networks. The concept of enrichment increasing the brain's resilience to stress, injury and disease processes (increasing brain and cognitive reserve) has been reviewed by Nithianantharajah and Hannan (2009).

Components of environmental enrichment

Environmental enrichment is made up of social and nonsocial components that both have a significant impact on mice.

Exercise and cognitive stimulation

There is substantial literature on the positive influence of exercise on rodent models of depression as well as in human studies (Bjornebekk et al., 2008; Duman et al., 2008; Greer and Trivedi, 2009; Lavretsky, 2009). In fact numerous studies have identified physical exercise as the single most beneficial component of rodent environmental enrichment. For example, comparing female C57BL/6 mice exposed to rodent toys (cognitive stimulation) or running wheels (exercise) or daily acrobatic training showed that only the exercise group improved their memory (Lambert et al., 2005). Likewise, a comparison of running only, enrichment only, and enrichment with running, showed that only mice with access to running benefited from increased BDNF and adult hippocampal neurogenesis (Kobilo et al., 2011). The nature of the exercise, voluntary versus forced, appears to be an important factor for rats and mice (van Praag et al., 1999; Leasure and Jones, 2008; Griesbach et al., 2012). This may be due, in part, to the suppression of BDNF protein and mRNA by the elevation of glucocorticoids in response to stress (Hansson et al., 2006). In cases where environmental enrichment shows benefits over voluntary running alone, this is most likely due to a synergistic effect of sensory, cognitive and physical stimulation. Furthermore a mouse running in a wheel experiences a qualitatively different type of physical exercise to a mouse negotiating its way around a three-dimensional cage full of enrichment objects (Nithianantharajah and Hannan, 2009). In the R6/1 mouse model of Huntington's disease, environmental enrichment improved motor coordination but running wheel access did not (van Dellen et al., 2000; Pang et al., 2006). Nevertheless, increased voluntary exercise in the HD mice did ameliorate specific motor, cognitive, and affective abnormalities (Pang et al., 2006; van Dellen et al., 2008; Renoir et al., 2012), reflecting some of the beneficial effects of environmental enrichment (van Dellen et al., 2000; Nithianantharajah et al., 2008; Pang et al., 2009). We saw a similar difference in response to enrichment and exercise (wheel running) in female Rett syndrome model mice, described later in this chapter.

Social interaction

Laboratory mice and rats are derived from generally social species that live in large colonies in the wild. Therefore social housing should be utilised to avoid phenotypes unrelated to the condition of interest. In fact, social manipulations such as maternal deprivation, social isolation and social defeat stress are experimental paradigms used to mimic the effects of human social stressors in rodent models (Buwalda et al., 2005; Niwa et al., 2011). Social isolation causes a range of negative physiological and behavioral effects (Lu et al., 2003; Ibi et al., 2008; Leasure and Jones, 2008; Pietropaolo et al., 2008). Social isolation, in combination with genetic mutations in mice, is used to model behavioral and neurochemical deficits associated with psychiatric disorders (Jiang et al., 2013; Niwa et al., 2013). Furthermore social isolation can eliminate the benefit of treatments including exercise. Stranahan and coworkers (2006) found that social isolation combined with voluntary running resulted in circadian dysregulation of corticosterone levels compared to control, group-housed male rats. Social isolation in both male and female rats prevented exercise-induced hippocampal adult neurogenesis, which was observed in the group-housed controls, and resulted in higher levels of corticosterone in response to stress (Stranahan et al., 2006; Leasure and Decker, 2009). Fuss and coworkers (2010) found that isolation-housed male mice exposed to voluntary wheel running displayed increased corticosterone levels and behavioral anxiety and showed no behavioral benefits despite increases in hippocampal neurogenesis and BDNF levels.

Molecular changes in response to environmental modulation

Environmental enrichment and physical exercise in rodents can change the mRNA and protein levels of a wide range of molecules, including neurotrophins and neuroimmune/inflammation-related molecules, that influence brain function by altering neural plasticity, particularly adult neurogenesis, synaptic plasticity, and neurotransmitter receptors (for reviews on this topic see Nithiananantharajah and Hannan (2006) and Singhal et al. (2014)). Here we will focus on brain-derived neurotrophic factor (BDNF) and glucocorticoids in the context of environmental modulation and affective disorders.

Brain-derived neurotrophic factor

Environmental enrichment increases the production of neurotrophins, including BDNF, which is essential for neuronal survival, differentiation, and synaptic plasticity during development and in adulthood (Falkenberg et al., 1992; Ickes et al., 2000; Lu, 2003; Spires et al., 2004; Branchi et al., 2006; Rossi et al., 2006). BDNF, which signals through two different cell surface receptors, the high affinity tyrosine receptor kinase B and the low affinity p75 neurotrophin receptor, is a complex protein that is regulated in a tissue-specific manner; alternative splicing of untranslated exons to the common 3′ protein coding exon, resulting in the same final product from multiple transcripts (Metsis et al., 1993; Timmusk et al., 1995; Liu et al., 2006; Aid et al., 2007). The transcripts are distributed to different brain regions and are regulated by diverse physiological stimuli, allowing independent regulation of the different transcripts (Martinowich and Lu, 2008). For consistency, we have used nomenclature from Aid and coworkers (2007) who demonstrated that the gene structure was more complex than previously thought, with eight untranslated exons.

BDNF protein levels appear to be regulated in an activity-dependent manner (Shieh et al., 1998; Tao et al., 1998). Although transcription from *Bdnf* exon 4 is activity dependent (Metsis et al., 1993; Tao et al., 2002), an enrichment effect on exon 4 is not always observed. The largest effects on gene expression tend to be seen in short-term enrichment studies, up to 2 weeks, but are less pronounced in mice that lived in enriched environments for extended periods of time (Rampon et al., 2000; Zajac et al., 2010). It is possible that the initial high levels of *Bdnf* expression are only required to initiate the development of dendrites, synapses and circuits associated with enrichment effects, and subside once these become established.

The hypothalamic-pituitary-adrenal axis

The hypothalamic-pituitary-adrenal (HPA) axis influences anxiety response, cognitive function, emotion/mood, as well as numerous aspects of brain development underlying these behaviors. Normally the HPA axis is tightly regulated: the hypothalamus secretes corticotropin-releasing hormone (CRH), which stimulates the pituitary to produce adrenocorticotropic hormone (ACTH) that signals the adrenal cortex to release glucocorticoids (cortisol in humans and corticosterone in mice) which negatively regulates the production of CRH and ACTH. The paraventricular nucleus of the hypothalamus (PVN) is a key site in the negative feedback control of the HPA axis by glucocorticoids. The PVN also integrates input from several brain regions that are highly susceptible to the effects of stressors, including the prefrontal cortex and hippocampus, via GABAergic interneurons. The presynaptic function of these GABAergic inputs is altered by chronic stress, contributing to the disinhibition of the HPA axis (Verkuyl et al., 2004; Jeanneteau and Chao, 2013). Excessive stress and HPA axis dysregulation have wide-reaching effects on the brain including pyramidal cell loss, dendritic atrophy and decreased neurogenesis (Sapolsky, 2000; Brummelte and Galea, 2010; Jutapakdeegul et al., 2010; Oomen et al., 2010).

Environment, BDNF, stress, and depression

Increased levels of the stress hormone cortisol and a dysregulated HPA axis are hallmarks of depression in humans (Owens and Nemeroff, 1991; Holsboer and Ising, 2008). HPA axis dysregulation appears to precede the onset of clinical symptoms, suggesting a mechanistic role in affective disorders (Modell et al., 1998). Studies in rodents have also shown that elevation of corticosterone, by stress-inducing regimes and by exogenous administration, induces depression-like behaviors including anhedonia, causes dysregulation of the HPA axis, and decreases BDNF levels (Sterner and Kalynchuk, 2010). Conversely, recovery from depression-like behaviors involves the normalization of corticosterone and rescue of BDNF mRNA and protein levels (Siuciak et al., 1997; Russo-Neustadt et al., 2001; Shirayama et al., 2002; Duman et al., 2008; Jeanneteau and Chao, 2013). Work in wild-type rodents has further shown that corticosterone regulates hippocampal BDNF in an exon-specific manner (Hansson et al., 2006). Loss of BDNF is though to be involved in vulnerability to depression with forebrain-specific *Bdnf* knockout mice replicating the sexual dichotomy observed in human depression (Monteggia et al., 2007).

Numerous studies have shown that both antidepressants and environmental enrichment increase the production of neurotrophins including BDNF (Falkenberg et al., 1992; Ickes et al., 2000; Spires et al., 2004; Branchi et al., 2006; Rossi et al., 2006). Increased BDNF in the hippocampus has been linked to an antidepressant-like effect and hippocampal neurogenesis has been shown to mediate the positive behavioral effects of antidepressants and enrichment (Shirayama et al., 2002; Santarelli et al., 2003; Hattori et al., 2007; Veena et al., 2009; Schloesser et al., 2010). Although the mechanism behind enrichment-derived benefits is not fully understood, it has been suggested that mouse hippocampal *Bdnf* expression is increased via sustained epigenetic modification of the promoters (Zajac et al., 2010; Kuzumaki et al., 2011) and may modify other genes in a similar way. Chronically stressed rats that experienced enrichment had lower corticosterone than chronically stressed rats that did not receive enrichment (Hutchinson et al., 2012). Basal plasma corticosterone was significantly lower in mice overexpressing BDNF in the forebrain compared to control animals, and forebrain BDNF overexpression prevented chronic stress-induced dendritic atrophy in the hippocampus (Govindarajan et al., 2006).

These studies highlight the important interaction between environment, BDNF, HPA axis function and depressive symptoms. In addition to lowered basal corticosterone and decreased anxiety, environmental enrichment in wild-type female mice was associated with lower *Crhr1* mRNA in the basolateral amygdala (Sztainberg et al., 2010). CRHR1, the receptor for CRH, is thought to modulate anxiety-related behavior independently of the HPA axis (Muller et al., 2003). Environmental modulation likely affects multiple components of the stress pathway and further work is needed to understand the molecules and brain regions involved in this complex relationship.

Epigenetics and environmental influence

Epigenetic regulation refers to long-term changes in gene expression potential without changes to the DNA sequence (Jaenisch and Bird, 2003). In multicellular eukaryotes DNA methylation, histone modifications and chromatin remodelling mediate epigenetic regulation (Jaenisch and Bird, 2003; Klose and Bird, 2006; Portela and Esteller, 2010). Positive and negative environmental experiences including diet, disease, social interaction, and physical activity can both lay down and alter epigenetic markings to dynamically influence gene expression, resulting in long-term behavioral, cognitive, and physical health effects (Figure 3.1).

Gene–environment interactions and epigenetics in psychiatric and neurodevelopmental disorders

Stress (particularly during critical developmental stages including prenatal, early life, and adolescence) is thought to be one of the environmental susceptibility factors for the development of psychiatric disorders (Bock et al., 2015). Early life stress in rodents, including lack of maternal care (low licking and grooming), can alter methylation patterns of genes involved in the stress response and influences hippocampal development and HPA axis function leading to later life susceptibility to anxiety-like and depression-like behaviors (Weaver et al., 2004;

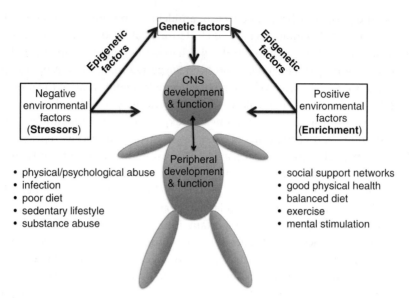

Figure 3.1 Positive and negative environmental experiences affect epigenetic markings and gene expression.

Meaney and Szyf, 2005; Weaver et al., 2005; Murgatroyd et al., 2009; Murgatroyd et al., 2010). Mice exposed to prenatal restraint stress displayed schizophrenia-like behavioral changes, a decrease in BDNF and glutamic acid decarboxylase 67, and an increase in DNA methyltransferase 1 (Matrisciano et al., 2012). Although early life insults can modify brain function in significant ways, encouragingly postweaning environmental enrichment in rats was found to reverse the effect of poor maternal care on the cognitive function of the adult pups by mediating changes in synaptic density and expression of NMDA and AMPA receptor subunits (Bredy et al., 2003; Bredy et al., 2004).

Despite popular categorization of certain environmental conditions as detrimental or beneficial to health, one of the challenges in psychiatric research is that not everyone reacts in the same way. For example stress in adolescence may have a significant pathological impact on one person while having minimal effect on another. A gene–environment interaction model for psychotic depression demonstrated that social isolation during adolescence in mice with a susceptible genotype, dominant-negative DISC1 (disrupted in schizophrenia 1) mutation, caused a decrease in dopamine in the frontal cortex that was not evident in mice with just the mutation or wild-type mice just exposed to isolation (Niwa et al., 2013). The psychosis-like and depression-like behavior and dopaminergic changes were caused by elevated levels of corticosterone, which altered methylation of the tyrosine hydroxylase gene (the rate-limiting step in the synthesis of dopamine) specifically in cells projecting from the ventral tegmental area to the frontal cortex. Studies like these highlight the importance of gene–environment interaction, in addition to genetic and environmental contributions, to epigenetic regulation of gene expression that may be involved in psychiatric disorders (Figure 3.2; for a review on the epigenomic contribution to psychiatric diseases, see Bredy et al., 2010). In the out-bred human population there are likely many gene combinations that increase susceptibility to or confer protection from psychiatric disorders. Therefore the balance of risk and protection in an individual's genetic makeup will likely affect their response to positive and negative environmental factors.

It is becoming apparent that mutations or variants in the same genes can increase the risk for several brain disorders (reviewed in Zhu et al. (2014)). Methyl-CpG-binding protein 2 (MeCP2), a multifunctional epigenetic regulator, may be a key player in developmental and psychiatric diseases, acting as a bridge between environmentally mediated methylation patterns and gene expression (Zimmermann et al., 2015). In addition to Rett syndrome, the prototypical disease resulting from a deficit of MeCP2 protein levels, MeCP2 dysregulation has been found in frontal cortex samples from patients with autism, Angelman syndrome, Prader-Willi syndrome, Down syndrome, and attention deficit hyperactive disorder (Nagarajan et al., 2006). Mutations, single nucleotide polymorphisms and copy number variation in *MECP2* have also been associated with neuropsychiatric conditions including schizophrenia, depression and anxiety (Ramocki et al., 2009; Wong et al., 2014). In the following sections we describe Rett syndrome and work done in mouse models of MeCP2 deficit that have helped us to understand the association between this gene, environmental modulation and neurodevelopmental/psychiatric disorders.

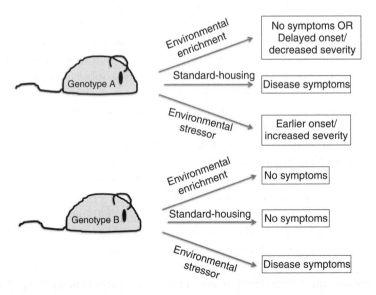

Figure 3.2 Role of genetic background in epigenetic regulation of gene expression that may be involved in psychiatric disorders.

Overview of Rett syndrome

Rett syndrome (RTT) is a debilitating childhood onset neurodevelopmental disorder that results in severe physical, cognitive, psychological, and autonomic disability (Hagberg et al., 1983; Hagberg and Witt-Engerstrom, 1986; Engerstrom, 1992; Kerr and Burford, 2001; Jellinger, 2003). The incidence is one in 10,000–15,000 live births and mutation in *MECP2* on Xq28 has been identified as the cause of 85–95% of classic RTT cases (Amir et al., 1999; Moretti and Zoghbi, 2006). The majority of patients are female since mutation of *MECP2* usually results in early lethality in males with only a single copy of the gene. Many *MECP2* mutations cause complete or partial loss of protein function and large deletions involving exons 3 and 4, which contain the methyl-CpG binding domain and the transcriptional repressor domain, are sometimes detected in classic RTT patients (Yusufzai and Wolffe, 2000; Erlandson et al., 2003). The mutations in the first *Mecp2*-null mouse models were designed to mimic these, with the null animals producing no MeCP2 mRNA or protein (Chen et al., 2001; Guy et al., 2001).

Genetic sources of phenotypic variation in Rett syndrome and other brain disorders

Although the genetic contribution to phenotype variation in complex brain disorders is often attributed to the different combinations of genes and mutation types involved, an additional factor may be genetic mosaicism. Females are a genetic mosaic, as normally one of the X chromosomes is randomly selected for inactivation in somatic cells. Therefore expression of genes located on the X-chromosome can be affected by stochastic processes during establishment of X-chromosome inactivation, or cell selection during subsequent development (Watson et al., 2005). Since *MECP2* is located on the X chromosome, the variable penetrance seen in RTT was originally thought to result from a combination of mutation type and individual differences in skewing of X-chromosome inactivation in female patients (Warby, 2002). Skewing has been found in carriers or mildly affected females; however, the majority of RTT patients appear to display random patterns of X-chromosome inactivation in blood and brain, showing no consistent correlation with symptom severity (Wan et al., 1999; Amir et al., 2000; Amir and Zoghbi, 2000; Young and Zoghbi, 2004; Watson et al., 2005; Vignoli et al., 2009). Another source of genetic variation in brain diseases that can affect both sexes is somatic mutation. Due to the rapid rate of cell proliferation during development, the brain may be particularly susceptible to postzygotic mutations that may play a role in the pathogenesis of neurodevelopmental and psychiatric disorders (Freed et al., 2014; Insel, 2014; O'Roak et al., 2014). The proportion and effect of somatic mosaic cells would depend on the developmental stage and location at which the mutation occurred. Along with epigenetics and environmental influences, mosaicism could help to explain the reports of discordant presentation and progression of symptoms in monozygotic twins with RTT, schizophrenia or bipolar disorder and may partially explain why similar mutations result in different disease severity (Migeon et al., 1995; Ogawa et al., 1997; De Bona et al., 2000; Scala et al., 2007; Dempster et al., 2011).

The functions of MeCP2

The MeCP2 protein is relatively well conserved across vertebrate species indicating its importance in biological functions (Lewis et al., 1992; Yusufzai and Wolffe, 2000; Weaving et al., 2005). The importance of tight regulation of MeCP2 levels *in vivo* was shown with mice expressing double the normal wild-type dose and half the normal dose, both displaying disease symptoms with increasing age (Collins et al., 2004; Samaco et al., 2008).

MeCP2 is a multifunctional protein. It is involved in methylation-dependent transcriptional regulation of target genes through chromatin remodelling by recruiting histone deacetylases and co-repressors, RNA splicing, repression of retrotransposons, and can bind to unmethylated DNA to remodel chromatin independently of histone modifying proteins (Jones et al., 1998; Yu et al., 2001; Georgel et al., 2003; Buschdorf and Stratling, 2004; Young et al., 2005; Nikitina et al., 2007a; Nikitina et al., 2007b; Yasui et al., 2007; Chahrour et al., 2008). The original idea of MeCP2 being a global transcriptional repressor has fallen out of favour due to the apparent lack of genome-wide transcriptional dysregulation in RTT patients or *Mecp2*-null mutant mice displaying overt disease symptoms (Tudor et al., 2002; Klose and Bird, 2003). Instead, the primary role of MeCP2 dysfunction in disease is thought to be transcriptional dysregulation of key neuronal activity-dependent target genes, including *Bdnf* and *Crh* (Chen et al., 2003; Martinowich et al., 2003; McGill et al., 2006; Zhou et al., 2006; Tao et al., 2009; De Filippis et al., 2013).

The brains of RTT patients and *Mecp2*-null mutant mice weigh less than normal at any given age and are described as having immature characteristics, such as decreased dendritic spine density and smaller or less complex arbours of pyramidal neurons, and altered expression of presynaptic proteins (Belichenko et al., 1994; Kishi and Macklis, 2004; Kishi and Macklis, 2005; Smrt et al., 2007). This is unsurprising as increasing levels of MeCP2 expression in the brain is associated with neuronal maturation, particularly in the hippocampus, cortex, cerebellum and brain stem, the regions primarily affected in RTT (Kishi and Macklis, 2004). MeCP2 protein levels were found to influence excitatory synaptic strength via regulation of glutamatergic synaptic density and may also be involved in maturation and/or pruning of synapses (Zoghbi, 2003; Kishi and

Macklis, 2005; Chao et al., 2007). A deficit of *Mecp2* in GABAergic neurons caused a reduction in miniature inhibitory postsynaptic current (mIPSC) quantal size in somatosensory cortex pyramidal neurons and striatal neurons (Chao et al., 2010). Indeed impaired long-term potentiation (LTP) has been reported in the hippocampus, primary motor cortex and primary somatosensory cortex of *Mecp2* mutant mice further supporting MeCP2's role in the induction of synaptic plasticity (Asaka et al., 2006; Moretti et al., 2006; Chao et al., 2010). MeCP2 has been associated with depression, schizophrenia, and bipolar disorder, in which GABAergic and glutamatergic dysfunction are also implicated (Cherlyn et al., 2010; Gao and Bao, 2011). Interestingly, antidepressants and psychostimulants were found to induce transcription of *Mecp2* in mice and phosphorylation of the protein at Ser421 (Cassel et al., 2006; Deng et al., 2010; Hutchinson et al., 2012). Following chronic social defeat stress, knockin mice with a nonphosphorylatable Ala residue at the 421 position (S421A) were unable to respond positively to chronic antidepressant treatment unlike MeCP2 wild-type mice (Hutchinson et al., 2012). The work in mice indicates that mutation and dysregulation of MeCP2 protein levels in the brain may result in a cycle of insufficient capacity to process neural input and insufficient neural plasticity, increasing the susceptibility to additional negative environmental or genetic factors.

Can disease progression in Rett syndrome be prevented?

There is currently no cure for RTT and treatment involves the management of symptoms to ease discomfort and maximise functionality (Budden, 1997). Although there have been reports of limited functional improvement, such as improved hand-use, language comprehension, and mobility from interventions including intensive physiotherapy, music therapy, and use of a modified tread-mill, the benefits have not been substantial (Piazza et al., 1993; Jacobsen et al., 2001; Yasuhara and Sugiyama, 2001; Lotan et al., 2004; Downs et al., 2009). Work in *Mecp2*-null male and heterozygous female mouse models, however, suggest that the neurons are not irrevocably damaged by the absence of MeCP2 during development, since transgenic re-expression of *Mecp2* in *Mecp2* mutant mice suppressed the disease phenotype (Giacometti et al., 2007; Guy et al., 2007; Jugloff et al., 2008). More recently, proof of concept for gene therapy in RTT was demonstrated in null and heterozygous mice using systemic delivery of MeCP2 cDNA via an adeno-associated viral vector (Gadalla et al., 2013; Garg et al., 2013). Although the mosaic nature of healthy and mutant cells in RTT patients, as well as the requirement for tight regulation of MeCP2 dosage, makes gene therapy challenging, the capacity to prevent symptom development and rescue mutant cells in mice suggests that an effective therapy in postnatal life could restore neuronal functionality and achieve symptomatic amelioration for RTT patients and others with a MeCP2 deficit.

Regulation of *Bdnf* and *Crh* by MeCP2

Using cultured neurons, two groups independently found that normal MeCP2 can regulate expression of rodent *Bdnf* exon 4 in a neuronal activity-dependent manner (Chen et al., 2003; Martinowich et al., 2003). Chang and coworkers (2006) conducted a series of experiments providing *in vivo* evidence for an inter- action between *Mecp2* and *Bdnf*, demonstrating the physiological significance of altered BDNF expression/signalling. *Bdnf* conditional mutant mice exhibit characteristics similar to those of symptomatic *Mecp2*-null mutant mice. Deletion of *Bdnf* in *Mecp2*-null mice caused an earlier onset of RTT-like symptoms, while BDNF overexpression in the *Mecp2* mutants extended the life span, rescued locomotion, dendritic morphology, and an electrophysiological deficit in layer 5 pyramidal neurons of the somatosensory cortex (Chang et al., 2006; Larimore et al., 2009). These results support the hypothesis that a moderate decrease in BDNF protein levels may mediate some of the deficits in *Mecp2* mutant mice and RTT patients. As described earlier, the neurological and behavioral deficits resulting from lack of MeCP2 are similar to those seen when BDNF is deficient and/or corticosterone is high. Studies using male mutant mice have also shown that *Mecp2* mutation causes abnormal regulation of stress response and stress-associated genes including *Crh*, serum glucocorticoid-inducible kinase 1 (*Sgk1*), FK506-binding protein 5 (*Fkbp5*), and pro-opiomelanocortin (*Pomc* – the polypeptide precursor of ACTH)(Nuber et al., 2005; McGill et al., 2006; De Filippis et al., 2013). Hence part of the reason for an "immature brain" may be due to HPA axis dysfunction and a deficit of neurotrophins to facilitate maturation of neuronal networks.

Effects of environmental enrichment in *Mecp2* mutant mice

Several mouse models of RTT have been developed with different types of muta- tions to the *Mecp2* gene (Chen et al., 2001; Guy et al., 2001; Shahbazian et al., 2002; Collins et al., 2004; Pelka et al., 2006). Our group used the *Mecp2*[tm1Tam] mouse, which lacks the entire methyl-CpG binding domain (exon 3 and part of exon 4) and produces no MeCP2 protein. The mixed genetic background (129sv x C57BL6) of this model slightly extends the life span of the hemizygous-null males, allowing some behavioral testing that was not possible in other null models due to the severity of symptoms (Chen et al., 2001; Guy et al., 2001).

The majority of RTT mouse studies have used male hemizygous mutants, which avoids the potentially problematic effect of X chromosome inactivation, providing a clean study of the consequence of MeCP2 deficit. However, in order to understand a disease that principally affects females heterozygous for *MECP2* mutations, we thought that it was important to examine the effects of environmental modulation in female heterozygous mice alongside the null male model.

The loss of ability to coordinate movements is one of the most debilitating symptoms of RTT and age-related cerebellar atrophy is thought to contribute to this (Hagberg et al., 1983; Engerstrom, 1992; Murakami et al., 1992). *Mecp2*[tm1Tam] hemizygous-null males also display severe motor coordination and cerebellar motor learning deficits (Pelka et al., 2006), which were not ameliorated by postweaning environmental enrichment from 4 weeks of age (Kondo et al., 2008). Standard-housed 10-week-old hemizygous mice had only 67% of the standard-housed wild-type levels of cerebellar BDNF. Consistent with the lack of improvement in coordination, BDNF levels remained low in environmentally enriched hemizygotes. An independent study also reported low BDNF protein levels in the cerebellum (59% of wild-type levels) in 6-8 week-old male *Mecp2* knockout mice (Chang et al., 2006). Thirty week-old standard-housed heterozygous female mice displaying impaired motor coordination had only 75% of standard-housed wild-type BDNF protein levels in the cerebellum, while the environmentally enriched heterozygous mice, with 85% of wild-type levels, displayed a dramatic improvement in the rotarod performance baseline and longitudinal rescue of motor coordination (Kondo et al., 2008). BDNF induced by enrichment is thought to facilitate cerebellar plasticity. Other groups have found that long-term postweaning enrichment significantly increased BDNF and NGF protein in the cerebellum of male Wistar rats as well as BDNF in cerebellar Purkinje neurons in mice (Angelucci et al., 2009; Vazquez-Sanroman et al., 2013).

Although not considered one of the severely disabling features, disturbed mood has been reported in children with RTT, with up to 70% displaying low mood and over 75% having frequent episodes of anxiety (Sansom et al., 1993; Mount et al., 2002; Robertson et al., 2006). In a follow-up study we found that female heterozygous *Mecp2*[tm1Tam] mice display deficits in the saccharin-preference test and novelty-suppressed feeding test, suggesting a previously unreported affective phenotype. The heterozygous mice also displayed decreased hippocampal BDNF protein, increased corticosterone and dysregulation of the HPA axis including significantly decreased levels of *Crh* mRNA (Kondo et al., 2015). Interestingly we found that increased voluntary exercise (on running wheels) rescued saccharin-preference performance but not novelty-suppressed feeding, while environmental enrichment normalised performance in both tests. Environmental enrichment also partially normalised basal serum corticosterone but not *Crh* expression. We also saw a rescue of hippocampal BDNF protein levels in the enriched heterozygous females suggesting that the beneficial effect on the depression-like symptoms may be due, at least partially, to upregulation of BDNF and downregulation of corticosterone.

Although we saw no positive effects of postweaning environmental enrichment from 4 weeks of age in the *Mecp2* null-males, other groups saw positive outcomes when enrichment was started earlier. Using an early environmental enrichment paradigm where multiple litters and dams were housed in a large cage with enrichment objects, Lonetti and coworkers (2010) found that the motor coordination of *Mecp2* null-males could be rescued. Preweaning enrichment has a larger capacity to compensate for MeCP2 deficits by influencing maternal licking and grooming behavior, hence methylation and epigenetic gene regulation in the pups during a critical developmental stage, in addition to providing direct enrichment of the pup. Postweaning enrichment of null males from 3 weeks of age resulted in improved locomotor activity and coordination as well as elevated-plus maze performance (Nag et al., 2009; Kerr et al., 2010). These studies demonstrate that despite a total lack of MeCP2, hemizygous mutants maintain the capacity to improve function if environmental intervention occurred early enough. Since abundant synaptogenesis and hippocampal development occur during the second postnatal week (preweaning) in rodents, an increase in BDNF near this time is more likely to be beneficial for mutants than later in life.

Summary

This research field is entering an exciting stage, with more genetic and environmental susceptibility factors being identified for a wide variety of neurodevelopmental and psychiatric disorders, providing new insights into both pathogenesis and novel therapeutic targets. However, there is still a long way to go before we have a good understanding of how all the genetic and environmental factors interact to produce the complex pathogenic pathways and symptomatology of each disorder. Here, we have explored the role of environmental enrichment and social stressors, and some of the downstream behavioral and molecular effects in the context of rodent models. Although we are not yet at the stage of employing sophisticated multigenic animal models that truly reflect the human disease condition, it is possible to gain some insight into complex brain disorders by utilising single gene mutation models that display relevant endophenotypes. We highlighted the example of *Mecp2* mutant mice for their potential to aid understanding of gene–environment interaction mechanisms in depression, autism and schizophrenia, in addition to Rett syndrome. It is hoped that such research will not only provide new insights into pathogenic mechanisms, but also pave the way for the development of badly needed new therapies for these and other devastating brain disorders.

References

Aid T, Kazantseva A, Piirsoo M, Palm K, Timmusk T. (2007). Mouse and rat BDNF gene structure and expression revisited. *J Neurosci Res* 85:525–535.

Amir RE, Van den Veyver IB, Wan M, Tran CQ, Francke U, Zoghbi HY. (1999). Rett syndrome is caused by mutations in X-linked MECP2, encoding methyl-CpG-binding protein 2. *Nat Genet* 23:185–188.

Amir RE, Van den Veyver IB, Schultz R, Malicki DM, Tran CQ, Dahle EJ, Philippi A, Timar L, Percy AK, Motil KJ, Lichtarge O, Smith EO, Glaze DG, Zoghbi HY. (2000). Influence of mutation type and X chromosome inactivation on Rett syndrome phenotypes. *Ann Neurol* 47:670–679.

Amir RE, Zoghbi HY. (2000). Rett syndrome: methyl-CpG-binding protein 2 mutations and phenotype-genotype correlations. *Am J Med Genet* 97:147–152.

Angelucci F, De Bartolo P, Gelfo F, Foti F, Cutuli D, Bossu P, Caltagirone C, Petrosini L. (2009). Increased concentrations of nerve growth factor and brain–derived neurotrophic factor in the rat cerebellum after-exposure to environmental enrichment. *Cerebellum* 8:499–506.

Asaka Y, Jugloff DG, Zhang L, Eubanks JH, Fitzsimonds RM. (2006). Hippocampal synaptic plasticity is impaired in the Mecp2-null mouse model of Rett syndrome. *Neurobiol Dis* 21:217–227.

Begenisic T, Spolidoro M, Braschi C, Baroncelli L, Milanese M, Pietra G, Fabbri ME, Bonanno G, Cioni G, Maffei L, Sale A. (2011). Environmental enrichment decreases GABAergic inhibition and improves cognitive abilities, synaptic plasticity, and visual functions in a mouse model of Down syndrome. *Front Cell Neurosci* 5:29.

Belichenko PV, Oldfors A, Hagberg B, Dahlstrom A. (1994). Rett syndrome: 3-D confocal microscopy of cortical pyramidal dendrites and afferents. *Neuroreport* 5:1509–1513.

Bjornebekk A, Mathe AA, Gruber SH, Brene S. (2008). Housing conditions modulate escitalopram effects on antidepressive-like behaviour and brain neurochemistry. *Int J Neuropsychopharmacol* 11:1135–1147.

Bock J, Wainstock T, Braun K, Segal M. (2015). Stress in utero: prenatal programming of brain plasticity and cognition. *Biol Psychiatry* 78:315–326.

Branchi I, D'Andrea I, Fiore M, Di Fausto V, Aloe L, Alleva E. (2006). Early social enrichment shapes social behavior and nerve growth factor and brain-derived neurotrophic factor levels in the adult mouse brain. *Biol Psychiatry* 60:690–696.

Bredy TW, Humpartzoomian RA, Cain DP, Meaney MJ. (2003). Partial reversal of the effect of maternal care on cognitive function through environmental enrichment. *Neuroscience* 118:571–576.

Bredy TW, Zhang TY, Grant RJ, Diorio J, Meaney MJ. (2004). Peripubertal environmental enrichment reverses the effects of maternal care on hippocampal development and glutamate receptor subunit expression. *Eur J Neurosci* 20:1355–1362.

Bredy TW, Sun YE, Kobor MS. (2010). How the epigenome contributes to the development of psychiatric disorders. *Dev Psychobiol* 52:331–342.

Brummelte S, Galea LA. (2010). Chronic high corticosterone reduces neurogenesis in the dentate gyrus of adult male and female rats. *Neuroscience* 168:680–690.

Budden SS. (1997). Rett syndrome: habilitation and management reviewed. *Eur Child Adolesc Psychiatry 6 Suppl* 1:103–107.

Burrows EL, McOmish CE, Hannan AJ. (2011). Gene–environment interactions and construct validity in preclinical models of psychiatric disorders. *Prog Neuropsychopharmacol Biol Psychiatry* 35:1376–1382.

Buschdorf JP, Stratling WH. (2004). A WW domain binding region in methyl-CpG-binding protein MeCP2: impact on Rett syndrome. *J Mol Med* 82:135–143.

Buwalda B, Kole MH, Veenema AH, Huininga M, de Boer SF, Korte SM, Koolhaas JM. (2005). Long-term effects of social stress on brain and behavior: a focus on hippocampal functioning. *Neurosci Biobehav Rev* 29:83–97.

Cancedda L, Putignano E, Sale A, Viegi A, Berardi N, Maffei L. (2004). Acceleration of visual system development by environmental enrichment. *J Neurosci* 24:4840–4848.

Cassel S, Carouge D, Gensburger C, Anglard P, Burgun C, Dietrich JB, Aunis D, Zwiller J. (2006). Fluoxetine and cocaine induce the epigenetic factors MeCP2 and MBD1 in adult rat brain. *Mol Pharmacol* 70:487–492.

Chahrour M, Jung SY, Shaw C, Zhou X, Wong ST, Qin J, Zoghbi HY. (2008). MeCP2, a key contributor to neurological disease, activates and represses transcription. *Science* 320:1224–1229.

Chang Q, Khare G, Dani V, Nelson S, Jaenisch R. (2006). The disease progression of Mecp2 mutant mice is affected by the level of BDNF expression. *Neuron* 49:341–348.

Chao HT, Zoghbi HY, Rosenmund C. (2007). MeCP2 controls excitatory synaptic strength by regulating glutamatergic synapse number. *Neuron* 56:58–65.

Chao HT, Chen H, Samaco RC, Xue M, Chahrour M, Yoo J, Neul JL, Gong S, Lu HC, Heintz N, Ekker M, Rubenstein JL, Noebels JL, Rosenmund C, Zoghbi HY. (2010). Dysfunction in GABA signalling mediates autism-like stereotypies and Rett syndrome phenotypes. *Nature* 468:263–269.

Chen RZ, Akbarian S, Tudor M, Jaenisch R. (2001). Deficiency of methyl-CpG binding protein-2 in CNS neurons results in a Rett-like phenotype in mice. *Nat Genet* 27:327–331.

Chen WG, Chang Q, Lin Y, Meissner A, West AE, Griffith EC, Jaenisch R, Greenberg ME. (2003). Derepression of BDNF transcription involves calcium-dependent phosphorylation of MeCP2. *Science* 302:885–889.

Cherlyn SY, Woon PS, Liu JJ, Ong WY, Tsai GC, Sim K. (2010). Genetic association studies of glutamate, GABA and related genes in schizophrenia and bipolar disorder: a decade of advance. *Neurosci Biobehav Rev* 34:958–977.

Collins AL, Levenson JM, Vilaythong AP, Richman R, Armstrong DL, Noebels JL, David Sweatt J, Zoghbi HY. (2004). Mild overexpression of MeCP2 causes a progressive neurological disorder in mice. *Hum Mol Genet* 13:2679–2689.

De Bona C, Zappella M, Hayek G, Meloni I, Vitelli F, Bruttini M, Cusano R, Loffredo P, Longo I, Renieri A. (2000). Preserved speech variant is allelic of classic Rett syndrome. *Eur J Hum Genet* 8:325–330.

De Filippis B, Ricceri L, Fuso A, Laviola G. (2013). Neonatal exposure to low dose corticosterone persistently modulates hippocampal mineralocorticoid receptor expression and improves locomotor/exploratory behaviour in a mouse model of Rett syndrome. *Neuropharmacology* 68:174–183.

Dempster EL, Pidsley R, Schalkwyk LC, Owens S, Georgiades A, Kane F, Kalidindi S, Picchioni M, Kravariti E, Toulopoulou T, Murray RM, Mill J. (2011). Disease-associated epigenetic changes in monozygotic twins discordant for schizophrenia and bipolar disorder. *Hum Mol Genet* 20:4786–4796.

Deng JV, Rodriguiz RM, Hutchinson AN, Kim IH, Wetsel WC, West AE. (2010). MeCP2 in the nucleus accumbens contributes to neural and behavioral responses to psychostimulants. *Nat Neurosci* 13:1128–1136.

Downs J, Bergman A, Carter P, Anderson A, Palmer GM, Roye D, van Bosse H, Bebbington A, Larsson EL, Smith BG, Baikie G, Fyfe S, Leonard H. (2009). Guidelines for management of scoliosis in Rett syndrome patients based on expert consensus and clinical evidence. *Spine* 34:E607–617.

Du X, Pang TY, Mo C, Renoir T, Wright DJ, Hannan AJ. (2015). The influence of the HPG axis on stress response and depressive-like behaviour in a transgenic mouse model of Huntington's disease. *Exp Neurol* 263:63–71.

Duffy SN, Craddock KJ, Abel T, Nguyen PV. (2001). Environmental enrichment modifies the PKA-dependence of hippocampal LTP and improves hippocampus-dependent memory. *Learn Mem* 8:26–34.

Duman CH, Schlesinger L, Russell DS, Duman RS. (2008). Voluntary exercise produces antidepressant and anxiolytic behavioral effects in mice. *Brain Res* 1199:148–158.

Engerstrom IW. (1992). Rett syndrome: the late infantile regression period – a retrospective analysis of 91 cases. *Acta Paediatr* 81:167–172.

Erlandson A, Samuelsson L, Hagberg B, Kyllerman M, Vujic M, Wahlstrom J. (2003). Multiplex ligation-dependent probe amplification (MLPA) detects large deletions in the MECP2 gene of Swedish Rett syndrome patients. *Genet Test* 7:329–332.

Falkenberg T, Mohammed AK, Henriksson B, Persson H, Winblad B, Lindefors N. (1992). Increased expression of brain-derived neurotrophic factor mRNA in rat hippocampus is associated with improved spatial memory and enriched environment. *Neurosci Lett* 138:153–156.

Fordyce DE, Wehner JM. (1993). Physical activity enhances spatial learning performance with an associated alteration in hippocampal protein kinase C activity in C57BL/6 and DBA/2 mice. *Brain Res* 619:111–119.

Fox C, Merali Z, Harrison C. (2006). Therapeutic and protective effect of environmental enrichment against psychogenic and neurogenic stress. *Behav Brain Res* 175:1–8.

Franceschelli A, Herchick S, Thelen C, Papadopoulou-Daifoti Z, Pitychoutis PM. (2014). Sex differences in the chronic mild stress model of depression. *Behav Pharmacol* 25:372–383.

Freed D, Stevens EL, Pevsner J. (2014). Somatic mosaicism in the human genome. *Genes* 5:1064–1094.

Fuss J, Ben Abdallah NM, Vogt MA, Touma C, Pacifici PG, Palme R, Witzemann V, Hellweg R, Gass P. (2010). Voluntary exercise induces anxiety–like behavior in adult C57BL/6J mice correlating with hippocampal neurogenesis. *Hippocampus* 20:364–376.

Gadalla KK, Bailey ME, Spike RC, Ross PD, Woodard KT, Kalburgi SN, Bachaboina L, Deng JV, West AE, Samulski RJ, Gray SJ, Cobb SR. (2013). Improved survival and reduced phenotypic severity following AAV9/MECP2 gene transfer to neonatal and juvenile male Mecp2 knockout mice. *Mol Ther* 21:18–30.

Gao SF, Bao AM. (2011). Corticotropin–releasing hormone, glutamate, and gamma–aminobutyric acid in depression. *Neuroscientist* 17:124–144.

Garg SK, Lioy DT, Cheval H, McGann JC, Bissonnette JM, Murtha MJ, Foust KD, Kaspar BK, Bird A, Mandel G. (2013). Systemic delivery of MeCP2 rescues behavioral and cellular deficits in female mouse models of Rett syndrome. *J Neurosci* 33:13612–13620.

Georgel PT, Horowitz–Scherer RA, Adkins N, Woodcock CL, Wade PA, Hansen JC. (2003). Chromatin compaction by human MeCP2. Assembly of novel secondary chromatin structures in the absence of DNA methylation. *J Biol Chem* 278:32181–32188.

Giacometti E, Luikenhuis S, Beard C, Jaenisch R. (2007). Partial rescue of MeCP2 deficiency by postnatal activation of MeCP2. *Proc Natl Acad Sci USA* 104:1931–1936.

Gonder JC, Laber K. (2007). A renewed look at laboratory rodent housing and management. *ILAR J* 48:29–36.

Gottesman, II, Gould TD. (2003). The endophenotype concept in psychiatry: etymology and strategic intentions. *Am J Psychiatry* 160:636–645.

Govindarajan A, Rao BS, Nair D, Trinh M, Mawjee N, Tonegawa S, Chattarji S. (2006). Transgenic brain–derived neurotrophic factor expression causes both anxiogenic and antidepressant effects. *Proc Natl Acad Sci USA* 103:13208–13213.

Greer TL, Trivedi MH. (2009). Exercise in the treatment of depression. *Curr Psychiatry Rep* 11:466–472.

Griesbach GS, Tio DL, Vincelli J, McArthur DL, Taylor AN. (2012). Differential effects of voluntary and forced exercise on stress responses after traumatic brain injury. *J Neurotrauma* 29:1426–1433.

Guy J, Hendrich B, Holmes M, Martin JE, Bird A. (2001). A mouse Mecp2–null mutation causes neurological symptoms that mimic Rett syndrome. *Nat Genet* 27:322–326.

Guy J, Gan J, Selfridge J, Cobb S, Bird A. (2007). Reversal of neurological defects in a mouse model of Rett syndrome. *Science* 315:1143–1147.

Hagberg B, Aicardi J, Dias K, Ramos O. (1983). A progressive syndrome of autism, dementia, ataxia, and loss of purposeful hand use in girls: Rett's syndrome: report of 35 cases. *Ann Neurol* 14:471–479.

Hagberg B, Witt–Engerstrom I. (1986). Rett syndrome: a suggested staging system for describing impairment profile with increasing age towards adolescence. *Am J Med Genet Suppl* 1:47–59.

Hansson AC, Sommer WH, Metsis M, Stromberg I, Agnati LF, Fuxe K. (2006). Corticosterone actions on the hippocampal brain–derived neurotrophic factor expression are mediated by exon IV promoter. *J Neuroendocrinol* 18:104–114.

Hattori S, Hashimoto R, Miyakawa T, Yamanaka H, Maeno H, Wada K, Kunugi H. (2007). Enriched environments influence depression–related behavior in adult mice and the survival of newborn cells in their hippocampi. *Behav Brain Res* 180:69–76.

Hockly E, Cordery PM, Woodman B, Mahal A, van Dellen A, Blakemore C, Lewis CM, Hannan AJ, Bates GP. (2002). Environmental enrichment slows disease progression in R6/2 Huntington's disease mice. *Ann Neurol* 51:235–242.

Holsboer F, Ising M. (2008). Central CRH system in depression and anxiety – evidence from clinical studies with CRH1 receptor antagonists. *Eur J Pharmacol* 583:350–357.

Horiuchi Y, Kano S, Ishizuka K, Cascella NG, Ishii S, Talbot CC, Jr., Jaffe AE, Okano H, Pevsner J, Colantuoni C, Sawa A. (2013). Olfactory cells via nasal biopsy reflect the developing brain in gene expression profiles: utility and limitation of the surrogate tissues in research for brain disorders. *Neurosci Res* 77:247–250.

Hutchinson AN, Deng JV, Cohen S, West AE. (2012). Phosphorylation of MeCP2 at Ser421 contributes to chronic antidepressant action. *J Neurosci* 32:14355–14363.

Hutchinson KM, McLaughlin KJ, Wright RL, Bryce Ortiz J, Anouti DP, Mika A, Diamond DM, Conrad CD. (2012). Environmental enrichment protects against the effects of chronic stress on cognitive and morphological measures of hippocampal integrity. *Neurobiol Learn Mem* 97:250–260.

Ibi D, Takuma K, Koike H, Mizoguchi H, Tsuritani K, Kuwahara Y, Kamei H, Nagai T, Yoneda Y, Nabeshima T, Yamada K. (2008). Social isolation rearing–induced impairment of the hippocampal neurogenesis is associated with deficits in spatial memory and emotion–related behaviors in juvenile mice. *J Neurochem* 105:921–932.

Ickes BR, Pham TM, Sanders LA, Albeck DS, Mohammed AH, Granholm AC. (2000). Long–term environmental enrichment leads to regional increases in neurotrophin levels in rat brain. *Exp Neurol* 164:45–52.

Insel TR. (2014). Brain somatic mutations: the dark matter of psychiatric genetics? *Mol Psychiatry* 19:156–158.

Jacobsen K, Viken A, von Tetzchner S. (2001). Rett syndrome and ageing: a case study. *Disabil Rehabil* 23:160–166.

Jaenisch R, Bird A. (2003). Epigenetic regulation of gene expression: how the genome integrates intrinsic and environmental signals. *Nat Genet* 33 Suppl:245–254.

Jeanneteau F, Chao MV. (2013). Are BDNF and glucocorticoid activities calibrated? *Neuroscience* 239:173–195.

Jellinger KA. (2003). Rett syndrome – an update. *J Neural Transm* 110:681–701.

Jiang Z, Rompala GR, Zhang S, Cowell RM, Nakazawa K. (2013). Social isolation exacerbates schizophrenia–like phenotypes via oxidative stress in cortical interneurons. *Biol Psychiatry* 73:1024–1034.

Jones PL, Veenstra GJ, Wade PA, Vermaak D, Kass SU, Landsberger N, Strouboulis J, Wolffe AP. (1998). Methylated DNA and MeCP2 recruit histone deacetylase to repress transcription. *Nat Genet* 19:187–191.

Jugloff DG, Vandamme K, Logan R, Visanji NP, Brotchie JM, Eubanks JH. (2008). Targeted delivery of an Mecp2 transgene to forebrain neurons improves the behavior of female Mecp2–deficient mice. *Hum Mol Genet* 17:1386–1396.

Jutapakdeegul N, Afadlal S, Polaboon N, Phansuwan–Pujito P, Govitrapong P. (2010). Repeated restraint stress and corticosterone injections during late pregnancy alter GAP–43 expression in the hippocampus and prefrontal cortex of rat pups. *Int J Dev Neurosci* 28:83–90.

Kendler KS. (2013). What psychiatric genetics has taught us about the nature of psychiatric illness and what is left to learn. *Mol Psychiatry* 18:1058–1066.

Kerr AM, Burford B. (2001). Towards a full life with Rett disorder. *Pediatr Rehabil* 4:157–168; discussion 155–156.

Kerr B, Silva PA, Walz K, Young JI. (2010). Unconventional transcriptional response to environmental enrichment in a mouse model of Rett syndrome. *PLoS One* 5:e11534.

Kishi N, Macklis JD. (2004). MECP2 is progressively expressed in post–migratory neurons and is involved in neuronal maturation rather than cell fate decisions. *Mol Cell Neurosci* 27:306–321.

Kishi N, Macklis JD. (2005). Dissecting MECP2 function in the central nervous system. *J Child Neurol* 20:753–759.

Klose R, Bird A. (2003). Molecular biology. MeCP2 repression goes nonglobal. *Science* 302:793–795.

Klose RJ, Bird AP. (2006). Genomic DNA methylation: the mark and its mediators. *Trends Biochem Sci* 31:89–97.

Kobilo T, Liu QR, Gandhi K, Mughal M, Shaham Y, van Praag H. (2011). Running is the neurogenic and neurotrophic stimulus in environmental enrichment. *Learn Mem* 18:605–609.

Kondo M, Gray LJ, Pelka GJ, Christodoulou J, Tam PP, Hannan AJ. (2008). Environmental enrichment ameliorates a motor coordination deficit in a mouse model of Rett syndrome – Mecp2 gene dosage effects and BDNF expression. *Eur J Neurosci* 27:3342–3350.

Kondo MA, Gray LJ, Pelka GJ, Leang S–K, Christodoulou J, Tam PPL, Hannan AJ. (2015). Affective dysfunction in a mouse model of Rett syndrome: therapeutic effects of environmental stimulation and physical activity. *Developmental Neurobiology*. Advance online publication. doi:10.1002/dneu.22308.

Kuzumaki N, Ikegami D, Tamura R, Hareyama N, Imai S, Narita M, Torigoe K, Niikura K, Takeshima H, Ando T, Igarashi K, Kanno J, Ushijima T, Suzuki T. (2011). Hippocampal epigenetic modification at the brain–derived neurotrophic factor gene induced by an enriched environment. *Hippocampus* 21:127–132.

Lambert TJ, Fernandez SM, Frick KM. (2005). Different types of environmental enrichment have discrepant effects on spatial memory and synaptophysin levels in female mice. *Neurobiol Learn Mem* 83:206–216.

Larimore JL, Chapleau CA, Kudo S, Theibert A, Percy AK, Pozzo–Miller L. (2009). Bdnf overexpression in hippocampal neurons prevents dendritic atrophy caused by Rett–associated MECP2 mutations. *Neurobiol Dis* 34:199–211.

Laviola G, Hannan AJ, Macri S, Solinas M, Jaber M. (2008). Effects of enriched environment on animal models of neurodegenerative diseases and psychiatric disorders. *Neurobiol Dis* 31:159–168.

Lavretsky H. (2009). Complementary and alternative medicine use for treatment and prevention of late–life mood and cognitive disorders. *Aging Health* 5:61–78.

Leasure JL, Decker L. (2009). Social isolation prevents exercise–induced proliferation of hippocampal progenitor cells in female rats. *Hippocampus* 19:907–912.

Leasure JL, Jones M. (2008). Forced and voluntary exercise differentially affect brain and behavior. *Neuroscience* 156:456–465.

Lewis JD, Meehan RR, Henzel WJ, Maurer–Fogy I, Jeppesen P, Klein F, Bird A. (1992). Purification, sequence, and cellular localization of a novel chromosomal protein that binds to
methylated DNA. *Cell* 69:905–914.

Liu QR, Lu L, Zhu XG, Gong JP, Shaham Y, Uhl GR. (2006). Rodent BDNF genes, novel
promoters, novel splice variants, and regulation by cocaine. *Brain Res* 1067:1–12.

Lonetti G, Angelucci A, Morando L, Boggio EM, Giustetto M, Pizzorusso T. (2010). Early
environmental enrichment moderates the behavioral and synaptic phenotype of MeCP2
null mice. *Biol Psychiatry* 67:657–665.

Lotan M, Isakov E, Merrick J. (2004). Improving functional skills and physical fitness in children
with Rett syndrome. *J Intellect Disabil Res* 48:730–735.

Lu B. (2003). BDNF and activity–dependent synaptic modulation. *Learn Mem* 10:86–98.

Lu L, Bao G, Chen H, Xia P, Fan X, Zhang J, Pei G, Ma L. (2003). Modification of hippocampal
neurogenesis and neuroplasticity by social environments. *Exp Neurol* 183:600–609.

Martinez–Cue C, Baamonde C, Lumbreras M, Paz J, Davisson MT, Schmidt C, Dierssen M, Florez
J. (2002). Differential effects of environmental enrichment on behavior and learning of male
and female Ts65Dn mice, a model for Down syndrome. *Behav Brain Res* 134:185–200.

Martinowich K, Lu B. (2008). Interaction between BDNF and serotonin: role in mood disorders.
Neuropsychopharmacology 33:73–83.

Martinowich K, Hattori D, Wu H, Fouse S, He F, Hu Y, Fan G, Sun YE. (2003). DNA
methylation–related chromatin remodeling in activity–dependent BDNF gene regulation.
Science 302:890–893.

Matrisciano F, Tueting P, Maccari S, Nicoletti F, Guidotti A. (2012). Pharmacological activation of
group–II metabotropic glutamate receptors corrects a schizophrenia–like phenotype induced
by prenatal stress in mice. *Neuropsychopharmacology* 37:929–938.

McGill BE, Bundle SF, Yaylaoglu MB, Carson JP, Thaller C, Zoghbi HY. (2006). Enhanced anxiety
and stress–induced corticosterone release are associated with increased Crh expression in a
mouse model of Rett syndrome. *Proc Natl Acad Sci USA* 103:18267–18272.

Meaney MJ, Szyf M. (2005). Maternal care as a model for experience–dependent chromatin
plasticity? *Trends Neurosci* 28:456–463.

Metsis M, Timmusk T, Arenas E, Persson H. (1993). Differential usage of multiple brain–derived
neurotrophic factor promoters in the rat brain following neuronal activation. *Proc Natl Acad
Sci USA* 90:8802–8806.

Meziane H, Ouagazzal AM, Aubert L, Wietrzych M, Krezel W. (2007). Estrous cycle effects on
behavior of C57BL/6J and BALB/cByJ female mice: implications for phenotyping strategies.
Genes Brain Behav 6:192–200.

Migeon BR, Dunn MA, Thomas G, Schmeckpeper BJ, Naidu S. (1995). Studies of X inactivation
and isodisomy in twins provide further evidence that the X chromosome is not involved in
Rett syndrome. *Am J Hum Genet* 56:647–653.

Modell S, Lauer CJ, Schreiber W, Huber J, Krieg JC, Holsboer F. (1998). Hormonal response
pattern in the combined DEX–CRH test is stable over time in subjects at high familial risk
for affective disorders. *Neuropsychopharmacology* 18:253–262.

Monteggia LM, Luikart B, Barrot M, Theobold D, Malkovska I, Nef S, Parada LF, Nestler EJ.
(2007). Brain–derived neurotrophic factor conditional knockouts show gender differences
in depression–related behaviors. *Biol Psychiatry* 61:187–197.

Moretti P, Zoghbi HY. (2006). MeCP2 dysfunction in Rett syndrome and related disorders. *Curr
Opin Genet Dev* 16:276–281.

Moretti P, Levenson JM, Battaglia F, Atkinson R, Teague R, Antalffy B, Armstrong D, Arancio
O, Sweatt JD, Zoghbi HY. (2006). Learning and memory and synaptic plasticity are impaired
in a mouse model of Rett syndrome. *J Neurosci* 26:319–327.

Mount RH, Charman T, Hastings RP, Reilly S, Cass H. (2002). The Rett Syndrome Behaviour
Questionnaire (RSBQ): refining the behavioural phenotype of Rett syndrome. *J Child Psychol
Psychiatry* 43:1099–1110.

Muller MB, Zimmermann S, Sillaber I, Hagemeyer TP, Deussing JM, Timpl P, Kormann MS, Droste SK, Kuhn R, Reul JM, Holsboer F, Wurst W. (2003). Limbic corticotropin–releasing hormone receptor 1 mediates anxiety–related behavior and hormonal adaptation to stress. *Nat Neurosci* 6:1100–1107.

Murakami JW, Courchesne E, Haas RH, Press GA, Yeung–Courchesne R. (1992). Cerebellar and cerebral abnormalities in Rett syndrome: a quantitative MR analysis. *AJR Am J Roentgenol* 159:177–183.

Murgatroyd C, Patchev AV, Wu Y, Micale V, Bockmuhl Y, Fischer D, Holsboer F, Wotjak CT, Almeida OF, Spengler D. (2009). Dynamic DNA methylation programs persistent adverse effects of early–life stress. *Nat Neurosci* 12:1559–1566.

Murgatroyd C, Wu Y, Bockmuhl Y, Spengler D. (2010). Genes learn from stress: How infantile trauma programs us for depression. *Epigenetics* 5.

Nag N, Moriuchi JM, Peitzman CG, Ward BC, Kolodny NH, Berger–Sweeney JE. (2009). Environmental enrichment alters locomotor behaviour and ventricular volume in Mecp2 1lox mice. *Behav Brain Res* 196:44–48.

Nagarajan RP, Hogart AR, Gwye Y, Martin MR, LaSalle JM. (2006). Reduced MeCP2 expression is frequent in autism frontal cortex and correlates with aberrant MECP2 promoter methylation. *Epigenetics* 1:e1–11.

Nikitina T, Ghosh RP, Horowitz–Scherer RA, Hansen JC, Grigoryev SA, Woodcock CL. (2007a). MeCP2–chromatin interactions include the formation of chromatosome–like structures and are altered in mutations causing Rett syndrome. *J Biol Chem* 282:28237–28245.

Nikitina T, Shi X, Ghosh RP, Horowitz–Scherer RA, Hansen JC, Woodcock CL. (2007b). Multiple modes of interaction between the methylated DNA binding protein MeCP2 and chromatin. *Mol Cell Biol* 27:864–877.

Nithianantharajah J, Hannan AJ. (2006). Enriched environments, experience–dependent plasticity and disorders of the nervous system. *Nat Rev Neurosci* 7:697–709.

Nithianantharajah J, Hannan AJ. (2009). The neurobiology of brain and cognitive reserve: mental and physical activity as modulators of brain disorders. *Prog Neurobiol* 89: 369–382.

Nithianantharajah J, Barkus C, Murphy M, Hannan AJ. (2008). Gene–environment interactions modulating cognitive function and molecular correlates of synaptic plasticity in Huntington's disease transgenic mice. *Neurobiol Dis* 29:490–504.

Niwa M, Matsumoto Y, Mouri A, Ozaki N, Nabeshima T. (2011). Vulnerability in early life to changes in the rearing environment plays a crucial role in the aetiopathology of psychiatric disorders. *Int J Neuropsychopharmacol* 14:459–477.

Niwa M, Jaaro–Peled H, Tankou S, Seshadri S, Hikida T, Matsumoto Y, Cascella NG, Kano S, Ozaki N, Nabeshima T, Sawa A. (2013). Adolescent stress–induced epigenetic control of dopaminergic neurons via glucocorticoids. *Science* 339:335–339.

Nuber UA, Kriaucionis S, Roloff TC, Guy J, Selfridge J, Steinhoff C, Schulz R, Lipkowitz B, Ropers HH, Holmes MC, Bird A. (2005). Up–regulation of glucocorticoid–regulated genes in a mouse model of Rett syndrome. *Hum Mol Genet* 14:2247–2256.

Ogawa A, Mitsudome A, Yasumoto S, Matsumoto T. (1997). Japanese monozygotic twins with Rett syndrome. *Brain Dev* 19:568–570.

Olsson IA, Dahlborn K. (2002). Improving housing conditions for laboratory mice: a review of "environmental enrichment." *Lab Anim* 36:243–270.

Oomen CA, Soeters H, Audureau N, Vermunt L, van Hasselt FN, Manders EM, Joels M, Lucassen PJ, Krugers H. (2010). Severe early life stress hampers spatial learning and neurogenesis, but improves hippocampal synaptic plasticity and emotional learning under high–stress conditions in adulthood. *J Neurosci* 30:6635–6645.

O'Roak BJ, Stessman HA, Boyle EA, Witherspoon KT, Martin B, Lee C, Vives L, Baker C, Hiatt JB, Nickerson DA, Bernier R, Shendure J, Eichler EE. (2014). Recurrent de novo mutations implicate novel genes underlying simplex autism risk. *Nat Commun* 5:5595.

Owens MJ, Nemeroff CB. (1991). Physiology and pharmacology of corticotropin–releasing factor. *Pharmacol Rev* 43:425–473.

Pang TY, Hannan AJ. (2013). Enhancement of cognitive function in models of brain disease through environmental enrichment and physical activity. *Neuropharmacology* 64: 515–528.

Pang TY, Stam NC, Nithianantharajah J, Howard ML, Hannan AJ. (2006). Differential effects of voluntary physical exercise on behavioral and brain–derived neurotrophic factor expression deficits in Huntington's disease transgenic mice. *Neuroscience* 141:569–584.

Pang TY, Du X, Zajac MS, Howard ML, Hannan AJ. (2009). Altered serotonin receptor expression is associated with depression–related behavior in the R6/1 transgenic mouse model of Huntington's disease. *Hum Mol Genet* 18:753–766.

Pelka GJ, Watson CM, Radziewic T, Hayward M, Lahooti H, Christodoulou J, Tam PP. (2006). Mecp2 deficiency is associated with learning and cognitive deficits and altered gene activity in the hippocampal region of mice. *Brain* 129:887–898.

Piazza CC, Anderson C, Fisher W. (1993). Teaching self–feeding skills to patients with Rett syndrome. *Dev Med Child Neurol* 35:991–996.

Pietropaolo S, Singer P, Feldon J, Yee BK. (2008). The postweaning social isolation in C57BL/6 mice: preferential vulnerability in the male sex. *Psychopharmacology* 197:613–628.

Plappert CF, Rodenbucher AM, Pilz PK. (2005). Effects of sex and estrous cycle on modulation of the acoustic startle response in mice. *Physiol Behav* 84:585–594.

Portela A, Esteller M. (2010). Epigenetic modifications and human disease. *Nat Biotechnol* 28:1057–1068.

Ramocki MB, Peters SU, Tavyev YJ, Zhang F, Carvalho CM, Schaaf CP, Richman R, Fang P, Glaze DG, Lupski JR, Zoghbi HY. (2009). Autism and other neuropsychiatric symptoms are prevalent in individuals with MeCP2 duplication syndrome. *Ann Neurol* 66:771–782.

Rampon C, Jiang CH, Dong H, Tang YP, Lockhart DJ, Schultz PG, Tsien JZ, Hu Y. (2000). Effects of environmental enrichment on gene expression in the brain. *Proc Natl Acad Sci USA* 97:12880–12884.

Renoir T, Pang TY, Zajac MS, Chan G, Du X, Leang L, Chevarin C, Lanfumey L, Hannan AJ. (2012). Treatment of depressive–like behaviour in Huntington's disease mice by chronic sertraline and exercise. *Br J Pharmacol* 165:1375–1389.

Restivo L, Ferrari F, Passino E, Sgobio C, Bock J, Oostra BA, Bagni C, Ammassari–Teule M. (2005). Enriched environment promotes behavioral and morphological recovery in a mouse model for the fragile X syndrome. *Proc Natl Acad Sci USA* 102:11557–11562.

Robertson L, Hall SE, Jacoby P, Ellaway C, de Klerk N, Leonard H. (2006). The association between behavior and genotype in Rett syndrome using the Australian Rett Syndrome Database. *Am J Med Genet B Neuropsychiatr Genet* 141B:177–183.

Rossi C, Angelucci A, Costantin L, Braschi C, Mazzantini M, Babbini F, Fabbri ME, Tessarollo L, Maffei L, Berardi N, Caleo M. (2006). Brain–derived neurotrophic factor (BDNF) is required for the enhancement of hippocampal neurogenesis following environmental enrichment. *Eur J Neurosci* 24:1850–1856.

Russo–Neustadt A, Ha T, Ramirez R, Kesslak JP. (2001). Physical activity–antidepressant treatment combination: impact on brain–derived neurotrophic factor and behavior in an animal model. *Behav Brain Res* 120:87–95.

Sale A, Maya Vetencourt JF, Medini P, Cenni MC, Baroncelli L, De Pasquale R, Maffei L. (2007). Environmental enrichment in adulthood promotes amblyopia recovery through a reduction of intracortical inhibition. *Nat Neurosci* 10:679–681.

Sale A, Berardi N, Maffei L. (2009). Enrich the environment to empower the brain. *Trends Neurosci* 32:233–239.

Samaco RC, Fryer JD, Ren J, Fyffe S, Chao HT, Sun Y, Greer JJ, Zoghbi HY, Neul JL. (2008). A partial loss of function allele of methyl–CpG–binding protein 2 predicts a human neurodevelopmental syndrome. *Hum Mol Genet* 17:1718–1727.

Sansom D, Krishnan VH, Corbett J, Kerr A. (1993). Emotional and behavioural aspects of Rett syndrome. *Dev Med Child Neurol* 35:340–345.

Santarelli L, Saxe M, Gross C, Surget A, Battaglia F, Dulawa S, Weisstaub N, Lee J, Duman R, Arancio O, Belzung C, Hen R. (2003). Requirement of hippocampal neurogenesis for the behavioral effects of antidepressants. *Science* 301:805–809.

Sapolsky RM. (2000). The possibility of neurotoxicity in the hippocampus in major depression: a primer on neuron death. *Biol Psychiatry* 48:755–765.

Scala E, Longo I, Ottimo F, Speciale C, Sampieri K, Katzaki E, Artuso R, Mencarelli MA, D'Ambrogio T, Vonella G, Zappella M, Hayek G, Battaglia A, Mari F, Renieri A, Ariani F. (2007). MECP2 deletions and genotype–phenotype correlation in Rett syndrome. *Am J Med Genet A* 143A:2775–2784.

Schizophrenia Working Group of the Psychiatric Genomics Consortium. (2014). Biological insights from 108 schizophrenia–associated genetic loci. *Nature* 511:421–427.

Schloesser RJ, Lehmann M, Martinowich K, Manji HK, Herkenham M. (2010). Environmental enrichment requires adult neurogenesis to facilitate the recovery from psychosocial stress. *Mol Psychiatry* 15:1152–1163.

Shahbazian M, Young J, Yuva–Paylor L, Spencer C, Antalffy B, Noebels J, Armstrong D, Paylor R, Zoghbi H. (2002). Mice with truncated MeCP2 recapitulate many Rett syndrome features and display hyperacetylation of histone H3. *Neuron* 35:243–254.

Shieh PB, Hu SC, Bobb K, Timmusk T, Ghosh A. (1998). Identification of a signaling pathway involved in calcium regulation of BDNF expression. *Neuron* 20:727–740.

Shirayama Y, Chen AC, Nakagawa S, Russell DS, Duman RS. (2002). Brain–derived neurotrophic factor produces antidepressant effects in behavioral models of depression. *J Neurosci* 22:3251–3261.

Singhal G, Jaehne EJ, Corrigan F, Baune BT. (2014). Cellular and molecular mechanisms of immunomodulation in the brain through environmental enrichment. *Front Cell Neurosci* 8:97.

Siuciak JA, Lewis DR, Wiegand SJ, Lindsay RM. (1997). Antidepressant–like effect of brain–derived neurotrophic factor (BDNF). *Pharmacol Biochem Behav* 56:131–137.

Smrt RD, Eaves–Egenes J, Barkho BZ, Santistevan NJ, Zhao C, Aimone JB, Gage FH, Zhao X. (2007). Mecp2 deficiency leads to delayed maturation and altered gene expression in hippocampal neurons. *Neurobiol Dis* 27:77–89.

Spires TL, Grote HE, Varshney NK, Cordery PM, van Dellen A, Blakemore C, Hannan AJ. (2004). Environmental enrichment rescues protein deficits in a mouse model of Huntington's disease, indicating a possible disease mechanism. *J Neurosci* 24:2270–2276.

Sterner EY, Kalynchuk LE. (2010). Behavioral and neurobiological consequences of prolonged glucocorticoid exposure in rats: relevance to depression. *Prog Neuropsychopharmacol Biol Psychiatry* 34:777–790.

Stranahan AM, Khalil D, Gould E. (2006). Social isolation delays the positive effects of running on adult neurogenesis. *Nat Neurosci* 9:526–533.

Sztainberg Y, Kuperman Y, Tsoory M, Lebow M, Chen A. (2010). The anxiolytic effect of environmental enrichment is mediated via amygdalar CRF receptor type 1. *Mol Psychiatry* 15:905–917.

Tao J, Hu K, Chang Q, Wu H, Sherman NE, Martinowich K, Klose RJ, Schanen C, Jaenisch R, Wang W, Sun YE. (2009). Phosphorylation of MeCP2 at Serine 80 regulates its chromatin association and neurological function. *Proc Natl Acad Sci USA* 106:4882–4887.

Tao X, Finkbeiner S, Arnold DB, Shaywitz AJ, Greenberg ME. (1998). Ca2+ influx regulates BDNF transcription by a CREB family transcription factor–dependent mechanism. *Neuron* 20:709–726.

Tao X, West AE, Chen WG, Corfas G, Greenberg ME. (2002). A calcium–responsive transcription factor, CaRF, that regulates neuronal activity–dependent expression of BDNF. *Neuron* 33:383–395.

Timmusk T, Lendahl U, Funakoshi H, Arenas E, Persson H, Metsis M. (1995). Identification of brain–derived neurotrophic factor promoter regions mediating tissue–specific, axotomy–, and neuronal activity–induced expression in transgenic mice. *J Cell Biol* 128:185–199.

Tudor M, Akbarian S, Chen RZ, Jaenisch R. (2002). Transcriptional profiling of a mouse model for Rett syndrome reveals subtle transcriptional changes in the brain. *Proc Natl Acad Sci USA* 99:15536–15541.

Tylee DS, Kawaguchi DM, Glatt SJ. (2013). On the outside, looking in: a review and evaluation of the comparability of blood and brain "–omes". *Am J Med Genet B Neuropsychiatr Genet* 162B:595–603.

van Dellen A, Blakemore C, Deacon R, York D, Hannan AJ. (2000). Delaying the onset of Huntington's in mice. *Nature* 404:721–722.

van Dellen A, Cordery PM, Spires TL, Blakemore C, Hannan AJ. (2008). Wheel running from a juvenile age delays onset of specific motor deficits but does not alter protein aggregate density in a mouse model of Huntington's disease. *BMC Neurosci* 9:34.

van Praag H, Kempermann G, Gage FH. (1999). Running increases cell proliferation and neurogenesis in the adult mouse dentate gyrus. *Nat Neurosci* 2:266–270.

van Praag H, Kempermann G, Gage FH. (2000). Neural consequences of environmental enrichment. *Nat Rev Neurosci* 1:191–198.

Vazquez–Sanroman D, Sanchis–Segura C, Toledo R, Hernandez ME, Manzo J, Miquel M. (2013). The effects of enriched environment on BDNF expression in the mouse cerebellum depending on the length of exposure. *Behav Brain Res* 243:118–128.

Veena J, Srikumar BN, Raju TR, Shankaranarayana Rao BS. (2009). Exposure to enriched environment restores the survival and differentiation of new born cells in the hippocampus and ameliorates depressive symptoms in chronically stressed rats. *Neurosci Lett* 455:178–182.

Verkuyl JM, Hemby SE, Joels M. (2004). Chronic stress attenuates GABAergic inhibition and alters gene expression of parvocellular neurons in rat hypothalamus. *Eur J Neurosci* 20:1665–1673.

Vignoli A, La Briola F, Canevini MP. (2009). Evolution of stereotypies in adolescents and women with Rett syndrome. *Mov Disord* 24:1379–1383.

Wan M, Lee SS, Zhang X, Houwink–Manville I, Song HR, Amir RE, Budden S, Naidu S, Pereira JL, Lo IF, Zoghbi HY, Schanen NC, Francke U. (1999). Rett syndrome and beyond: recurrent spontaneous and familial MECP2 mutations at CpG hotspots. *Am J Hum Genet* 65: 1520–1529.

Warby S. (2002). Modeling classic female Rett Syndrome in male mice. *Clin Genet* 62:368–370.

Watson CM, Pelka GJ, Radziewic T, Shahbazian MD, Christodoulou J, Williamson SL, Tam PP. (2005). Reduced proportion of Purkinje cells expressing paternally derived mutant Mecp2308 allele in female mouse cerebellum is not due to a skewed primary pattern of X–chromosome inactivation. *Hum Mol Genet* 14:1851–1861.

Weaver IC, Cervoni N, Champagne FA, D'Alessio AC, Sharma S, Seckl JR, Dymov S, Szyf M, Meaney MJ. (2004). Epigenetic programming by maternal behavior. *Nat Neurosci* 7:847–854.

Weaver IC, Champagne FA, Brown SE, Dymov S, Sharma S, Meaney MJ, Szyf M. (2005). Reversal of maternal programming of stress responses in adult offspring through methyl supplementation: altering epigenetic marking later in life. *J Neurosci* 25:11045–11054.

Weaving LS, Ellaway CJ, Gecz J, Christodoulou J. (2005). Rett syndrome: clinical review and genetic update. *J Med Genet* 42:1–7.

Willner P. (1984). The validity of animal models of depression. *Psychopharmacology* 83:1–16.

Wong EH, So HC, Li M, Wang Q, Butler AW, Paul B, Wu HM, Hui TC, Choi SC, So MT, Garcia–Barcelo MM, McAlonan GM, Chen EY, Cheung EF, Chan RC, Purcell SM, Cherny SS, Chen RR, Li T, Sham PC. (2014). Common variants on Xq28 conferring risk of schizophrenia in Han Chinese. *Schizophr Bull* 40:777–786.

Yasuhara A, Sugiyama Y. (2001). Music therapy for children with Rett syndrome. *Brain Dev 23 Suppl* 1:S82–84.

Yasui DH, Peddada S, Bieda MC, Vallero RO, Hogart A, Nagarajan RP, Thatcher KN, Farnham PJ, Lasalle JM. (2007). Integrated epigenomic analyses of neuronal MeCP2 reveal a role for long–range interaction with active genes. *Proc Natl Acad Sci USA* 104:19416–19421.

Young JI, Zoghbi HY. (2004). X–chromosome inactivation patterns are unbalanced and affect the phenotypic outcome in a mouse model of rett syndrome. *Am J Hum Genet* 74:511–520.

Young JI, Hong EP, Castle JC, Crespo–Barreto J, Bowman AB, Rose MF, Kang D, Richman R, Johnson JM, Berget S, Zoghbi HY. (2005). Regulation of RNA splicing by the methylation–dependent transcriptional repressor methyl–CpG binding protein 2. *Proc Natl Acad Sci USA* 102:17551–17558.

Yu F, Zingler N, Schumann G, Stratling WH. (2001). Methyl–CpG–binding protein 2 represses LINE–1 expression and retrotransposition but not Alu transcription. *Nucleic Acids Res* 29:4493–4501.

Yusufzai TM, Wolffe AP. (2000). Functional consequences of Rett syndrome mutations on human MeCP2. *Nucleic Acids Res* 28:4172–4179.

Zajac MS, Pang TY, Wong N, Weinrich B, Leang LS, Craig JM, Saffery R, Hannan AJ. (2010). Wheel running and environmental enrichment differentially modify exon–specific BDNF expression in the hippocampus of wild–type and pre–motor symptomatic male and female Huntington's disease mice. *Hippocampus* 20:621–636.

Zhou Z, Hong EJ, Cohen S, Zhao WN, Ho HY, Schmidt L, Chen WG, Lin Y, Savner E, Griffith EC, Hu L, Steen JA, Weitz CJ, Greenberg ME. (2006). Brain–specific phosphorylation of MeCP2 regulates activity–dependent Bdnf transcription, dendritic growth, and spine maturation. *Neuron* 52:255–269.

Zhu X, Need AC, Petrovski S, Goldstein DB. (2014). One gene, many neuropsychiatric disorders: lessons from Mendelian diseases. *Nat Neurosci* 17:773–781.

Zimmermann CA, Hoffmann A, Raabe F, Spengler D. (2015). Role of mecp2 in experience–dependent epigenetic programming. *Genes* 6:60–86.

Zoghbi HY. (2003). Postnatal neurodevelopmental disorders: meeting at the synapse? *Science* 302:826–83.

CHAPTER 4

Critical periods and neurodevelopmental brain disorders

Rhiannon M. Meredith

Center for Neurogenomics & Cognitive Research (CNCR), VU University Amsterdam, Amsterdam, The Netherlands

Introduction

Developing a brain is not a simple process at consistent speeds of growth but rather a series of time-limited developmental stages, beautifully integrated from early blastocyst postfertilization to the fully formed adult brain. These early developmental stages are guided and directed by specific molecular cues arising from early gene expression and later influenced by both intrinsic neuronal activity and external factors, such as maternal influences upon the neuronal circuitry forming in the developing brain (Spitzer, 2006; Marin et al., 2010; Zimmerman and Connors, 2010). During mammalian development, there are periods of heightened change in both the brain and in animal behavior that are restricted to distinct developmental stages, commonly referred to as critical or sensitive periods. Critical and sensitive periods exist across many vertebrate species both during pre- and postnatal stages of development (Clancy et al., 2007; Workman et al., 2013). In the last decade, dysregulation of synaptic, neuronal, and behavioral phenotypes in neurodevelopmental brain disorders (NDDs) has been increasingly observed during known critical and sensitive periods for brain development and behavior (LeBlanc and Fagiolini, 2011; Martin and Huntsman, 2012; Meredith et al., 2012; Kroon et al., 2013; Wang et al., 2014; Meredith, 2015). These observations have formed a concept that there are sensitive time windows during brain development for the onset and manifestation of impairments that underlie neurodevelopmental disorders. Existence of such time windows has three key implications for NDDs: (1) that these developmental stages mark the earliest known onset periods for phenotypic alterations in known NDDs, (2) that time windows act as indicators of when the brain may be more vulnerable to genetic or environmental insults

Environmental Experience and Plasticity of the Developing Brain, First Edition.
Edited by Alessandro Sale.
© 2016 John Wiley & Sons, Inc. Published 2016 by John Wiley & Sons, Inc.

that could trigger the onset of a disorder, and (3) that during these periods, the brain may be more amenable to therapeutic intervention to correct phenotypes directly arising or to prevent those developing as a consequence of the original insult. This chapter will review the key ideas that led to the hypothesis of critical and sensitive period dysregulation and further discuss the implications for our understanding of early stages of development in NDDs.

Developmental aspects of NDDs

As their name suggests, NDDs are caused by alteration or impairment during growth and maturation of the central nervous system leading to dysfunction at multiple levels from neurons to behavior (Goldstein and Reynolds, 1999). They are characterised by age-regulated onset of symptoms including motor control, language, emotion and cognitive ability and in some cases regression of newly acquired abilities during early periods of life (Zoghbi and Bear, 2012). NDDs encompass a wide range of syndromes and conditions, thus for the purpose of this chapter, evidence for dysregulation of critical periods is restricted to NDDs of intellectual disability (ID) and autistic spectrum disorders (ASDs). Although age of symptom onset can vary between these disorders, in all cases cognitive and behavioral alterations must have manifest before the age of 18 and not be due to physical injury or be part of a neurodegenerative process. For many disorders including ID syndromes and ASDs, the onset and progression of symptoms can be striking with children missing key developmental milestones and delays in motor, social and language skill acquisition (Geschwind and Levitt, 2007; Abbeduto et al., 2014). During early developmental stages, hypotonia and motor skill impairments are often reported in many NDDs including Fragile X and Angelman syndromes (Kau et al., 2000; Clayton-Smith and Laan, 2003; Williams et al., 2006). Impairments in speech and language acquisition skills, difficulties with social communication and social interaction are also reported for some individuals with Fragile X and Angelman syndromes, in which they may be defined as core symptoms, or these impairments can be categorised as part of an associated ASD for certain disorders (Gillberg and Billstedt, 2000; Amiet et al., 2008). Although the exact symptoms of NDDs can differ significantly between individual syndromes, high comorbidity exists between ID, ASDs and epilepsy: 40% of those diagnosed with ID will also have ASD and 30% of children who have epilepsy will be diagnosed with a form of ASD and/or ID (Tuchman et al., 2009). Furthermore for people with ASD, the lower the IQ, the significantly greater the likelihood that they will also have epilepsy at some stage of their development (Amiet et al., 2008).

The common patterns of symptoms across syndromes and their onset at specific developmental periods have led to the idea of a common set of aetiologies underlying many NDDs. The inclusion of NDDs is not restricted to purely syndromic conditions since many nonsyndromic disorders that likely arise from genetic mutations as well as disorders caused by environmental insults show age-dependent symptom manifestations at similar developmental stages (see "Implications of misregulated critical periods and future directions" section). Disregarding the genetic or environmental cause of the NDD, early postnatal symptom onset and developmental delays in key skills are prominent for both syndromic and nonsyndromic disorders. In order to understand the neurobiological mechanisms underlying brain development in NDDs, our knowledge on both neurotypical and aberrant development at the synaptic and neuronal levels in the brain has largely been acquired through use of genetically engineered animal models for monogenic disorders – predominantly flies and mice.

Brain development and critical periods

During the early developmental stages of an organism, there are critical and sensitive periods of time when an organism undergoes significant functional and structural modifications and is more susceptible to change during these periods (Hensch, 2004; Hensch, 2005; Johnson, 2005; Michel and Tyler, 2005). During these periods, the brain and behavioral outputs of the organism undergo a state of heightened plasticity relative to other developmental stages, with changes either being driven by intrinsic factors such as molecular cues or modulated by external factors such as visual experience. Usage of the terms "critical" and "sensitive" period is often intertwined but historically, critical periods were used to describe brain circuit phenotypes in the sensory systems such as ocular dominance formation in the visual system or plasticity of synaptic connections in the brain in forming the somatosensory cortex corresponding to sensory information from a rodent's whiskers (Fox et al., 2000; Hensch, 2005). Critical periods are restricted windows of time during which a system or organism is most responsive to an essential developmental change, the lack of which causes a permanent modification in the system itself or the behavior of the organism. Later modification outside these critical periods is not classically thought possible but more recent findings have shown that subtle alterations in adulthood can be induced (e.g., Pizzorusso et al., 2002; Oberlaender et al., 2012). Sensitive periods refer to periods of time during which the exposure of the organism to external factors modulates its behavior at the time and has influence later in life. These time windows have often been thought to be less stringent than critical periods but what is more apparent is that absence of a sensitive period, whilst having lifelong consequences for an organism's behavior, does not usually lead to critical changes in the brain that are essential for further development. The classical example of a sensitive period is that for filial imprinting, whereby young animals such as chicks form social attachments to their parents or main carers (Lorenz, 1935; Horn, 2004).

Documentation of critical and sensitive periods provides a framework for mapping developmental stages when a system, such as part of the brain, or behavior of the organism undergoes heightened plasticity and remodelling. During brain formation and maturation, functional connections between individual neurons and between entire brain regions are made in a typical pattern from cell migration guided by molecular cues to axonal and dendritic outgrowths, followed by formation of filopodia and eventually strong, stable synapses (Katz and Shatz, 1996; Ethell and Pasquale, 2005; Lohmann and Kessels, 2014). The pattern of forming and remodelling connections at the synaptic level continues during adulthood (Grutzendler et al., 2002; Trachtenberg et al., 2002; Holtmaat et al., 2005). However, in the vertebrate brain, the peak of synapse formation and remodelling occurs during early postnatal periods of development (Pan and Gan, 2008). A well-documented set of critical periods for synaptic formation and remodelling has been described in the rodent somatosensory system. Beginning in the embryonic brain, axons grow out from trigeminal nuclei along lemniscal and paralemniscal pathways to project to regions of the thalamus, with its distinctive barreloid patterning, followed by thalamic axonal outgrowth from the thalamus to somatosensory cortex where the barrels are formed (Fox, 2002; Lopez-Bendito and Molnar, 2003; Feldmeyer et al., 2013). These sequential stages of development and plastic modification of the somatosensory system from brainstem to cortical layers occur within restricted critical periods of time. For example, thalamocortical excitatory projections from thalamus to layer 4 in the cortex only undergo synaptic plasticity during postnatal days 3 to 7 in rodents (Crair and Malenka, 1995). The target neurons in layer 4 make functional connections with cortical neurons in layers 2 and 3 from postnatal day 5 onwards and then undergo a period of heightened synaptic plasticity during the second postnatal week, ending a week later (Bender et al., 2003; Maravall et al., 2004; Mierau et al., 2004). Thus, critical periods can occur in a sequential wave-like fashion as related circuits across the brain wire up and modify their connections. What is clear is that critical and sensitive periods mark epochs of time during development of an organism when systems from the molecular through to synaptic and behavioral levels exhibit heightened plasticity and are more susceptible to modification.

Dysregulation of brain development in NDDs: a framework for misregulated timing

Whilst the early onset of symptoms and developmental delays in behavioral milestones are known and reported in the clinic for individuals with NDDs, significantly less is known regarding the potential underlying neurobiological mechanisms during early developmental stages of the brain. The use of genetically engineered animal models for monogenic NDD syndromes, particularly mouse models, has provided evidence for early developmental dysregulation of neurons and synaptic connections leading to the notion of misregulated timing of critical and sensitive periods in these disorders. Key to this notion is the idea that the temporal onset and progression of symptoms characteristic for a disorder may be caused by misregulation of time windows for synaptic circuit development that subsequently alter or impede sensitive periods for behavior.

From postmortem fetal and neonatal human brain tissue and from embryonic to early postnatal mouse brain tissue samples, alterations in neuronal circuit formation and neuron morphology strongly support the hypothesis that synaptic and neuronal alterations are a *causal* stage in the development of a NDD, due to their presence in the brain before significant cognitive and behavioral dysfunctions (Purpura, 1974; Kaufmann and Moser, 2000; La Fata et al.; 2014, Pucilowska et al., 2015). This does not rule out later *consequential* changes upon synapses and neurons as a result of behavioral and sensory processing impairments but emphasises their underlying initial roles as elements in the aetiology of NDDs.

Upon what evidence is the framework for misregulated timing of brain development in NDDs based? Aberrant synapse morphology, particularly that of dendritic spines, is common to individuals with NDDs, as observed in postmortem brain tissue and in genetic mouse models for corresponding syndromic disorders of ID and ASD (Kaufmann and Moser, 2000; Ramakers, 2002; Portera–Cailliau, 2012). From the variety of different genetic mouse models for NDDs, studies have consistently observed dendritic spine dysmorphologies and significant alterations in the pattern of spine formation along neuronal dendrites (Meng et al., 2002; Galvez and Greenough, 2005; Dolen et al., 2007; Meikle et al., 2007; Yashiro et al., 2009; Cruz-Martin et al., 2010; Sato and Stryker, 2010; Maynard and Stein, 2012; Powell et al., 2012). Such changes have been documented both during adulthood, coincident with phenotypic impairments of behavior, and during a period of juvenile development between 2-3 postnatal weeks in rodents, corresponding to periods when hippocampal and cortical brain regions undergo heightened synaptic plasticity and refinement (Portera-Cailliau, 2012). More recently, an increasing number of longitudinal experimental studies report alterations in synapse morphology and functional synaptic phenotypes such as plasticity along developmental trajectories from neonatal through to adolescent and adult developmental stages in rodents (for complete review see Kroon et al.; 2013, Meredith, 2015). A prominent example to illustrate developmentally regulated synaptic phenotypes in a mouse model for a monogenic NDD is that of the somatosensory system in the Fmr1-gene knockout (KO) mouse for Fragile X syndrome, a leading known cause of ID with comorbidity for ASD in some individuals, and with spine dysmorphology in cortical and hippocampal brain regions (Bagni and Greenough, 2005; Pfeiffer and Huber, 2009).

During the first postnatal month, alterations in synaptic function, plasticity and spine morphology are observed in the Fmr1-KO mouse (detailed coverage in Meredith et al., 2012). In the first postnatal week, increased NMDA:AMPA ratios are observed along with altered synaptic plasticity of thalamocortical excitatory inputs to layer 4 neurons (Harlow et al., 2010; see Figure 4.1). However, these differences are transient and normalize by the end of the second postnatal week. Local GABAergic inhibition is also altered within Fmr1-KO mice, with delayed maturation of inhibition to layer 4 neurons at postnatal day 10, which again normalizes by day 15 (Daw et al., 2007; He et al., 2014).

Such phenotypes are not restricted to sensory cortex but are observed in the amygdala, prefrontal cortex and hippocampus of the Fmr1-KO mouse

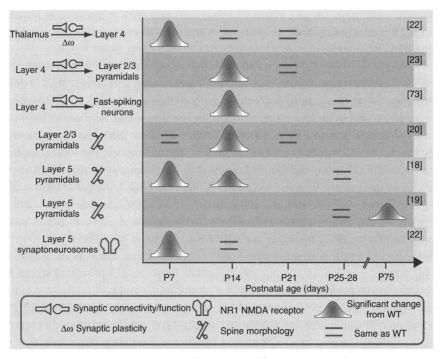

Figure 4.1 Developmentally regulated time windows in the Fmr1-KO mouse model. Several morphological and functional impairments in synapse properties are observed in the somatosensory cortex and specifically the barrel region of the Fmr1-KO model for Fragile X syndrome (FXS) (Nimchinsky et al., 2001; Bureau et al., 2008; Gibson et al., 2008; Cruz-Martin et al., 2010; Harlow et al., 2010). Many of these functional alterations are transient, occurring only during restricted periods of early postnatal development. Another developmentally regulated phenotype is spine morphology in layer 5 pyramidal neurons, where the alteration disappears at P28 but reappears in later adulthood around P75 (Nimchinsky et al., 2001; Galvez and Greenough, 2005). (Taken from Meredith et al., 2012.)

during postnatal development (Meredith et al., 2011; Testa-Silva et al., 2012; Vislay et al., 2013; summarized in Meredith et al., 2012). Developmental delays in synaptic phenotypes or transient alterations in synaptic function and morphology are not unique to the Fmr1-KO mouse. Transient alterations in spine morphology are reported in layer 5 cortical pyramidal neurons in the Down syndrome cell adhesion molecule (DSCAMdel17) mouse model, with an immature spine phenotype re-emerging postweaning (Maynard and Stein, 2012), similar to that observed in the Fmr1-KO mouse model (Galvez and Greenough, 2005).

In addition to critical periods for synaptic circuit formation and refinement, misregulated phenotypes are also reported for classical critical periods of adaption to sensory re-mapping. In rodent visual cortex, ocular dominance and experience-dependent plasticity in response to monocular deprivation (MD) are well documented during a postnatal period from juvenile to adolescent development (Hensch, 2005). Using Fmr1-KO mice, a short period of MD induced only a small reduction in response to the deprived eye and an enhanced response in the cortex to the open eye, in comparison to remodelling responses in unaffected littermate mice (Dolen et al., 2007). Such a lack of plasticity to sensory deprivation was also seen in maternal-UBE3A KO mice, a genetic mouse model for Angelman syndrome where the maternal copy of the gene is absent (Yashiro et al., 2009; Sato and Stryker, 2010). In these latter mice, the effect was not due to a shifted critical period profile since no change in the response to MD was observed if the protocol was performed before, during or after the neurotypical critical period known for this response (Sato and Stryker, 2010).

Mis-timing of synapse maturation during early brain development may also have significant consequences if dysregulation occurs in the opposite direction, that is the phenotype has a precocial onset and closure in the NDD model (Figure 4.2). Indeed, heterozygous mutant mice for Syngap1, a gene where mutations are documented in a spectrum of NDDs including ID, ASD, epilepsy, and schizophrenia (Rauch et al., 2012; Carvill et al., 2013; Stefansson et al., 2014), show precocial maturation of thalamocortical NMDA:AMPA ratios and plasticity (Clement et al., 2013) and premature dendritic growth, accelerated spine formation and pruning with emergence of abnormally large spines (Aceti et al., 2015). A similar precocial maturation of NMDA:AMPA ratios along with matured NMDA receptor subunit composition was also observed in the developing hippocampus only in the first two postnatal weeks of mice with deleted MET receptor tyrosine kinase, a molecular risk factor for ASD (Qiu et al., 2014). Thus, opposing phenotypes of developmental delays or precocial maturation may lead in both cases to disrupted timing of synapse formation and plasticity during the neurotypical critical period for that synaptic circuit, and ultimately play a role in later emergence and development of NDD phenotypes.

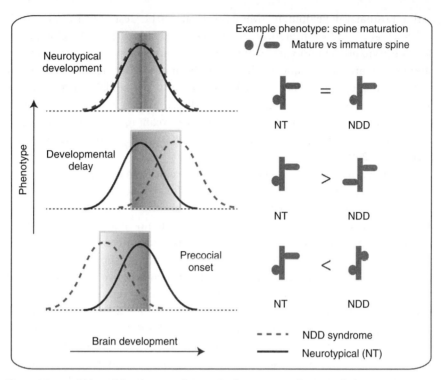

Figure 4.2 Regulation of developmental synaptic phenotypes and potential alteration in neurodevelopmental brain disorders (NDDs). (Left) Developmental profiles of synaptic phenotypes illustrating neurotypical development (top), developmental delay (middle), and precocial phenotypic onset (bottom). Gray bars indicate critical periods for phenotype plasticity. (Right) An example of a developmentally regulated synapse phenotype, spine morphology with longer, thinner filopodia-like spines observed in the immature state and shorter, stubbier spines in the mature state. Predicted phenotypic differences for developmental delay and precocial onset differences illustrated at phenotypic peak for neurotypical profile (black curves in lefthand panel). (Adapted from Meredith et al., 2012.) (See insert for color representation of this figure.)

Potential mechanisms underlying critical period dysregulation in NDDs

Given the variety of different genetic targets underlying neurodevelopmental conditions of ID and ASD, it is perhaps not surprising that no single mechanism has yet emerged to account for all alterations in the brain. Of the many genes underlying monogenic syndromes and those identified as risk factors from large genome-wide assays, a large proportion are identified as being expressed at the pre- and/or postsynaptic compartments of a neuron, or directly regulating synaptic function (Ruano et al., 2010; Kang et al., 2011; van Bokhoven, 2011; Voineagu et al., 2011; Parikshak et al., 2013; Willsey et al., 2013; De Rubeis et al., 2014; Iossifov et al., 2014). Conditions such as ID and ASD are collectively referred to as "synaptopathies" because of their effects at the synapse, although this term is not exclusive to NDDs (Brose et al., 2010). Many of the genes linked directly to NDDs interact in signalling pathways connected to the Rho family of GTPases (Ramakers, 2002; Ethell and Pasquale, 2005; Figure 4.3). This family of small GTPases comprises the ras homolog gene family member A (RhoA), ras-related C3 botulinum toxin substrate (Rac1), and cell division cycle 42 (Cdc42), which can all dynamically regulate the structure of dendritic

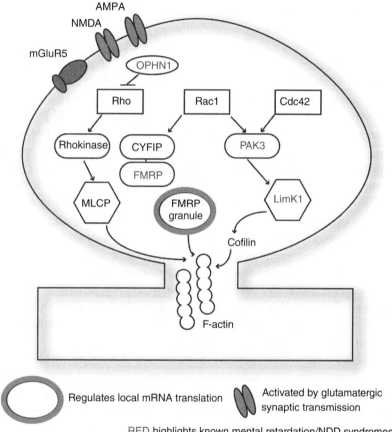

Figure 4.3 Many NDD-associated and linked genes function at the synapse to alter spine morphology. Many monogenic syndrome-associated genes (red) function at the synapse, illustrated here postsynaptically, to mediate changes in spine morphology via small GTPase-mediated signalling pathways and F-actin in response to synaptic activation (receptors highlighted in green). Abbreviations: AMPA, 2-amino-3-(3-hydroxy-5-methyl-isoxazol-4-yl) propanoic acid receptor; Cdc42, cell division cycle 42; CYFIP, cytoplasmic binding partner of Fragile X protein; FMRP, Fragile X Mental Retardation Protein; LimK1, LIM domain kinase 1; mGluR5 metabotropic glutamate receptor subunit 5; NMDA, N-Methyl-D-aspartic acid or N-Methyl-D-aspartate Receptor; OPHN1, oligophrenin-1; PAK, serine/threonine-protein kinase; Rac1, ras-related C3 botulinum toxin substrate; RhoA, ras homolog gene family, member A; MLCP, Myosin light-chain phosphatise. (Modified from Kroon et al., 2013.) (See insert for color representation of this figure.)

spines via remodelling of the actin cytoskeleton (Tashiro et al., 2000; Ethell and Pasquale, 2005). FMRP targets distinct mRNAs with a key group of these regulating GTPase activity, including Rac1 (Darnell et al., 2011). For the syndromic oligophrenin 1(OPHN1) ID, its effects on spine morphology are mediated via regulation of RhoA, which functions as a GTPase-activating protein (Govek et al., 2004). The ID Williams syndrome is linked to the LIM domain kinase 1 (LIMK1) gene, which can mediate changes in the actin cytoskeleton and hence spine morphology via Cdc42 and Rac1 signalling pathways (Edwards et al., 1999). LIMK1 also interacts with the family of P21-activated kinases (PAKs), some of which are mutated in nonsyndromic ID cases (Allen and Walsh, 1999).

In addition to direct effects on spine morphology and actin remodelling, many genes implicated in NDDs also regulate gene transcription and mRNA translation and thereby influence protein synthesis (Nan et al., 1997; Bagni and Greenough, 2005; Kelleher and Bear, 2008; Guy et al., 2011). Misregulated protein synthesis, particularly for specific synaptic proteins, is proposed to underlie many of the synaptopathies observed in disorders and syndromes affecting FMRP (Fragile X syndrome), ubiquitin-protein ligase E3A (cases of Angelman syndrome), Eukaryotic translation initiation factor 4E (EiF4E, nonsyndromic ASDs), tuberous sclerosis genes 1 and 2 (Tuberous sclerosis), and, most recently, genes affected on chromosome 16p11.2 microdeletion-associated with ASD (Auerbach et al., 2011; Zoghbi and Bear, 2012; Santini et al., 2013; Tian et al., 2015). Thus, genes implicated in many syndromic and nonsyndromic NDDs directly affect synaptic structure and function as well as regulating protein synthesis in the developing and adult brain. This convergence of genes to affect related signalling pathways, such as GTPase regulatory activity, may explain why different genetic mutations can give rise to similar synaptic phenotypes in experimental mouse models for these disorders during formation and refinement of synapses in the developing brain.

On a broad level, we can propose that there are two routes whereby critical period disruption can be tightly linked to NDDs. The first of these is through aberrant interactions between the target NDD gene itself and mechanisms that are known to regulate critical periods in the brain during neurotypical development [indirect regulation, Figure 4.4(a), taken from Kroon et al., 2013]. Using the Fmr1-KO mouse model and dysregulated sensory plasticity as an example, both the strength of response and the timing of onset may be indirectly regulated via the Fmr1 product, Fragile X Mental Retardation Protein (FMRP). Ocular dominance and auditory frequency mapping occur within well-defined critical periods in rodents and aspects are misregulated in the Fmr1-KO mouse model (Dolen et al., 2007; Kim et al., 2013). FMRP activity is coupled to activation of metabotropic glutamate receptor subtype 5 (mGluR5) (Weiler et al., 1997), a key molecule for specific forms of synaptic plasticity (Huber et al., 2000; Raymond et al., 2000). Blockade of mGluR5 dysregulated synaptic plasticity in adult rodent visual cortex (Tsanov and Manahan-Vaughan,

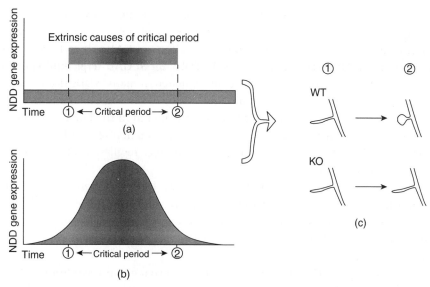

Figure 4.4 Illustrated hypothesis of how dysfunction of NDD-associated genes may dysregulate critical periods. A critical period is shown here as the timeframe between "1" and "2" (a). In this scenario, the critical period is caused by changing genetic expression (blue bar), such as expression of the GABA-synthesising enzyme, GAD65. Expression of the NDD gene (red bar) during neurotypical development is constant before, during, and after the critical period. Expression of genes that determine the dynamics of the critical period does not directly regulate the "NDD gene." Rather, the NDD gene role can indirectly regulate the critical period via its interaction with molecules that mediate synaptic changes during the critical period; for example, expression of GABAergic receptor subunits necessary to mediate synaptic inhibition. FMRP is able to interact with other 800 different mRNA targets in the adult brain, including many proteins with synaptic function and localization (Darnell et al., 2011). Hence dysfunction of the NDD gene can lead to an impaired critical period by indirect regulation. (b) Increased NDD gene expression changes during a restricted developmental stage (red curve) and directly regulates the occurrence of a critical period, independent of external factors. Such dynamic patterns of upregulated "NDD gene" expression, coincident with timing of thalamic and cortical critical periods, occur for many genes including Fmr1, neurofibromin (NF1), and ubiquitin-protein ligase E3A (UBE3A) (Figure 3 Kroon et al., 2013, Allen developing mouse brain atlas: http://developingmouse.brain-map.org). Therefore, dysfunction of the NDD gene causes the critical period to be absent completely. (c) In both scenarios, the NDD gene is necessary for the phenotypic change that takes place during the critical period ("WT" vs. "KO"), represented here by maturation of spine morphology. (Figure taken from Kroon et al., 2013.) (See insert for color representation of this figure.)

2009). Thus, the absence or downregulation of FMRP could indirectly alter synaptic plasticity during visual critical periods via mGluR5-mediated plasticity mechanisms, thereby affecting ocular dominance responsiveness via other extrinsic factors in the Fmr1-KO mouse.

The timing of the critical period for ocular dominance in rodents is strongly regulated by GABAergic inhibition: its onset can be quickened by application of benzodiazepines to enhance GABAergic transmission or conversely delayed, by preventing GABAergic maturation via deletion of the GAD65 synthesising enzyme or interference with the depolarising effects of GABA in early development (Hensch, 2005; Deidda et al., 2015). Imbalanced GABAergic inhibition is a key signalling system proposed to be misregulated in many NDDs (Rubenstein and Merzenich, 2003; Chattopadhyaya and Cristo, 2012). Molecular and electrophysiological aspects of GABAergic function are altered in the Fmr1-KO mouse model (Paluszkiewicz et al., 2011a). Thus, downregulation of FMRP could also alter the timing of visual critical periods via indirect regulation of GABAergic circuit function in the cortex.

The second route by which NDDs are linked to critical period disruption is via the expression profile of the target NDD gene itself [direct regulation, Figure 4.4(b)]. In this manner, the change in expression level of an individual gene underlying a NDD during a restricted period of time could constitute a critical period in itself.

Expression patterns in the brain of genes underlying many syndromic NDDs are strongly regulated both spatially and temporally (Hawrylycz et al., 2012; Allen Developing mouse brain atlas: http://developingmouse.brain-map.org). Mutation or dysregulation of the NDD gene could thereby directly misregulate a phenotype emergent during the critical period.

Corrective strategies for NDDs: genetic and pharmacological interventions

Although there is no known universal set of mechanisms that underlie all ID and ASD conditions, candidate targets for treatment have been discovered and tested for monogenic syndromes using data gathered in animal models and in some cases, leading to clinical trials in individuals with corresponding syndromes (Levenga et al., 2010; Ghosh et al., 2013). Using mouse models with the same genetic mutations corresponding to specific syndromes, synaptic, neuronal, and behavioral phenotypes have been corrected, albeit partially, for disorders ranging from Fragile X syndrome (Michalon et al., 2012) and tuberous sclerosis (Ehninger et al., 2008), Angelman syndrome (van Woerden et al., 2007) to Down syndrome (Fernandez et al., 2007; Deidda et al., 2015). For ASDs, phenotypic corrections are also observed following pharmacological treatments including benzodiazepines in an inbred mouse strain for idiopathic autism (Gogolla et al., 2014), bumetanide in a valproic acid–induced model (Tyzio et al., 2014), and oxytocin in a Cntnap2 mouse model for ASD in cortical dysplasia and focal epilepsy syndrome (Penagarikano et al., 2015). However, in many cases corrections are only partial and some impairments or altered phenotypes remain uncorrected in the mouse models.

Translation of some of these findings from mouse models has already begun with a prominent recent example being the testing of negative allosteric modulators for mGluR5 in individuals with Fragile X syndrome. Following promising results in initial phases (Jacquemont et al., 2011), larger scale trials were initiated in both adolescents and adults. These trials, however, failed and were halted in 2014 due to lack of efficacy. One key factor proposed to significantly contribute to the lack of efficacy was the age of trial participants (Mullard, 2015). Pharmaceutical intervention was being tested in these individuals with Fragile X syndrome years after diagnosis, symptom onset and closure of many of their brain's critical periods for development of synapses and functional connections in the brain.

The framework of misregulated timing of critical periods in the brain in NDDs proposes the idea that greater efficacy of potential therapeutic compounds could be observed if treatment was tested at earlier developmental stages. That is to say that during critical periods for brain development, the brain may be more amenable to therapeutic intervention to correct phenotypes directly arising or to prevent those developing as a consequence of the original insult. The importance of brain development and timing of interventions to rescue phenotypes is well illustrated using a rodent model for *in utero* knockdown of the Dcx gene, the mutation of which impairs neuronal migration resulting in subcortical heterotopia or double cortex syndrome (Bai et al., 2003). Reintroduction of the Dcx gene was able to partly rescue phenotypic impairments in the mouse but only if intervention was timed to occur before postnatal day (P)5 and not at later timepoints (Manent et al., 2009). This strategy of timed pharmaceutical or genetic intervention has not been extensively tested to-date in mouse models for monogenic syndromes. In Fmr1-KO mice, pharmacological intervention targeting mGluR5 signalling in the brain was more efficient in correcting spine morphology if administered to pups compared with adult mice (Su et al., 2011). An early intervention strategy was also tested in TS65Dn mice, a model for Down syndrome, where administration of an agonist for the Sonic hedgehog pathway in newborn mouse pups corrected specific hippocampal and cerebellar phenotypes as well as behavior (Das et al., 2013), although again this correction was incomplete and other cerebellar phenotypes remained unchanged (Gutierrez-Castellanos et al., 2013). A newer strategy has been to test pharmaceutical interventions antenatally, using compounds that are demonstrated to cross the blood-brain barrier and the placenta of the pregnant dam. Administration of bumetanide, an antagonist for NKCC1 interfering with the polarity of GABAergic synaptic transmission, corrected hippocampal neuronal activity, hippocampal oscillations and pup vocalisations when given one day pre-delivery to Fmr1-Hz pregnant female mice and to valproic acid treated pregnant rats (Tyzio et al., 2014). Bumetanide administration from embryonic day (E)17 to P7 in wildtype mouse pups has been documented to cause a long-term disruption of excitatory synaptic transmission, a developmental delay and altered sensorimotor gating (Wang and Kriegstein, 2011). Hence, caution is needed in advocating pharmaceutical interventions during critical periods of early brain development, particularly for nonsyndromic disorders, but it could indicate that timing an intervention to a relevant critical period for development could be a therapeutically relevant strategy in the future.

The implementation of this approach, even if there is a clear target molecule identified in the brain for a specific syndrome, is not straightforward. First, the brain exhibits multiple critical periods for specific phenotypes across different brain regions that do not necessarily occur simultaneously but rather in sequential and overlapping fashion. Second, within one brain circuit, the neurons may undergo a succession of critical periods for different aspects of synapse and neuron maturation, each supported by different neurotransmitter and molecular mechanisms. The visual system demonstrates a defined sequence of critical periods for synchronous network activity during prenatal and early postnatal development in rodents: retinal activity is first supported by gap junction coupling, followed by cholinergic supporting mechanisms and finally glutamatergically mediated properties (reviewed in Blankenship and Feller, 2010). Third, not all synapses may be affected in the same manner throughout the brain for a specific NDD syndrome and the phenotype could be synapse- or brain region-specific. To illustrate this phenomenon, the ILRAP1 mouse model for ID shows synapse-specific alterations of thalamic projections on to principal amygdala neurons but not on to neighbouring interneurons in the amygdala at the same developmental stage (Houbaert et al., 2013). And finally, reintroduction strategies for specific protein expression need careful fine-tuning to re-establish levels of expression in the brain. The importance of a balanced protein expression level can be seen in the Shank gene family whose members encode for scaffolding proteins and are implicated in a number of ASDs including Shank3 in Phelan-McDermid (22q13 deletion) syndrome (Grabrucker et al., 2011). In mouse models, absence of Shank3 causes stereotypy, alterations in social interactions and synapse dysmorphology (Peca et al., 2011). Yet, Shank3 overexpression designed to mimic a Shank3 duplication in an individual with ASD, caused manic behaviors and seizures in mice (Han et al., 2013). A similar phenomenon of phenotypic impairments arises from gene deletion of chromosome 15q11-q13 associated with cognitive impairments in Angelman and Prader-Willi syndromes (Nicholls and Knepper, 2001) and gene duplication in "dup15 syndrome," which leads to cognitive delay, sensory processing impairments, and autistic behaviors (Chamberlain and Lalande, 2010). Thus, translation of early intervention strategies from animal models to individuals in the clinic should proceed with great caution since interference during critical stages of brain development is a complex and delicate procedure.

Syndrome-specific molecules or common signalling hubs? Targets for future pharmacotherapeutic interventions

In fundamental research studies using animal models and in translational studies leading to clinical trials, the focus of potential therapeutic interventions has been targeted to molecules or signalling pathways specific to an individual NDD syndrome with a monogenic cause. However, it is increasingly clear that for both syndromic and nonsyndromic NDDs, the variety of different underlying genes can be grouped or clustered based, for example, on functional signalling pathway interactions (Ruano et al., 2010), spatial location in synapses or cortical layers (van Bokhoven, 2011; Parikshak et al., 2013; Willsey et al., 2013) and developmental expression in the brain (Willsey et al., 2013; De Rubeis et al., 2014). These studies points towards the idea of shared signalling "hubs" that may be dysregulated across many different ID and ASD conditions (Bill and Geschwind, 2009; Voineagu et al., 2011; Zoghbi and Bear, 2012). In a handful of studies using mouse models, these shared signalling pathways have proved to be important in establishing whether there are shared axes of synaptic pathophysiology between different NDD syndromes, where over- or under-regulation of a molecular signalling process can result in separate disorders but with overlapping symptoms (Auerbach et al., 2011; Baudouin et al., 2012; Tian et al., 2015).

At a genetic level, there are at least 450 genes known to associate with ID disorders and many hundreds of de novo and inherited mutations implicated in ASDs (Betancur, 2011; Mitchell, 2011; van Bokhoven, 2011; State and Sestan, 2012). The great variety of genes underlying NDDs is a major source of difficulty for industry searching for new pharmaceutical targets for NDDs, since clinical testing for drug targets unique to individual syndromes is costly financially and takes significant time to support through clinical trials (Ghosh et al., 2013). Identifying unifying signalling mechanisms or potential molecular target hubs that are implicated in multiple NDDs is a highly desirable strategy and if feasible, would potentially benefit not only individuals with recognised syndromes but those diagnosed with nonsyndromic disorders with similar ID and ASD phenotypes.

Dysregulated critical period framework as a unifying hypothesis for prominent NDD theories

Aside from a newer focus on clustering genes into spatio-temporal expression patterns and finding dysregulated signalling pathways common to different NDDs, there are three prominent mechanistic hypotheses that have arisen from both clinical and nonclinical data collected from animal models and studies of individuals with ID and ASDs. The first is that of an altered connectivity in the brain at both short-range and long-range distances between neurons or between different brain regions (NDD Hypothesis 1) (Belmonte et al., 2004; Just et al., 2004; Courchesne et al., 2005). For ASDs, an excessive number of functional connections, neuronal hyperconnectivity, is proposed to occur over short-range distances in the brain whereas long-range connections between more distant neurons or brain regions is proposed to be weaker or hypo-connected in adults (Belmonte et al., 2004; Just et al., 2004). In children, evidence shows that hyperconnectivity may be prevalent at both short- and long-range connections between brain regions, with a greater hyperconnectivity being correlated with more severe ASD impairments (Supekar et al., 2013). In genetic mouse models, hyperconnectivity of local excitatory synaptic connections is observed in medial prefrontal cortex of Fmr1-KO mice (Testa-Silva et al., 2012). A hyperconnectivity excitatory phenotype may correlate with increased synchrony and up-state network activity observed in somatosensory neocortex of juvenile Fmr1-KO mice (Goncalves et al., 2013), in line with that of decreased excitatory drive to interneurons and increased up-state duration in thalamic-driven networks of the same mouse model (Gibson et al., 2008). These phenotypes point towards the second working hypothesis, namely that of hyperexcitability of neuronal networks in the brain of Fmr1-KO mice, and potentially other NDD models (NDD Hypothesis 2). Like many other NDDs, Fragile X syndrome has comorbidity with epileptic seizures with uncontrolled excitatory brain activity in a proportion of individuals and is strongly linked to epileptoform activity in the Fmr1-KO mouse model (Chuang et al., 2005; Zhao et al., 2011). Such a dysregulation in network activity may not be solely due to a hyperexcitability phenotype however. Imbalances in the levels of excitation and inhibition in the brain are also hypothesised to underlie many NDDs and their corresponding mouse models, particularly ASDs and those IDs with ASD comorbidity (NDD Hypothesis 3) (Rubenstein and Merzenich, 2003; Chattopadhyaya and Cristo, 2012). For Fragile X syndrome, downregulations in GABAergic receptor subunits and alterations in inhibitory transmission are observed in amygdala, hippocampal and cortical brain regions in the Fmr1-KO mouse (D'Hulst et al., 2006; Olmos-Serrano et al., 2011; Paluszkiewicz et al., 2011b; Vislay et al., 2013).

It is clear that these three hypotheses are not mutually exclusive in NDDs but rather co-occur or may share overlapping mechanisms. Placing these theories into the context of a dysregulated critical period framework does not contradict the original theories but could explain many of the developmental aspects of documented phenotypes in both animal models and humans (Figure 4.5). It is during critical developmental periods that the synaptic networks of the brain are established and refined, thus alterations in connectivity and imbalances in excitation relative to inhibition will likely arise during these periods and in some cases, only transiently appear before re-emerging in early adulthood.

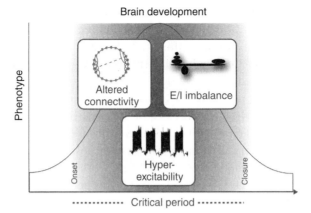

Figure 4.5 Framework of dysregulated critical periods and time windows during brain development as unifying theory for temporal aspects of mechanisms underlying many NDDs of ID and ASD, and prominently illustrated in this article with the Fmr1-KO mouse model for Fragile X syndrome. The three prominent hypotheses for the neurobiological bases of NDDs are shown, namely (1) altered connectivity at short- and long-range distances between neurons, (2) a relative imbalance between excitation (E) and inhibition (I) within brain circuitry, and (3) hyperexcitability of neurons with specific networks in the brain. Neuronal connectivity and both excitatory and inhibitory synaptic strength undergo heightened plasticity during early critical periods in the brain. It is likely that dysregulated phenotypes, such as an imbalance in the levels of synaptic excitation and inhibition, first arise during these critical periods in NDD models. Therefore, the use of known critical periods for cortical and hippocampal circuits may predict when these phenotypes first occur and how long they remain. (See insert for color representation of this figure.)

Implications of misregulated critical periods and future directions

In recent years, the number of genes associated with ID and ASDs has increased significantly, implicating a multitude of signalling pathways and functional groups of molecules, many of which are synaptic, in the mechanisms underlying these specific types of NDDs (Zoghbi and Bear, 2012). Current theories regarding the mechanistic basis of these NDDs have focused on altered synaptic connectivity between individual neurons and across brain regions, with an emphasis on hyper-excitation but also a potential imbalance in excitation relative to inhibition in neuronal networks. The placing of these theories within a framework of misregulated critical periods, which arose from observations in both the clinic and at the lab bench, provides spatioemporal markers of where and when to look for dysregulated phenotypes in the brain. Knowledge of the critical period for synapse development and plasticity could provide a useful strategy to first look for onset of synaptic phenotypes in syndromic mouse models for specific disorders. The framework also emphasises the developmental aspects of underlying aetiology of these disorders. Whereas many genetic mouse models have been traditionally studied at one juvenile stage around the second postnatal week or during stages of adulthood to correlate with behavioral symptoms, a study of critical period misregulation requires a longitudinal series of observations to fully document the onset, duration and in some cases, transient nature of the phenotypic impairment before compensatory mechanisms potentially set in (Meredith et al., 2012).

The application of misregulated critical periods may also be extended to nongenetic causes of NDDs, such as those induced by environmental toxins (Marco et al., 2011). For example, a single exposure to perfluorinated compounds or to an industry-used flame retardant at postnatal day 10 in rodents, significantly altered synaptic proteins and behaviors in adulthood (Johansson et al., 2009; Viberg, 2009; Viberg et al., 2011). This potential for developmental consequences is similar to that observed already in the offspring of mothers who took the antiepileptic drug valproic acid during pregnancy (Christensen et al., 2013). Here, the level of malformations in the foetus was highest if exposure to the drug occurred within the first trimester of gestation (Lindhout and Omtzigt, 1992). This effect is replicated in a rodent model of valproic acid exposure, whereby injection at embryonic day 12.5 in the mother caused an increased incidence of neural tube closure deficits in the offspring and, during adolescence, pups showed increased autistic behavioral patterns of hyperactivity and stereotypy (Schneider and Przewlocki, 2005; Dawson et al., 2006). Thus, future application of potential environmental toxins at a range of specific developmental stages could indicate time windows of vulnerability during neuronal development where contaminants have the greatest consequences upon brain development and later behavior.

What are the consequences of dysregulated synaptic phenotypes and altered critical periods in the brain? An example to illustrate the effects of disrupting an early critical period is taken from retinotopic map development in the visual system: disruption of retinal synaptic activity during an early critical period alters later patterns of connectivity within the visual system (Eglen et al., 2003). Early retinal waves were desynchronised in mouse pups that lacked the beta2 nicotinic acetylcholine receptor subunit during the first week of postnatal development. This desynchrony correlated with an altered refinement of axons projecting into the brainstem (Grubb et al., 2003; McLaughlin et al., 2003), altered geniculocortical projections (Cang et al., 2005) and a decrease in visual activity in later life (Rossi et al., 2001). Thus, disruption of an early critical period can alter both structure and function of connections in later life not only in the affected brain region but also in other connected regions of the sensory processing pathways to alter perception. If this principle is applied to NDDs, an early disruption of a critical period during brain development could be causal for later aberrations in synaptic and neuronal function, leading to behavioral impairments that characterise many ID and ASDs.

In conclusion, recent work demonstrates the critical aspects of early development for the onset and transient patterning of phenotypic impairments in the brain in NDDs. By studying known critical periods and their underlying mechanisms, our understanding of the neurobiological bases of NDDs may be enhanced by investigating the full trajectory of brain development with the later consequences upon brain circuitry and behavior in ID and ASDs.

Acknowledgments

Research and ideas on this topic have been funded in the lab by an NWO VIDI fellowship (917.10.372), Hersenstichting NL, Fondation Jérôme LeJeune, and the Marie Curie Framework 7 ITN, "Braintrain." Thanks to Julia Dawitz, Ioannis Kramvis, and Tim Kroon for useful discussions on the topic that led to the formulation of this framework.

References

Abbeduto L, Ozonoff S, Thurman AJ, McDuffie A, Schweitzer J. (2014). Neurodevelopmental disorders. In: *The American Psychiatric Publishing Textbook of Psychiatry*. Arlington, VA: American Psychiatric Publishing.

Aceti M, Creson TK, Vaissiere T, Rojas C, Huang WC, Wang YX, Petralia RS, Page DT, Miller CA, Rumbaugh G. (2015). Syngap1 haploinsufficiency damages a postnatal critical period of pyramidal cell structural maturation linked to cortical circuit assembly. *Biol Psychiatry* 77:805–815.

Allen KM, Walsh, CA. (1999). Genes that regulate neuronal migration in the cerebral cortex. *Epilepsy Res* 36:143–154.

Amiet C, Gourfinkel-An I, Bouzamondo A, Tordjman S, Baulac M, Lechat P, Mottron L, Cohen D. (2008). Epilepsy in autism is associated with intellectual disability and gender: evidence from a meta–analysis. *Biol Psychiatry* 64:577–582.

Auerbach BD, Osterweil EK, Bear MF. (2011). Mutations causing syndromic autism define an axis of synaptic pathophysiology. *Nature* 480:63–68.

Bagni C, Greenough WT. (2005). From mRNP trafficking to spine dysmorphogenesis: the roots of Fragile X syndrome. *Nat Rev Neurosci* 6:376–387.

Bai J, Ramos RL, Ackman JB, Thomas AM, Lee RV, Loturco JJ. (2003). RNAi reveals doublecortin is required for radial migration in rat neocortex. *Nat Neurosci* 6:1277–1283.

Baudouin SJ, Gaudias J, Gerharz S, Hatstatt L, Zhou K, Punnakkal P, Tanaka KF, Spooren W, Hen R, de Zeeuw CI, Vogt K, Scheiffele P. (2012). Shared synaptic pathophysiology in syndromic and nonsyndromic rodent models of autism. *Science* 338:128–132.

Belmonte MK, Allen G, Beckel–Mitchener A, Boulanger LM, Carper RA, Webb SJ. (2004). Autism and abnormal development of brain connectivity. *J Neurosci* 24:9228–9231.

Bender KJ, Rangel J, Feldman DE. (2003). Development of columnar topography in the excitatory layer 4 to layer 2/3 projection in rat barrel cortex. *J Neurosci* 23:8759–8770.

Betancur C. (2011). Etiological heterogeneity in autism spectrum disorders: more than 100 genetic and genomic disorders and still counting. *Brain Res* 1380:42–77.

Bill BR, Geschwind DH. (2009). Genetic advances in autism: heterogeneity and convergence on shared pathways. *Curr Opin Genet Dev* 19:271–278.

Blankenship AG, Feller MB. (2010). Mechanisms underlying spontaneous patterned activity in developing neural circuits. *Nat Rev Neurosci* 11:18–29.

Brose, N, O'Connor V, Skehel P. (2010). Synaptopathy: dysfunction of synaptic function? *Biochem Soc Trans* 38:443–444.

Bureau I, Shepherd GM, Svoboda K. (2008). Circuit and plasticity defects in the developing somatosensory cortex of FMR1 knock–out mice. *J Neurosci* 28:5178–5188.

Cang J, Renteria RC, Kaneko M, Liu X, Copenhagen DR, Stryker MP. (2005). Development of precise maps in visual cortex requires patterned spontaneous activity in the retina. *Neuron* 48:797–809.

Carvill GL, Heavin SB, Yendle SC, McMahon JM, et al. (2013). Targeted resequencing in epileptic encephalopathies identifies de novo mutations in CHD2 and SYNGAP1. *Nat Genet* 45:825–830.

Chamberlain SJ, Lalande M. (2010). Neurodevelopmental disorders involving genomic imprinting at human chromosome 15q11–q13. *Neurobiol Dis* 39:13–20.

Chattopadhyaya B, Cristo GD. (2012). GABAergic circuit dysfunctions in neurodevelopmental disorders. *Front Psychiatry* 3:51.

Christensen J, Gronborg TK, Sorensen MJ, Schendel D, Parner ET, Pedersen LH, Vestergaard M. (2013). Prenatal valproate exposure and risk of autism spectrum disorders and childhood autism. *JAMA* 309:1696–1703.

Chuang SC, Zhao W, Bauchwitz R, Yan Q, Bianchi R, Wong RK. (2005). Prolonged epileptiform discharges induced by altered group I metabotropic glutamate receptor–mediated synaptic responses in hippocampal slices of a Fragile X mouse model. *J Neurosci* 25:8048–8055.

Clancy B, Finlay BL, Darlington RB, Anand KJ. (2007). Extrapolating brain development from experimental species to humans. *Neurotoxicology* 28:931–937.

Clayton–Smith J, Laan L. (2003). Angelman syndrome: a review of the clinical and genetic aspects. *J Med Genet* 40:87–95.

Clement JP, Ozkan ED, Aceti M, Miller CA, Rumbaugh G. (2013). SYNGAP1 links the maturation rate of excitatory synapses to the duration of critical–period synaptic plasticity. *J Neurosci* 33:10447–10452.

Courchesne E, Redcay E, Morgan JT, Kennedy DP. (2005). Autism at the beginning: microstructural and growth abnormalities underlying the cognitive and behavioral phenotype of autism. *Dev Psychopathol* 17:577–597.

Crair MC, Malenka RC. (1995). A critical period for long–term potentiation at thalamocortical synapses. *Nature* 375:325–328.

Cruz–Martin A, Crespo M, Portera–Cailliau C. (2010). Delayed stabilization of dendritic spines in Fragile X mice. *J Neurosci* 30:7793–7803.

Darnell JC, Van Driesche SJ, Zhang C, Hung KY, et al. (2011). FMRP stalls ribosomal translocation on mRNAs linked to synaptic function and autism. *Cell* 146:247–261.

Das I, Park JM, Shin JH, Jeon SK, Lorenzi H, Linden DJ, Worley PF, Reeves RH. (2013). Hedgehog agonist therapy corrects structural and cognitive deficits in a Down syndrome mouse model. *Science Translational Medicine* 5:201ra120.

Daw MI, Ashby MC, Isaac JT. (2007). Coordinated developmental recruitment of latent fast spiking interneurons in layer IV barrel cortex. *Nat Neurosci* 10:453–461.

Dawson JE, Raymond AM, Winn LM. (2006). Folic acid and pantothenic acid protection against valproic acid–induced neural tube defects in CD–1 mice. *Toxicol Appl Pharmacol* 211:124–132.

Deidda G, Parrini M, Naskar S, Bozarth IF, Contestabile A, Cancedda L. (2015). Reversing excitatory GABAAR signaling restores synaptic plasticity and memory in a mouse model of Down syndrome. *Nat Med* 21:318–326.

De Rubeis S, He X, Goldberg AP, Poultney CS, et al. (2014). Synaptic, transcriptional and chromatin genes disrupted in autism. *Nature* 515:209–215.

D'Hulst C, De Geest N, Reeve SP, Van Dam D, De Deyn PP, Hassan BA, Kooy RF. (2006). Decreased expression of the GABA(A) receptor in Fragile X syndrome. *Brain Res* 1121:238–245.

Dolen G, Osterweil E, Rao BSS, Smith GB, Auerbach BD, Chattarji S, Bear MF. (2007). Correction of Fragile X syndrome in mice. *Neuron* 56:955–962.

Edwards DC, Sanders LC, Bokoch GM, Gill GN. (1999). Activation of LIM–kinase by Pak1 couples Rac/Cdc42 GTPase signalling to actin cytoskeletal dynamics. *Nat Cell Biol* 1:253–259.

Eglen SJ, Demas J, Wong RO. (2003). Mapping by waves. Patterned spontaneous activity regulates retinotopic map refinement. *Neuron* 40:1053–1055.

Ehninger D, Li W, Fox K, Stryker MP, Silva AJ. (2008). Reversing Neurodevelopmental Disorders in Adults. *Neuron* 60:950–960.

Ethell IM, Pasquale EB. (2005). Molecular mechanisms of dendritic spine development and remodeling. *Prog Neurobiol* 75:161–205.

Feldmeyer D, Brecht M, Helmchen F, Petersen CC, Poulet JF, Staiger JF, Luhmann HJ, Schwarz C. (2013). Barrel cortex function. *Prog Neurobiol* 103:3–27.

Fernandez F, Morishita W, Zuniga E, Nguyen J, Blank M, Malenka RC, Garner CC. (2007). Pharmacotherapy for cognitive impairment in a mouse model of Down syndrome. *Nat Neurosci* 10:411–413.

Fox K. (2002). Anatomical pathways and molecular mechanisms for plasticity in the barrel cortex. *Neuroscience* 111:799–814.

Fox K, Glazewski S, Schulze S. (2000). Plasticity and stability of somatosensory maps in thalamus and cortex. *Curr Opin Neurobiol* 10:494–497.

Galvez R, Greenough WT. (2005). Sequence of abnormal dendritic spine development in primary somatosensory cortex of a mouse model of the Fragile X mental retardation syndrome. *Am J Med Genet A* 135:155–160.

Geschwind DH, Levitt P. (2007). Autism spectrum disorders: developmental disconnection syndromes. *Curr Opin Neurobiol* 17:103–111.

Ghosh A, Michalon A, Lindemann L, Fontoura P, Santarelli L. (2013). Drug discovery for autism spectrum disorder: challenges and opportunities. *Nat Rev Drug Discov* 12:777–790.

Gibson JR, Bartley AF, Hays SA, Huber KM. (2008). Imbalance of neocortical excitation and inhibition and altered UP states reflect network hyperexcitability in the mouse model of Fragile X syndrome. *J Neurophysiol* 100:2615–2626.

Gillberg C, Billstedt E. (2000). Autism and Asperger syndrome: coexistence with other clinical disorders. *Acta Psychiatr Scand* 102:321–330.

Gogolla N, Takesian AE, Feng G, Fagiolini M, Hensch TK. (2014). Sensory integration in mouse insular cortex reflects GABA circuit maturation. *Neuron* 83:894–905.

Goldstein S, Reynolds CR. (1999). *Handbook of Neurodevelopmental and Genetic Disorders in Children*. New York: Guilford Press.

Goncalves JT, Anstey JE, Golshani P, Portera–Cailliau C. (2013). Circuit level defects in the developing neocortex of Fragile X mice. *Nat Neurosci* 16:903–909.

Govek EE, Newey SE, Akerman CJ, Cross JR, Van Der Veken L, Van Aelst L. (2004). The X–linked mental retardation protein oligophrenin–1 is required for dendritic spine morphogenesis. *Nat Neurosci* 7:364–372.

Grabrucker AM, Schmeisser MJ, Schoen M, Boeckers TM. (2011). Postsynaptic ProSAP/Shank scaffolds in the cross–hair of synaptopathies. *Trends Cell Biol* 21:594–603.

Grubb MS, Rossi FM, Changeux JP, Thompson ID. (2003). Abnormal functional organization in the dorsal lateral geniculate nucleus of mice lacking the beta 2 subunit of the nicotinic acetylcholine receptor. *Neuron* 40:1161–1172.

Grutzendler J, Kasthuri N, Gan WB. (2002). Long–term dendritic spine stability in the adult cortex. *Nature* 420:812–816.

Gutierrez–Castellanos N, Winkelman BH, Tolosa–Rodriguez L, Devenney B, Reeves RH, De Zeeuw CI. (2013). Size does not always matter: Ts65Dn Down syndrome mice show cerebellum–dependent motor learning deficits that cannot be rescued by postnatal SAG treatment. *J Neurosci* 33:15408–15413.

Guy J, Cheval H, Selfridge J, Bird A. (2011). The role of MeCP2 in the brain. *Annu Rev Cell Dev Biol* 27:631–652.

Han K, Holder JL Jr, Schaaf CP, Lu H, Chen H, Kang H. (2013). SHANK3 overexpression causes manic–like behaviour with unique pharmacogenetic properties. *Nature* 503:72–77.

Harlow EG, Till SM, Russell TA, Wijetunge LS, Kind P, Contractor A. (2010). Critical period plasticity is disrupted in the barrel cortex of FMR1 knockout mice. *Neuron* 65:385–398.

Hawrylycz MJ, Lein ES, Guillozet–Bongaarts AL, et al. (2012). An anatomically comprehensive atlas of the adult human brain transcriptome. *Nature* 489:391–399.

He Q, Nomura T, Xu J, Contractor A. (2014). The developmental switch in GABA polarity is delayed in Fragile X mice. *J Neurosci* 34:446–450.

Hensch TK. (2004). Critical period regulation. *Annu Rev Neurosci* 27:549–479.

Hensch TK. (2005). Critical period plasticity in local cortical circuits. *Nat Rev Neurosci* 6:877–888.

Holtmaat AJ, Trachtenberg JT, Wilbrecht L, Shepherd GM, Zhang X, Knott GW, Svoboda K. (2005). Transient and persistent dendritic spines in the neocortex in vivo. *Neuron* 45:279–291.

Horn G. (2004). Pathways of the past: the imprint of memory. *Nat Rev Neurosci* 5:108–120.

Houbaert X, Zhang CL, Gambino F, Lepleux M, Deshors M, et al. (2013). Target–specific vulnerability of excitatory synapses leads to deficits in associative memory in a model of intellectual disorder. *J Neurosci* 33:13805–13819.

Huber KM, Kayser MS, Bear MF. (2000). Role for rapid dendritic protein synthesis in hippocampal mGluR–dependent long–term depression. *Science* 288:1254–1257.

Iossifov I, O'Roak BJ, Sanders SJ, Ronemus M, et al. (2014). The contribution of de novo coding mutations to autism spectrum disorder. *Nature* 515:216–221.

Jacquemont S, Curie A, Des Portes V, Torrioli MG, et al. (2011). Epigenetic modification of the FMR1 gene in Fragile X syndrome is associated with differential response to the mGluR5 antagonist AFQ056. *Sci Transl Med* 3:64ra1.

Johansson N, Eriksson P, Viberg H. (2009). Neonatal exposure to PFOS and PFOA in mice results in changes in proteins which are important for neuronal growth and synaptogenesis in the developing brain. *Toxicol Sci* 108:412–418.

Johnson MH. (2005). Sensitive periods in functional brain development: problems and prospects. *Dev Psychobiol* 46:287–292.

Just MA, Cherkassky VL, Keller TA, Minshew NJ. (2004). Cortical activation and synchronization during sentence comprehension in high–functioning autism: evidence of underconnectivity. *Brain* 127:1811–1821.

Kang HJ, Kawasawa YI, Cheng F, Zhu Y, Xu X, Li M, et al. (2011). Spatio–temporal transcriptome of the human brain. *Nature* 478:483–289.

Katz LC, Shatz CJ. (1996). Synaptic activity and the construction of cortical circuits. *Science*, 274, 1133–8.

Kau AS, Reider EE, Payne L, Meyer WA, Freund L. (2000). Early behavior signs of psychiatric phenotypes in Fragile X syndrome. *Am J Ment Retard* 105:286–299.

Kaufmann WE, Moser HW. (2000). Dendritic anomalies in disorders associated with mental retardation. *Cereb Cortex* 10:981–991.

Kelleher RJ 3rd, Bear MF. (2008). The autistic neuron: troubled translation? *Cell* 135:401–406.

Kim H, Gibboni R, Kirkhart C, Bao S. (2013). Impaired critical period plasticity in primary auditory cortex of Fragile X model mice. *J Neurosci* 33:15686–15692.

Kroon T, Sierksma MC, Meredith RM. (2013). Investigating mechanisms underlying neurodevelopmental phenotypes of autistic and intellectual disability disorders: a perspective. *Front Syst Neurosci* 7:75.

La Fata G, Gartner A, Dominguez–Iturza N, Dresselaers T, et al. (2014). FMRP regulates multipolar to bipolar transition affecting neuronal migration and cortical circuitry. *Nat Neurosci* 17:1693–1700.

Leblanc JJ, Fagiolini M. (2011). Autism: a "critical period" disorder? *Neural Plast* 2011:921680.

Levenga J, De Vrij FM, Oostra BA, Willemsen R. (2010). Potential therapeutic interventions for Fragile X syndrome. *Trends Mol Med* 16:516–527.

Lindhout D, Omtzigt JG. (1992). Pregnancy and the risk of teratogenicity. *Epilepsia 33 Suppl* 4:S41–48.

Lohmann C, Kessels HW. (2014). The developmental stages of synaptic plasticity. *J Physiol* 592:13–31.

Lopez–Bendito G, Molnar Z. (2003). Thalamocortical development: how are we going to get there? *Nat Rev Neurosci* 4:276–289.

Lorenz K. (1935). Der Kumpan in der Umwelt des Vogels: der Artgenosse als auslosendes Moment sozialer Verhaltungsweisen. *J fur Ornithologie* 83:37–215; 289–413.

Manent JB, Wang Y, Chang Y, Paramasivam M, Loturco JJ. (2009). Dcx reexpression reduces subcortical band heterotopia and seizure threshold in an animal model of neuronal migration disorder. *Nat Med* 15:84–90.

Maravall M, Stern EA, Svoboda K. (2004). Development of intrinsic properties and excitability of layer 2/3 pyramidal neurons during a critical period for sensory maps in rat barrel cortex. *J Neurophysiol* 92:144–156.

Marco EM, Macri S, Laviola G. (2011). Critical age windows for neurodevelopmental psychiatric disorders: evidence from animal models. *Neurotox Res* 19:286–307.

Marin O, Valiente M, Ge X, Tsai LH. (2010). Guiding neuronal cell migrations. *Cold Spring Harb Perspect Biol* 2:a001834.

Martin BS, Huntsman MM. (2012). Pathological plasticity in Fragile X syndrome. *Neural Plast* 2012:275630.

Maynard KR, Stein E. (2012). DSCAM contributes to dendrite arborization and spine formation in the developing cerebral cortex. *J Neurosci* 32:16637–16650.

McLaughlin T, Torborg CL, Feller MB, O'Leary DD. (2003). Retinotopic map refinement requires spontaneous retinal waves during a brief critical period of development. *Neuron* 40:1147–1160.

Meikle L, Talos DM, Onda H, Pollizzi K, Rotenberg A, Sahin M, Jensen FE, Kwiatkowski DJ. (2007). A mouse model of tuberous sclerosis: neuronal loss of Tsc1 causes dysplastic and ectopic neurons, reduced myelination, seizure activity, and limited survival. *J Neurosci* 27:5546–5558.

Meng Y, Zhang Y, Tregoubov V, Janus C, Cruz L, et al. (2002). Abnormal spine morphology and enhanced LTP in LIMK–1 knockout mice. *Neuron* 35:121–133.

Meredith RM. (2015). Sensitive and critical periods during neurotypical and aberrant neurodevelopment: A framework for neurodevelopmental disorders. *Neurosci Biobehav Rev* 50C:180–188.

Meredith RM, De Jong R, Mansvelder HD. (2011). Functional rescue of excitatory synaptic transmission in the developing hippocampus in Fmr1–KO mouse. *Neurobiol Dis* 41: 104–110.

Meredith RM, Dawitz J, Kramvis I. (2012). Sensitive time–windows for susceptibility in neurodevelopmental disorders. *Trends Neurosci* 35:335–344.

Michalon A, Sidorov M, Ballard TM, Ozmen L, Spooren W, et al. (2012). Chronic pharmacological mGlu5 inhibition corrects Fragile X in adult mice. *Neuron* 74:49–56.

Michel GF, Tyler AN. (2005). Critical period: a history of the transition from questions of when, to what, to how. *Dev Psychobiol* 46:156–162.

Mierau SB, Meredith RM, Upton AL, Paulsen O. (2004). Dissociation of experience–dependent and –independent changes in excitatory synaptic transmission during development of barrel cortex. *Proc Natl Acad Sci USA* 101:15518–15523.

Mitchell KJ. (2011). The genetics of neurodevelopmental disease. *Curr Opin Neurobiol* 21:197–203.

Mullard A. (2015). Fragile X disappointments upset autism ambitions. *Nat Rev Drug Discov* 14:151–153.

Nan X, Campoy FJ, Bird A. (1997). MeCP2 is a transcriptional repressor with abundant binding sites in genomic chromatin. *Cell* 88:471–481.

Nicholls RD, Knepper JL. (2001). Genome organization, function, and imprinting in Prader–Willi and Angelman syndromes. *Annu Rev Genomics Hum Genet* 2:153–175.

Nimchinsky EA, Oberlander AM, Svoboda K. (2001). Abnormal development of dendritic spines in FMR1 knock–out mice. *J Neurosci* 21:5139–5146.

Oberlaender M, Ramirez A, Bruno RM. (2012). Sensory experience restructures thalamocortical axons during adulthood. *Neuron* 74:648–655.

Olmos–Serrano JL, Corbin JG, Burns MP. (2011). The GABA(A) receptor agonist THIP ameliorates specific behavioral deficits in the mouse model of Fragile X syndrome. *Dev Neurosci* 33:395–403.

Paluszkiewicz SM, Martin BS, Huntsman MM. (2011a). Fragile X syndrome: the GABAergic system and circuit dysfunction. *Dev Neurosci* 33:349–364.

Paluszkiewicz SM, Olmos–Serrano JL, Corbin JG, Huntsman MM. (2011b). Impaired inhibitory control of cortical synchronization in Fragile X syndrome. *J Neurophysiol* 106:2264–2272.

Pan F, Gan WB. (2008). Two–photon imaging of dendritic spine development in the mouse cortex. *Dev Neurobiol* 68:771–778.

Parikshak NN, Luo R, Zhang A, Won H, et al. (2013). Integrative functional genomic analyses implicate specific molecular pathways and circuits in autism. *Cell* 155:1008–1021.

Peca J, Feliciano C, Ting JT, Wang W, Wells MF, et al. (2011). Shank3 mutant mice display autistic–like behaviours and striatal dysfunction. *Nature* 472:437–442.

Penagarikano O, Lazaro MT, Lu XH, Gordon A, Dong H, Lam HA, et al. (2015). Exogenous and evoked oxytocin restores social behavior in the Cntnap2 mouse model of autism. *Sci Transl Med* 7:271ra8.

Pfeiffer BE, Huber KM. (2009). The state of synapses in Fragile X syndrome. *Neuroscientist* 15: 549–567.

Pizzorusso T, Medini P, Berardi N, Chierzi S, Fawcett JW, Maffei L. (2002). Reactivation of ocular dominance plasticity in the adult visual cortex. *Science* 298:1248–1251.

Portera–Cailliau C. (2012). Which comes first in Fragile X syndrome, dendritic spine dysgenesis or defects in circuit plasticity? *Neuroscientist* 18:28–44.

Powell AD, Gill KK, Saintot PP, Jiruska P, et al. (2012). Rapid reversal of impaired inhibitory and excitatory transmission but not spine dysgenesis in a mouse model of mental retardation. *J Physiol* 590:763–776.

Pucilowska J, Vithayathil J, Tavares EJ, Kelly C, et al. (2015). The 16p11.2 deletion mouse model of autism exhibits altered cortical progenitor proliferation and brain cytoarchitecture linked to the ERK MAPK pathway. *J Neurosci* 35:3190–3200.

Purpura DP. (1974). Dendritic spine "dysgenesis" and mental retardation. *Science* 186:1126–1128.

Qiu S, Lu Z, Levitt P. (2014). MET receptor tyrosine kinase controls dendritic complexity, spine morphogenesis, and glutamatergic synapse maturation in the hippocampus. *J Neurosci* 34: 16166–16179.

Ramakers GJ. (2002). Rho proteins, mental retardation and the cellular basis of cognition. *Trends Neurosci* 25:191–199.

Rauch A, Wieczorek D, Graf E, Wieland T, Endele S, et al. (2012). Range of genetic mutations associated with severe non–syndromic sporadic intellectual disability: an exome sequencing study. *Lancet* 380:1674–1682.

Raymond CR, Thompson VL, Tate WP, Abraham WC. (2000). Metabotropic glutamate receptors trigger homosynaptic protein synthesis to prolong long–term potentiation. *J Neurosci* 20:969–976.

Rossi FM, Pizzorusso T, Porciatti V, Marubio LM, et al. (2001). Requirement of the nicotinic acetylcholine receptor beta 2 subunit for the anatomical and functional development of the visual system. *Proc Natl Acad Sci USA,* 98:6453–6458.

Ruano D, Abecasis GR, Glaser B, Lips ES, et al. (2010). Functional gene group analysis reveals a role of synaptic heterotrimeric G proteins in cognitive ability. *Am J Hum Genet* 86: 113–125.

Rubenstein JL, Merzenich MM. (2003). Model of autism: increased ratio of excitation/inhibition in key neural systems. *Genes Brain Behav* 2:255–267.

Santini E, Huynh TN, Macaskill AF, Carter AG, et al. (2013). Exaggerated translation causes synaptic and behavioural aberrations associated with autism. *Nature* 493:411–415.

Sato M, Stryker MP. (2010). Genomic imprinting of experience–dependent cortical plasticity by the ubiquitin ligase gene Ube3a. *Proc Natl Acad Sci USA* 107:5611–5616.

Schneider T, Przewlocki R. (2005). Behavioral alterations in rats prenatally exposed to valproic acid: animal model of autism. *Neuropsychopharmacology* 30:80–89.

Spitzer NC. (2006). Electrical activity in early neuronal development. *Nature* 444:707–712.

State MW, Sestan N. (2012). Neuroscience. The emerging biology of autism spectrum disorders. *Science* 337:1301–1303.

Stefansson H, Meyer–Lindenberg A, Steinberg S, et al. (2014). CNVs conferring risk of autism or schizophrenia affect cognition in controls. *Nature* 505:361–366.

Su T, Fan HX, Jiang T, Sun WW, Den WY, Gao MM, et al. (2011). Early continuous inhibition of group 1 mGlu signaling partially rescues dendritic spine abnormalities in the Fmr1 knockout mouse model for Fragile X syndrome. *Psychopharmacology* 215:291–300.

Supekar K, Uddin LQ, Khouzam A, Phillips J, et al. (2013). Brain hyperconnectivity in children with autism and its links to social deficits. *Cell Rep* 5:738–747.

Tashiro A, Minden A, Yuste R. (2000). Regulation of dendritic spine morphology by the Rho family of small GTPases: antagonistic roles of Rac and Rho. *Cereb Cortex* 10:927–938.

Testa–Silva G, Loebel A, Giugliano M, De Kock CP, Mansvelder HD, Meredith RM. (2012). Hyperconnectivity and slow synapses during early development of medial prefrontal cortex in a mouse model for mental retardation and autism. *Cereb Cortex* 22:1333–1342.

Tian D, Stoppel LJ, Heynen AJ, Lindemann L, et al. (2015). Contribution of mGluR5 to patho-physiology in a mouse model of human chromosome 16p11.2 microdeletion. *Nat Neurosci* 18:182–184.

Trachtenberg JT, Chen BE, Knott GW, Feng G, et al. (2002). Long–term in vivo imaging of experience–dependent synaptic plasticity in adult cortex. *Nature* 420:788–794.

Tsanov M, Manahan–Vaughan D. (2009). Synaptic plasticity in the adult visual cortex is regulated by the metabotropic glutamate receptor, mGluR5. *Exp Brain Res* 199:391–399.

Tuchman R, Moshe SL, Rapin I. (2009). Convulsing toward the pathophysiology of autism. *Brain Dev* 31:95–103.

Tyzio R, Nardou R, Ferrari DC, Tsintsadze T, et al. (2014). Oxytocin–mediated GABA inhibition during delivery attenuates autism pathogenesis in rodent offspring. *Science* 343:675–679.

Van Bokhoven H. (2011). Genetic and epigenetic networks in intellectual disabilities. *Annu Rev Genet* 45:81–104.

Van Woerden GM, Harris KD, Hojjati MR, Gustin RM, et al. (2007). Rescue of neurological deficits in a mouse model for Angelman syndrome by reduction of [alpha]CaMKII inhibitory phosphorylation. *Nature Neurosci* 10:280–282.

Viberg H. (2009). Exposure to polybrominated diphenyl ethers 203 and 206 during the neonatal brain growth spurt affects proteins important for normal neurodevelopment in mice. *Toxicol Sci* 109:306–311.

Viberg H, Fredriksson A, Buratovic S, Eriksson P. (2011). Dose–dependent behavioral disturbances after a single neonatal Bisphenol A dose. *Toxicology* 290:187–194.

Vislay RL, Martin BS, Olmos–Serrano JL, Kratovac S, et al. (2013). Homeostatic responses fail to correct defective amygdala inhibitory circuit maturation in Fragile X syndrome. *J Neurosci* 33:7548–7558.

Voineagu I, Wang X, Johnston P, Lowe JK, Tian Y, et al. (2011). Transcriptomic analysis of autistic brain reveals convergent molecular pathology. *Nature* 474:380–384.

Wang DD, Kriegstein AR. (2011). Blocking early GABA depolarization with bumetanide results in permanent alterations in cortical circuits and sensorimotor gating deficits. *Cereb Cortex* 21:574–587.

Wang SS, Kloth AD, Badura A. (2014). The cerebellum, sensitive periods, and autism. *Neuron* 83:518–532.

Weiler IJ, Irwin SA, Klintsova AY, Spencer CM, et al. (1997). Fragile X mental retardation protein is translated near synapses in response to neurotransmitter activation. *Proc Natl Acad Sci USA* 94:5395–5400.

Williams CA, Beaudet AL, Clayton–Smith J, Knoll JH, et al. (2006). Angelman syndrome 2005: updated consensus for diagnostic criteria. *Am J Med Genet A* 140:413–418.

Willsey AJ, Sanders SJ, Li M, Dong S, et al. (2013). Coexpression networks implicate human midfetal deep cortical projection neurons in the pathogenesis of autism. *Cell* 155:997–1007.

Workman AD, Charvet CJ, Clancy B, Darlington RB, Finlay BL. (2013). Modeling transformations of neurodevelopmental sequences across mammalian species. *J Neurosci* 33:7368–7383.

Yashiro K, Riday TT, Condon KH, Roberts AC, et al. (2009). Ube3a is required for experience–dependent maturation of the neocortex. *Nat Neurosci* 12:777–783.

Zhao W, Chuang SC, Bianchi R, Wong RK. (2011). Dual regulation of Fragile X mental retardation protein by group I metabotropic glutamate receptors controls translation–dependent epileptogenesis in the hippocampus. *J Neurosci* 31:725–734.

Zimmerman AW, Connors SL. (2010). *Maternal Influences on Fetal Neurodevelopment*. New York: Springer.

Zoghbi HY, Bear MF. (2012). Synaptic dysfunction in neurodevelopmental disorders associated with autism and intellectual disabilities. *Cold Spring Harb Perspect Biol* 4. doi:10.1101/cshperspect.a009886.

CHAPTER 5

Maternal care and DNA methylation

Moshe Szyf

Department of Pharmacology and Therapeutics, McGill University, Montreal, Quebec, Canada

Introduction

The relationship between genotype and phenotype has been at the center of our understanding of biology in the last 150 years. However, it is obvious that differences in genotype cannot explain all phenotypic differences. The most striking example is cellular differentiation during embryonal development; in multicellular organisms one genotype encodes multiple phenotypes in different cell types that make up the organism. To address the question of how one genome could encode a variety of phenotypes, Waddington coined the term "epigenetics" more than six decades ago (Waddington, 1959). He fused the concepts of "epigenesis" and "genetics" into the new term of "epigenetics," implying that genes are sculpted by unknown factors during embryogenesis and are canalized into an array of different genetic programs (Van Speybroeck, 2002). Biochemistry has been characterizing during the last three decades many levels of such "epigenetic" mechanisms that include chromatin structure and histone modification that gate the access of transcriptional machinery to genes (Strahl and Allis, 2000; Jenuwein, 2001), noncoding RNAs including microRNA that regulate gene expression through altering chromatin configuration, inhibition of translation, and degradation of RNA (Bergmann and Lane, 2003), and modifications of cytosines in DNA by methylation and hydroxymethylation (Kriaucionis and Heintz, 2009; Jin et al., 2011). DNA methylation is a remarkable "epigenetic" layer of information that is part of the covalent chemistry of DNA. Therefore, the DNA that a child possesses at birth contains two layers of information and two kinds of identities, the genetic information inherited from the ancestors and identical in all tissues, as well as a pattern of DNA methylation and hydroxymethylation that varies from cell type to cell type and reveals the cellular identity of the DNA (Razin and Szyf, 1984). DNA methylation is a mechanism that confers different identities on the same identical DNA in cellular differentiation.

Environmental Experience and Plasticity of the Developing Brain, First Edition.
Edited by Alessandro Sale.
© 2016 John Wiley & Sons, Inc. Published 2016 by John Wiley & Sons, Inc.

For example, the emergence of cell-type specific DNA methylation patterns has been recently mapped in both humans and mice. The changes in DNA methylation that occur during differentiation are highly programmed and predictable and driven by developmental programs (Guo et al., 2013; Hirabayashi et al., 2013; Lister et al., 2013). The big question is whether the same mechanism that confers different cell-type identities to DNA during cellular differentiation would provide differential identities to people bearing the same DNA but exposed to different social and environmental experiences. A related question is whether such a mechanism operates to adapt genotypes to environmental cues transmitted by the mother during early life mother–infant interactions. Observations in rodents and nonhuman primates have suggested that quality of maternal care defines several behaviors in the offspring that remain into adulthood such as stress responsiveness and anxiety. DNA methylation has been proposed as a mechanism that mediates these effects serving as a mechanism for conferring experiential "identity" to DNA and playing an important role in generation of interindividual phenotypic differences that are triggered by "nurture."

DNA methylation

Methyl moieties are added to DNA by DNA methyltransferase (DNMT) enzymes that transfer a methyl group from the methyl donor S-adenosylmethionine (SAM) to the 5′ position on the cytosine ring (Adams and Burdon, 1982; Adams et al., 1984; Adams, 1995). In vertebrate genomes the main methylated dinucleotide sequence is CG; 60 to 80 % of this sequence is methylated in vertebrate DNA. However, it is clear that nonCG methylation exists and it is abundant in stem cells (Lister et al., 2009) as well as in the postmitotic brain (Lister et al., 2013). A CG dinucleotide in double stranded DNA is a "palindrome"; across a 5′CG3′ site in the paternal strand there is a 3′GC5′ site in the nascent daughter strand. DNMT1 is highly efficient in methylating a C in a CG dinucleotide of the daughter strand when the C on the complementary CG dinucleotide on the parental template is methylated, while it is highly inefficient in adding a methyl group to the nascent strands of DNA when the template is unmethylated (Gruenbaum et al., 1982). This maintenance mechanism ensures faithful copying of methylated cytosines while protecting from spurious addition of new methylation events and is believed to be responsible for faithful maintenance of the DNA methylation pattern and for conserving cell-type specific gene expression (Gruenbaum et al., 1982). *De novo* DNMTs that catalyze DNA methylation of CG and possibly nonCG sequences independent of the "template" DNA methylation are DNMT3A and DNMT3B (Hsieh, 1999; Okano, 1999). Several studies have shown that the *de novo* methyltransferase DNMT3A is present in postmitotic neurons (Feng et al., 2005; Brown et al., 2008; Feng et al., 2010) suggesting that postmitotic cells have the potential to alter the DNA methylation pattern by adding methyl moieties to new sites in DNA including into nonCG sites.

What makes DNA methylation particularly interesting as an "epigenetic" mechanism is the fact that during development different DNA methylation patterns are generated in different cell types (Razin and Riggs, 1980). This fact has led to the hypothesis that DNA methylation plays an important role in regulating cell-type specific gene expression (Razin and Riggs, 1980). The idea that DNA methylation distribution in the genome is sculpted during cellular differentiation and exhibits tissue specificity in the adult (Razin and Szyf, 1984) has been proposed more than three decades ago and was confirmed recently by next-generation genome-wide mapping of DNA methylation in the developing human and mouse brain (Guo et al., 2013; Hirabayashi et al., 2013; Lister et al., 2013). DNA methylation is therefore a mechanism that diversifies DNA molecule identities without altering the genetic sequence.

DNA methylation and regulation of gene expression

DNA methylation can alter gene expression and gene function in absence of a change in the sequence. The same sequence of DNA could either be expressed or silenced based on its state of methylation. Methylation of critical regulatory regions of genes can silence gene expression by either blocking the interaction of transcription factors with their recognition elements in genes (Comb and Goodman, 1990′ Inamdar et al., 1991) or through recruitment of methylated DNA binding factors such as the Rett syndrome protein Methyl CpG binding protein 2 (MeCP2). Methylated DNA binding proteins in turn recruit enzymes such as histone deacetylases (HDACs) and histone methyltransferases (HMTase) that modify the chromatin and precipitate an "inactive" chromatin structure (Nan et al., 1997). However, the role of methylated DNA binding proteins in regulating expression of methylated genes is unclear since MeCP2 as well as other methylated DNA binding proteins (MBD1-3) were found to interact with both methylated and silenced genes as well as unmethylated and active genes (Baubec et al., 2015). I believe that DNA methylation plays its main role through interfering with the binding of methylation sensitive transcription factors to DNA in enhancers, promoters and other regulatory elements, as we have shown to be the case with the regulation of the glucocorticoid receptor (*NR3C1*) by DNA methylation in response to maternal care (Weaver et al., 2007). Similarly DNA methylation might potentially play a role in gene suppression if it interferes with binding of repressors or if loss of DNA methylation in a promoter of a microRNA leads to increased expression of the microRNA and suppression of downstream targets (Alvarado et al., 2013).

Reversibility of DNA methylation

The role of DNA methylation in guarding cellular identify led to the idea that DNA methylation is fixed after differentiation and is unaltered in postmitotic cells such as neurons. It is possible to integrate into this concept the idea that stress during gestation would alter DNA methylation during times in development when new patterns of methylation are generated. However, if indeed DNA methylation is fixed after cellular differentiation is completed and cell division is halted, how it is then possible that postnatal experience such as maternal care would change the DNA methylation pattern? If DNA methylation plays a role in responding to experience in fully differentiated tissue it must be biochemically reversible. The presence of a *de novo* methylase such as DNMT3A can explain *de novo* methylation in postmitotic neurons but is it possible that methylated genes become demethylated in postmitotic tissue? If DNA methylation is a biological signal that responds to ongoing cues in early childhood and later in life it has to be reversible. However, the idea that the DNA could be biochemically reversed has encountered extremely heavy-handed resistance.

We proposed 15 years ago that the methyl moiety is released by a DNA demethylase/MBD2 in the form of methanol and that this DNA methylation is a true reversible biological signal (Bhattacharya et al., 1999; Ramchandani et al., 1999). The idea that a true removal of methyl groups is catalyzed enzymatically was seriously challenged (Ng et al., 1999) and alternative mechanisms that involve repair activity that removes the methyl cytosine and replaces it with a cytosine were proposed. Two decades ago Razin et al., proposed that a glycosylase cleaves the bond between the methylated base and the sugar and the abasic site is then repaired with unmethylated cytosines (Razin et al., 1986) and such a glycosylase activity was later identified by Jost (Jost, 1993). Other mechanisms included deamination of the methylated cytosine followed by repair as well as hydroxylation of the methylcytosine base to 5-hydroxymethylcytosine (Guo et al., 2011) followed by repair and replacement of the methylated cytosines with an unmethylated cytosines. Different complexes that included repair proteins (Barreto et al., 2007), cytosine deaminases such as AID (Rai et al., 2008) and C/T mismatch repair proteins such as MBD4 (Rai et al., 2008) were proposed to be involved in these demethylation events. More recently a mechanism for removal of the hydroxymethyl group by de novo DNMT3a and DNMT3b was demonstrated *in vitro* (Chen et al., 2012). Such a mechanism could participate in demethylation of methyl cytosines following their hydroxylation by (ten-eleven translocation family proteins) Tet enzymes. This mechanism is particularly relevant to the brain since Guo et al. have shown that neuronal activity induces demethylation in the dentate gyrus that is dependent on Tet1-induced oxidation of the methyl group, which is followed by deamination (Guo et al., 2011; see Figure 5.1 for scheme of methylation and demethylation equilibrium).

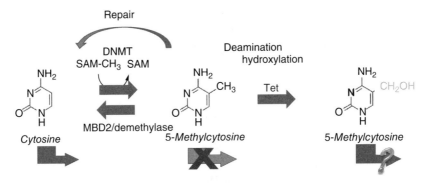

Figure 5.1 DNA methylation and demethylation reactions. DNA methylation reactions require the methyl donor SAM and are catalyzed by DNMT. Demethylation was suggested to be catalyzed by a bona fide demethylase (MBD2-demethylase), which removes a methyl group from DNA and releases it as methanol. Alternative mechanisms for demethylation involve either hydroxylation of the methyl group by TET enzymes or deamination by deaminase enzymes followed with repair. The methyl group is further modified to hydroxymethylcytosine by TET enzymes. Methylation at critical 5′ regulatory sites blocks transcription (X) while it is unclear whether hydroxylation might relieve this repression.

DNA methylation changes triggered by differences in maternal care in the *nr3c1* gene

The feasibility of reversing DNA methylation in postmitotic tissues led us to hypothesize that DNA methylation could be altered in response to changes in the social environment and that different DNA methylation identities of similar DNAs could be established not only by cellular differentiation but also by different experiences. The postnatal mother-neonate interaction is the earliest social environment encountered by the developing mammal and it plays an important role in its future health. In the rat, maternal care involves pup licking and grooming by the mother (LG) and there is a natural distribution of the intensity of LG across the population. Importantly, the adult offspring of mothers that exhibit increased levels of pup licking/grooming (i.e., High LG mothers) over the first week of life develop different behavioral phenotypes than offspring of low LG mothers and these differences are maintained into adulthood. These phenotypic differences are not transmitted by the germ line since cross fostering experiments show that the offspring phenotype is defined by the fostering and not the biological mother (Francis et al., 1999). This serves as a perfect example of the impact that postnatal social environment has on establishment of stable phenotypes independent of germ line transmission (Figure 5.2). Interestingly these phenotypes are transmitted across generations since female offspring of low LG mothers will develop to low LG mothers. Maternal behavior thus serves as a vector of inheritance. Unraveling mechanisms that mediate this seemingly magical impact of social environment on phenotypes provided one of the first examples

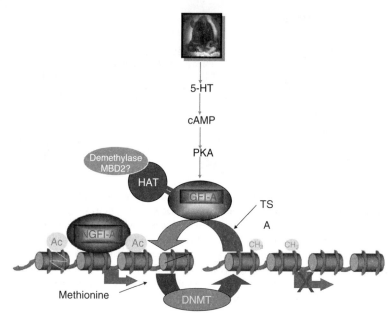

Figure 5.2 Epigenetic programming by maternal care. Maternal care causes activation of serotonin (5-HT) receptors, increases cAMP activation of protein kinase A followed by activation of NGFIA, which interacts with the *nr3c1* promoter and recruits chromatin modifying enzymes and MBD2/demethylase. Increased LG results in decreased methylation of DNA (CH3), increased histone acetylation (AC), and increased gene expression. The DNA methylation reaction is potentially reversible: histone deacetylase inhibitor TSA causes demethylation and activation of the gene, while methionine causes increased methylation and silencing of the gene. (See insert for color representation of this figure.)

of epigenetic programming of stable phenotypes independent of genomic and gamete transmission (Francis et al., 1999).

We therefore used this model of maternal care to test whether DNA methylation that fashions cell-type specific identities is also involved in conferring experience identity onto DNA. One phenotype that is characteristic of low LG adult offspring is heightened stress responsivity (Liu et al., 1997). Therefore, initial studies focused on a candidate gene, the glucocorticoid receptor (*nr3c1*) in the hippocampus. The glucocorticoid receptor in the hippocampus plays an important role in negative feedback regulation of the HPA axis. Increased expression of the receptor in the hippocampus results in enhanced feedback down regulation of ACTH release and lower levels of released glucocorticoids (Meaney et al., 1991). Adult offspring of high LG mothers show increased hippocampal GR expression, enhanced glucocorticoid feedback sensitivity, and decreased hypothalamic corticotrophin releasing factor (Liu et al., 1997; Francis et al., 1999). Cross-fostering studies suggest direct effects of the fostering mother rather than the biological mother on expression of *nr3c1* in the offspring (Francis et al., 1999) which pointed to the possibility that maternal behavior programs offspring genes epigenetically. Weaver et al. therefore compared the state of methylation of CG sites contained in the *nr3c1* exon 1_7 promoter, which is specifically expressed in the hippocampus, in hippocampi of adult offspring of low and high LG. Weaver et al., demonstrated a higher level of DNA methylation in the low LG in a CG site that is contained in the binding recognition element for the transcription factor NGFIA (Weaver et al., 2004). Differences in DNA methylation between the groups were associated with differences in histone acetylation and binding of the transcription factor NGFIA (Weaver et al., 2004). Like the effects of maternal behavior on the heightened stress responsivity phenotype, the DNA methylation differences emerged after birth during the early period of the pups being exposed to maternal licking and grooming, which is consistent with the hypothesis that they were programmed by maternal behavior and not by maternal genetics. High LG resulted in demethylation of the NGFIA binding sites in the offspring. These differences in DNA methylation in response to variations in maternal LG remain stable into adulthood (Weaver et al., 2004). Importantly, cross-fostering experiments demonstrated that the changes in DNA methylation are not transmitted by the biological mother but by the fostering mother, demonstrating that DNA methylation differences are introduced by maternal behavior (Weaver et al., 2004).

Molecular conduit between experience and DNA: signaling cascade leading from maternal care to epigenetic programming

In difference from in utero epigenetic effects that could be explained by direct exposure of the developing embryo to molecules released by the mother, the fact that maternal behavior results in a change in the chemical covalent modification of a specific gene in the brain of the offspring is seemingly very difficult to explain. What links an exposure to maternal behavior and chemical modification of a specific gene in a particular brain region? A plausible hypothesis that we had tested is that the response of the offspring to maternal care triggers a signaling pathway in the brain that leads through a cascade of protein-protein cross-talk to recruitment of DNA modifying enzymes to specific genes. This hypothesis is supported by data derived from the rat maternal care model. Maternal behavior triggers a signaling pathway that involves the serotonin receptor, increase in cAMP, recruitment of the transcription factor NGFI-A, which in turn recruits the histone acetyltransferase CBP, and the methylated DNA binding protein and candidate DNA demethylase MBD2 (Weaver et al., 2007) to the *nr3c1* exon 1_7 promoter (Figure 5.2). Weaver et al showed recently that binding of MBD2/demethylase to the *nr3c1* promoter is targeted by binding of the transcription factor NGFIA (Weaver et al., 2014); mutation in the binding site for NGFIA inhibits NGFIA binding, MBD2 binding and demethylation (Weaver et al., 2014). These data chart a molecular conduit between maternal behavior and epigenetic modification of a specific gene in the brain and serve as a paradigm for other changes in DNA methylation in the brain and possibly other tissues in response to behavioral exposures and experiences.

Reversibility of epigenetic programming by maternal care

The changes in DNA methylation in the postnatal brain in response to behavioral experiences suggest that DNA methylation in postmitotic brain is dynamic to a certain extent and is not fixed by cellular differentiation. The DNA methylation reaction is bidirectional as discussed above and therefore either pharmacological or behavioral interventions should potentially reverse these DNA methylation changes and alter the phenotype (Szyf, 2009). This is a fundamental difference between phenotypes fixed by genetic changes and those determined by epigenetic changes. A critical question is therefore whether it is possible to reverse the effects of a socially adverse early life environment using pharmacological interventions. Weaver et al. injected a histone deacetylase inhibitor Trichostatin A (TSA) into the ventricles of adult offspring of low and high LG maternal care. This compound increases histone acetylation but also enables DNA demethylation (Cervoni et al., 2001; Cervoni et al., 2002). TSA treatment of the low LG offspring reversed the epigenetic programming of the $nr3c1$ exon 1_7 promoter as well as stress responsivity and anxiety phenotypes of low LG offspring (Weaver et al., 2004). The behavioral phenotype could be changed in the other direction as well by increasing DNA methylation. To increase DNA methylation Weaver et al., injected into the ventricle the amino acid methionine (Weaver et al., 2005), the precursor of S-adenosyl methionine, the donor of methyl moiety in DNA methyltransferase catalyzed reactions and an inhibitor of active demethylation (Detich et al., 2003). Methionine treatment of adult offspring of high LG mothers increased DNA methylation of the $nr3c1$ gene and down regulated its expression as well as heightened stress responsivity and exhibited an open field behavior that was indistinguishable from the adult offspring of low LG mothers (Weaver et al., 2005). These data establish that not only the neonate brain but also the adult brain is epigenetically dynamic and amenable to epigenetic modulation. Thus, although DNA methylation and other epigenetic processes play an important role in setting up highly stable cellular differentiation states (Razin and Riggs, 1980), nevertheless they maintain a certain level of dynamic freedom that allows "adjusting" epigenetic states to external exposures throughout life.

These data also illustrate two fundamental properties of the effect of maternal care on offspring behavioral phenotype. First, behavioral experiences after birth can define a stable phenotype through epigenetic programming that includes changes in DNA methylation. Second, these phenotypes could be changed using epigenetic manipulations. This has obviously very important implications for psychiatry first, by pointing to epigenetic origins of psychiatric disorders, but even more, indicating that epigenetic therapeutics might be used to reverse adverse epigenetic programming behind psychiatric disorders.

Epigenetic programming by early life experience in humans; rRNA genes are hypermethylated in suicide victims who were abused as children

It is almost impossible to define a causal relationship between maternal care and offspring phenotype in humans in the same way that it is done in animals. Thus, there are formidable challenges in trying to determine whether early life experiences cause DNA methylation changes. Particularly, it is very difficult to tease apart epigenetic changes that are determined genetically from those that are defined by the experience of maternal care. However, the results in rat provide evolutionary justification for testing whether DNA methylation in adult humans is associated with early life adverse experiments. McGowan et al. examined brains of suicide victims who were abused as children and compared them with control brains. The first study examined the promoter of the rRNA genes. rRNA forms the skeleton of the ribosome, the protein synthesis machinery. Protein synthesis is essential for building new memories and creating new synapses in the brain. Our genome contains around 400 copies of the genes encoding rRNA. One possible way to control the protein synthesis capacity of a cell is through changing the fraction of active rRNA alleles in a cell (Brown and Szyf, 2007). We have previously shown that the fraction of rRNA genes that is active and is associated with the RNA Pol1 transcription machinery is unmethylated while the fraction that is inactive is methylated (Brown and Szyf, 2007). McGowan et al. showed that the suicide victims who experienced childhood abuse had higher overall methylation in their rRNA genes and expressed less rRNA (McGowan et al., 2008). This difference in methylation was region specific: it was specific to the hippocampus and was not observed in the cerebellum. Importantly, although significant methylation differences were observed between the controls and the suicide victims, no sequence differences were observed (McGowan et al., 2008).

McGowan et al. then examined in postmortem hippocampi the state of methylation of *nr3c1* exon 1_f promoter that is homologous to the promoter affected by maternal care in the rat. Remarkably, site-specific differences in DNA methylation were observed in the *nr3c1* exon 1_f promoter between suicide completers who had reported social adversity early in life and suicide completers who did not experience social adversity early in life (McGowan et al., 2009). Like in the rat the changes in DNA methylation affected the NGFIA binding site, interfered with binding of NGFIA and were associated with reduced expression of the *nr3c1* gene (McGowan et al., 2009). Although these data were just associations, the fact that an extremely similar epigenetic change occurs in rats where causality is demonstrated (Weaver et al., 2004) supports the hypothesis that these DNA methylation changes were caused by postnatal early life experience and that they in turn caused a change in *nr3c1* expression. These data are a first demonstration of evolutionary conservation of the epigenetic responses to early life.

The response to early life adversity is broad and involves several gene networks

The initial approach to the epigenetic response to the social environment involved "candidate" genes. Since one of the most striking phenotypic differences between high and low LG offspring was stress responsivity, the *nr3c1* gene in the hippocampus was an obvious candidate (Liu et al., 1997; Francis et al., 1999). However, it is clear that the impact of early life adversity on adult human health is broad (Power and Hertzman, 1997; Power et al., 2006). We therefore addressed the question of how broad the epigenetic response to maternal care was. Weaver et al., examined the transcriptome of the hippocampi of low and high LG adult offspring and revealed nine hundred genes whose expression was different between the groups. Importantly, a fraction of these changes in gene expression were reversed by TSA and methionine (Weaver et al., 2006). To determine whether DNA methylation and histone acetylation changes are also broad McGowan et al. performed a detailed mapping of DNA methylation histone H3K9 acetylation and transcription in 5 megabase of DNA upstream and downstream to the *nr3c1* locus in the hippocampus and identified broad and clustered differences in DNA methylation between the high and low LG animals. Interestingly, the study showed a broad cluster that includes the entire family of the *protocadherin* genes that is epigenetically programmed by maternal care; the cluster exhibited reduced expression, increased DNA methylation and reduced histone acetylation in low LG adult offspring (McGowan et al., 2011). Interestingly, members of the *protocadherin* gene family play a role in synaptogenesis (Weiner et al., 2005) and *protocadherin* genes were previously shown to be regulated by DNA methylation (Kawaguchi et al., 2008).

This broad response of the epigenome to early life experience is evolutionary conserved. McGowan et al examined the brains of human adults who were exposed to child abuse focusing on a region syntenic to that examined in rats, discovering similar broad and clustered differences in DNA methylation between the groups. Although the particular identity of specific differentially methylated regions within this genomic cluster differed, the overall picture was strikingly similar (Suderman, 2012). Importantly, the *protocadherin* gene family cluster that showed cluster-wide DNA methylation differences between high and low LG offspring adult rats is differentially methylated between adults who were abused as children and control adults as well. This remarkable evolutionary conservation of the epigenetic response presents a strong argument that early life experience alters epigenetic programming in the brain.

In summary, data from both rats and humans support the hypothesis that the response in DNA methylation to early life experience involves many genes in the hippocampus. The breadth of the change and its functional organization support the hypothesis that these changes represent an organized evolutionary conserved response that generates specific DNA methylation patterns as a function of early life experience such as maternal care.

System-wide responses to maternal deprivation; the impact of rearing differences in nonhuman primates

Any progress in incorporating epigenetic studies in behavioral studying of live humans will be limited to examining DNA methylation in the periphery. The critical question is whether the broad responses that we had reported in DNA methylation in the hippocampus in response to differences in maternal care in rodents (Weaver et al., 2004) or early life abuse in humans (McGowan et al., 2009) are limited to the brain. We hypothesized that the response to maternal care involves a system-wide change in DNA methylation and that the immune system, which is highly impacted by the HPA axis (Bakker et al., 1997), will be also affected by maternal care. It is impossible in humans to establish causality between maternal care quality and DNA methylation since it is impossible to randomize maternal care in humans for obvious ethical reasons. Moreover, it is not feasible in humans to obtain blood and brain samples from the same individual. In difference from rodents, nonhuman primates exhibit many of the complex maternal behaviors observed in humans. We therefore examined the effects of differential rearing on DNA methylation in adult rhesus macaque monkeys in both the prefrontal cortex and peripheral T cells concurrently. The monkeys were randomly separated early after birth to either a maternal-rearing group or to a surrogate peer-rearing group (Suomi et al., 1976) and blood and prefrontal cortex were isolated from adult monkeys. Provencal et al. showed that differential rearing leads to differential DNA methylation in both prefrontal cortex and T cells (Provencal et al., 2012). These differentially methylated promoters were clustered by both chromosomal region and gene function. Interestingly, although differences were observed in the rearing specific differentially methylated region in both tissues, there were striking similarities as well. Clustered regions as well individual genes were similarly differentially methylated in both tissues (Provencal et al., 2012). Sixteen promoters were different in both tissues and at the probe level at least five probes identified significant methylation differences between rearing groups in both tissues, a statistically significant overlap (Provencal et al., 2012). Interestingly, a site upstream of *A2D681*, the homologue of *NR3C1* in human was found to be more methylated in surrogate-peer-reared in both tissues (Provencal et al., 2012). The broad impact of maternal rearing on DNA methylation in both the brain and T cells supports the hypothesis that the response to maternal care is not limited to one tissue or one brain regions but that it is system-wide as well as genome-wide and that it persists to adulthood. The genome-wide changes in DNA methylation are consistent with the observations in hippocampi from rodents and humans discussed above. These data support the idea that different tissues show distinct DNA methylation differences in response to maternal deprivation; however, there are also responses that are similar across tissues (Provencal et al., 2012). We propose that these data might also suggest that the phenotypic impact of maternal deprivation will not be limited to the brain and involves other tissues such as the immune system (Coe and Lubach, 2000). These data provide proof of principle for the feasibility of studying the impact of the social environment in peripheral T-cell DNA methylation, which should have an important implication for progress in social and behavioral epigenetics (Provencal et al., 2012).

These changes in DNA methylation were detected in adults. How early are these changes established? A related question is whether the changes in DNA methylation that are triggered by maternal deprivation are stable into adulthood or whether they exhibit a developmental trajectory. Our preliminary data suggest first that DNA methylation differences between rearing conditions emerge early after maternal separation and that they are subjected to a developmental trajectory. While some of the differences remain into adulthood, others change during development.

Natural disasters as a model to study the impact of maternal stress on child DNA methylation

It is extremely difficult to determine causality between early life adversity, DNA methylation and the phenotype in humans since it is impossible to tease apart genetic and environmental or historical or other unknown exposures. In spite of a wealth of epidemiological data that correlated prenatal maternal stress and postnatal maternal care and emerging phenotypes, the main challenge is lack of randomization of early life adversity in most study designs. Natural disasters are a random source of adversity that offer unique opportunity for a "natural experiment" that tests the impact of early life adversity on emergence of phenotypic consequences in the developing human.

Cao et al. examined DNA methylation in T cells from 36 13-year-old children whose mothers were exposed to the 1998 Quebec ice storm during their pregnancy 13 years earlier. King et al. recruited women who had been pregnant during the disaster and assessed their degrees of objective hardship and subjective distress (King and Laplante, 2005). Cao et al. determined whether prenatal maternal stress was correlated with the state of DNA methylation of specific CG sites across the genome using an Illumina 450K array. 1675 CGs affiliated with 957 genes predominantly related to immune function were correlated with prenatal stress. Importantly, DNA methylation changes in *SCG5* and *LTA*, both highly correlated with maternal objective stress, were comparable in T cells, peripheral blood mononuclear cells (PBMCs) and saliva cells. These data support the hypothesis that social stress of the mother is transmitted to the offspring and trigger lasting broad changes in DNA methylation in the children in several cell types and tissues. These changes in DNA methylation are hypothesized to mediate a spectrum of behavioral and physical phenotypes (Cao-Lei et al., 2014). These data are the only evidence that we have to date that maternal stress is causally related to DNA methylation changes in the offspring, an effect including peripheral T cells.

In a related study, Cao et al. determined whether the effects of prenatal maternal stress on DNA methylation in human offspring are determined by the cognitive negative appraisal of the stressor by the mother or whether the DNA methylation alterations are solely determined by objective stress levels. The authors correlated DNA methylation profile in T cells from 34 adolescents with maternal cognitive appraisal of the 1998 Quebec ice storm's consequences as positive or negative (Cao-Lei et al., 2015). The methylation levels of 2872 CGs affiliated with 1564 different genes and with 408 different biological pathways, which are prominently featured in immune function, were significantly different between children whose mother rated their ice storm experience as positive or negative. These results suggest that during pregnancy maternal cognitive appraisal of a randomized adverse experience may have widespread effects on DNA methylation across the entire genome of the unborn children's' T cells. These data show a molecular signature of maternal cognitive appraisal of adverse experiences in the child's DNA and highlights the importance of mother's cognitive appraisal of experiences in addition to the objective experience itself in defining epigenetic programming in the offspring (Cao-Lei et al., 2015).

Summary

Studies on the epigenetic consequences of maternal care pioneered the field of behavioral epigenetics and the idea that experience, particularly early in life, could trigger epigenetic changes that stably alter the phenotype. These studies and others in the field of behavioral epigenetics suggest a mechanism explaining how interindividual differences in experience might trigger interindividual phenotypic differences. The studies provided evidence that DNA methylation patterns reflect dynamic interindividual differences in experience in addition to conserved programs of cellular differentiation. Overall the studies highlight the molecular and potentially phenotypic impact of maternal care on the offspring and the role of cognitive appraisal of mothers as a driving epigenetic force. However, many questions remain concerning the translational potential of these data. Would it be possible to use DNA methylation differences in peripheral white blood cells to early identify children who are at high risk of developing neurobehavioral problems? Are there behavioral interventions that could reverse adverse epigenetic programming early in life and target these high-risk children? Could DNA methylation markers be used to follow up the progress of interventions? What is the effect of gender and how do epigenetic responses triggered by early exposures interact with gender and development? How could we translate these epigenetic concepts to policy in prenatal care aimed at protecting the mother and creating "positively appraised" maternal conditions?

Mechanistically, the maternal care model in rodents provided a possible explanation for how experiential signals trigger a chain of events leading to changes in DNA methylation in the hippocampus. Many questions remain to be answered however. How general are these mechanisms for other experience driven DNA methylation changes? We have extremely limited understanding of how maternal stress or cognitive appraisals thereof are translated into gene-specific DNA methylation changes. How are these changes coordinated across the genome and across tissues? Do DNA methylation changes in peripheral tissues play a role in the behavioral phenotype or are they limited to peripheral phenotypes? It is important to differentiate between causal DNA methylation differences and downstream consequences. It is still unclear how particular changes in DNA methylation relate to either constitutive or inducible gene programming events and the biochemical mechanisms of regulation of gene expression need to be further explored. An important question is whether these epigenetic concepts could be translated into novel interventions to detect and reverse psychopathologies that are believed to be rooted in early life hardships. Animal models of maternal deprivation could be used to test novel behavioral and pharmacological epigenetic interventions (Szyf, 2014).

Acknowledgments

Work in Moshe Szyf's laboratory is supported by the Canadian Institute of Health Research and the Sackler Program in psychobiology and epigenetics at McGill University.

References

Adams RL. (1995). Eukaryotic DNA methyltransferases – structure and function. *Bioessays* 17(2): 139–145.

Adams RL, Burdon, RH. (1982). DNA methylation in eukaryotes. *CRC Crit Rev Biochem* 13(4): 349–384.

Adams RL, Davis T, Fulton J, Kirk D, Qureshi M, Burdon RH. (1984). Eukaryotic DNA methylase – properties and action on native DNA and chromatin. *Curr Top Microbiol Immunol* 108:142–156.

Alvarado S, Wyglinski J, Suderman M, Andrews SA, Szyf M. (2013). Methylated DNA binding domain protein 2 (MBD2) coordinately silences gene expression through activation of the microRNA has-mir-496 promoter in breast cancer cell line. *PLoS One* 8(10):e74009.

Bakker JM, Schmidt ED, Kroes H, Kavelaars A, Heijnen CJ, Tilders FJ, van Rees EP. (1997). Effects of neonatal dexamethasone treatment on hypothalamo–pituitary adrenal axis and immune system of the rat. *J Neuroimmunol* 74(1–2):69–76.

Barreto G, Schafer A, Marhold J, Stach D, Swaminathan SK, Handa V, Doderlein G, Maltry N, Wu W, Lyko F, Niehrs C. (2007). Gadd45a promotes epigenetic gene activation by repair-mediated DNA demethylation. *Nature* 445(7128):671–675.

Baubec T, Colombo DF, Wirbelauer C, Schmidt J, Burger L, Krebs AR, Akalin A, Schubeler D. (2015). Genomic profiling of DNA methyltransferases reveals a role for DNMT3B in genic methylation. *Nature*.

Bergmann A, Lane ME. (2003). HIDden targets of microRNAs for growth control. *Trends Biochem Sci* 28(9):461–463.

Bhattacharya SK, Ramchandani S, Cervoni N, Szyf M. (1999). A mammalian protein with specific demethylase activity for mCpG DNA [see comments]. *Nature* 397(6720):579–583.

Brown SE, Szyf M. (2007). Epigenetic programming of the rRNA promoter by MBD3. *Mol Cell Biol* 27(13):4938–4952.

Brown SE, Weaver IC, Meaney MJ, Szyf M. (2008). Regional–specific global cytosine methylation and DNA methyltransferase expression in the adult rat hippocampus. *Neurosci Lett* 440(1):49–53.

Cao–Lei L, Massart R, Suderman MJ, et al. (2014). DNA methylation signatures triggered by prenatal maternal stress exposure to a natural disaster: project ice storm. *PLoS One* 9(9):e107653.

Cao–Lei L, Elgbeili G, Massart R, et al. (2015). Pregnant women's cognitive appraisal of a natural disaster affects DNA methylation in their children 13 years later: project ice storm. *Transl Psychiatry* 5:e515.

Cervoni N, Sang–beom S, Chakravarti D, Szyf M. (2001). A novel regulatory role for Set/TAF–Iß oncoprotein integrating histone hypoacetylation and DNA hypermethylation in transcriptional silencing. submitted for publication.

Cervoni N, Detich N, Seo SB, et al. (2002). The oncoprotein Set/TAF–1beta, an inhibitor of histone acetyltransferase, inhibits active demethylation of DNA, integrating DNA methylation and transcriptional silencing. *J Biol Chem* 277(28):25026–25031.

Chen CC, Wang KY, Shen CK. (2012). The mammalian de novo DNA methyltransferases DNMT3A and DNMT3B are also DNA 5–hydroxymethylcytosine dehydroxymethylases. *J Biol Chem* 287(40):33116–33121.

Coe CL, Lubach GR. (2000). Prenatal influences on neuroimmune set points in infancy. *Ann NY Acad Sci* 917:468–477.

Comb M, Goodman HM. (1990). CpG methylation inhibits proenkephalin gene expression and binding of the transcription factor AP–2. *Nucleic Acids Res* 18(13):3975–3982.

Detich N, Hamm S, Just G, et al. (2003). The methyl donor S–adenosylmethionine inhibits active demethylation of DNA: a candidate novel mechanism for the pharmacologial effects of S-adenosylmethionine. *J Biol Chem* 278(23):20812–20820.

Feng J, Chang H, Li E, Fan G. (2005). Dynamic expression of de novo DNA methyltransferases Dnmt3a and Dnmt3b in the central nervous system. *J Neurosci Res* 79(6):734–746.

Feng J, Zhou Y, Campbell SL, et al. (2010). Dnmt1 and Dnmt3a maintain DNA methylation and regulate synaptic function in adult forebrain neurons. *Nat Neurosci* 13(4):423–430.

Francis D, Diorio J, Liu D, Meaney MJ. (1999). Nongenomic transmission across generations of maternal behavior and stress responses in the rat. *Science* 286(5442):1155–1158.

Gruenbaum Y, Cedar H, Razin A. (1982). Substrate and sequence specificity of a eukaryotic DNA methylase. *Nature* 295(5850):620–622.

Guo JU, Su Y, Zhong C, et al. (2011). Hydroxylation of 5–methylcytosine by TET1 promotes active DNA demethylation in the adult brain. *Cell* 145(3):423–434.

Guo JU, Su Y, Shin JH, et al. (2013). Distribution, recognition and regulation of non–CpG methylation in the adult mammalian brain. *Nat Neurosci* 17:215–222.

Hirabayashi K, Shiota K, Yagi S. (2013). DNA methylation profile dynamics of tissue–dependent and differentially methylated regions during mouse brain development. *BMC Genomics* 14:82.

Hsieh CL. (1999). In vivo activity of murine de novo methyltransferases, Dnmt3a and Dnmt3b. *Mol Cell Biol* 19(12):8211–8218.

Inamdar NM, Ehrlich KC, Ehrlich M. (1991). CpG methylation inhibits binding of several sequence–specific DNA– binding proteins from pea, wheat, soybean and cauliflower. *Plant Mol Biol* 17(1):111–123.

Jenuwein T. (2001). Re–SET–ting heterochromatin by histone methyltransferases. *Trends Cell Biol* 11(6):266–273.

Jin SG, Wu X, Li AX, Pfeifer GP. (2011). Genomic mapping of 5–hydroxymethylcytosine in the human brain. *Nucleic Acids Res* 39(12):5015–5024.

Jost JP. (1993). Nuclear extracts of chicken embryos promote an active demethylation of DNA by excision repair of 5–methyldeoxycytidine. *Proc Natl Acad Sci USA* 90(10):4684–4688.

Kawaguchi M, Toyama T, Kaneko R, et al. (2008). Relationship between DNA methylation states and transcription of individual isoforms encoded by the protocadherin–alpha gene cluster. *J Biol Chem* 283(18):12064–12075.

King S, Laplante DP. (2005). The effects of prenatal maternal stress on children's cognitive development: project ice storm. *Stress* 8(1):35–45.

Kriaucionis S, Heintz N. (2009). The nuclear DNA base 5–hydroxymethylcytosine is present in Purkinje neurons and the brain. *Science* 324(5929):929–930.

Lister R, Pelizzola M, Dowen RH, et al. (2009). Human DNA methylomes at base resolution show widespread epigenomic differences. *Nature* 462(7271):315–322.

Lister R, Mukamel EA, Nery JR, et al. (2013). Global epigenomic reconfiguration during mammalian brain development. *Science* 341(6146):1237905.

Liu D, Diorio J, Tannenbaum B, et al. (1997). Maternal care, hippocampal glucocorticoid receptors, and hypothalamic-pituitary-adrenal responses to stress. *Science* 277(5332):1659–1662.

McGowan PO, Sasaki A, Huang TC, et al. (2008). Promoter–wide hypermethylation of the ribosomal RNA gene promoter in the suicide brain. *PLoS ONE* 3(5):e2085.

McGowan PO, Sasaki A, D'Alessio AC, et al. (2009). Epigenetic regulation of the glucocorticoid receptor in human brain associates with childhood abuse. *Nat Neurosci* 12(3):342–348.

McGowan PO, Suderman M, Sasaki A, et al. (2011). Broad epigenetic signature of maternal care in the brain of adult rats. *PLoS One* 6(2):e14739.

Meaney MJ, Viau V, Bhatnagar S, et al. (1991). Cellular mechanisms underlying the development and expression of individual differences in the hypothalamic–pituitary–adrenal stress response. *J Steroid Biochem Mol Biol* 39(2):265–274.

Nan X, Campoy FJ, Bird A. (1997). MeCP2 is a transcriptional repressor with abundant binding sites in genomic chromatin. *Cell* 88(4):471–481.

Ng HH, Zhang Y, Hendrich B, et al. (1999). MBD2 is a transcriptional repressor belonging to the MeCP1 histone deacetylase complex. *Nat Genet* 23(1):58–61.

Okano M, Bell DW, Haber DA, Li E. (1999). DNA methyltransferases Dnmt3a and Dnmt3b are essential for de novo methylation and mammalian development. *Cell* 99(3):247–257.

Power C, Hertzman C. (1997). Social and biological pathways linking early life and adult disease. *Br Med Bull* 53(1):210–221.

Power C, Jefferis BJ, Manor O, Hertzman C. (2006). The influence of birth weight and socioeconomic position on cognitive development: does the early home and learning environment modify their effects? *J Pediatr* 148(1):54–61.

Provencal N, Suderman MJ, Guillemin C, et al. (2012). The signature of maternal rearing in the methylome in rhesus macaque prefrontal cortex and T cells. *J Neurosci* 32(44):15626–15642.

Rai K, Huggins IJ, James SR, et al. (2008). DNA demethylation in zebrafish involves the coupling of a deaminase, a glycosylase, and gadd45. *Cell* 135(7):1201–1212.

Ramchandani S, Bhattacharya SK, Cervoni N, Szyf M. (1999). DNA methylation is a reversible biological signal. *Proc Natl Acad Sci USA* 96(11):6107–6112.

Razin A, Riggs AD. (1980). DNA methylation and gene function. *Science* 210(4470):604–610.

Razin A, Szyf M. (1984). DNA methylation patterns. Formation and function. *Biochim Biophys Acta* 782(4):331–342.

Razin A, Szyf M, Kafri T, et al. (1986). Replacement of 5–methylcytosine by cytosine: a possible mechanism for transient DNA demethylation during differentiation. *Proc Natl Acad Sci USA* 83(9):2827–2831.

Strahl BD, Allis CD. (2000). The language of covalent histone modifications. *Nature* 403(6765):41–45.

Suderman MM, Sasaki PO, Huang A, et al. (2012). Conserved epigenetic sensitivity to early life experience in the rat and human hippocampus. *Proc Natl Acad Sci USA* 109 Suppl 2:17266–17272.

Suomi SJ, Collins ML, Harlow HF, Ruppenthal GC. (1976). Effects of maternal and peer separations on young monkeys. *J Child Psychol Psychiatry* 17(2):101–112.

Szyf M. (2009). Epigenetics, DNA methylation, and chromatin modifying drugs. *Annu Rev Pharmacol Toxicol* 49:243–263.

Szyf M. (2014). Epigenetics, a key for unlocking complex CNS disorders? Therapeutic implications. *Eur Neuropsychopharmacol*.

Van Speybroeck L. (2002). From epigenesis to epigenetics: the case of C. H. Waddington. *Ann NY Acad Sci* 981:61–81.

Waddington CH. (1959). Canalization of development and genetic assimilation of acquired characters. *Nature* 183(4676):1654–1655.

Weaver IC, Cervoni N, Champagne FA, et al. (2004). Epigenetic programming by maternal behavior. *Nat Neurosci* 7(8):847–854.

Weaver IC, Champagne FA, Brown SE, et al. (2005). Reversal of maternal programming of stress responses in adult offspring through methyl supplementation: altering epigenetic marking later in life. *J Neurosci* 25(47):11045–11054.

Weaver IC, Meaney MJ, Szyf M. (2006). Maternal care effects on the hippocampal transcriptome and anxiety–mediated behaviors in the offspring that are reversible in adulthood. *Proc Natl Acad Sci USA* 103(9):3480–3485.

Weaver IC, D'Alessio AC, Brown SE, et al. (2007). The transcription factor nerve growth factor–inducible protein a mediates epigenetic programming: altering epigenetic marks by immediate–early genes. *J Neurosci* 27(7):1756–1768.

Weaver IC, Hellstrom IC, Brown SE, et al. (2014). The methylated–DNA binding protein MBD2 enhances NGFI–A (egr–1)–mediated transcriptional activation of the glucocorticoid receptor. *Philos Trans R Soc Lond B Biol Sci* 369(1652).

Weiner JA, Wang X, Tapia JC, Sanes JR. (2005). Gamma protocadherins are required for synaptic development in the spinal cord. *Proc Natl Acad Sci USA* 102(1):8–14.

CHAPTER 6

Neurobiology and programming capacity of attachment learning to nurturing and abusive caregivers

Tania L. Roth[1], Gordon A. Barr[2,3], Michael J. Lewis[4,5], and Regina M. Sullivan[6,7]

[1] Department of Psychological and Brain Sciences, University of Delaware, Newark, Delaware, USA
[2] Department of Anesthesiology and Critical Care Medicine, The Children's Hospital of Philadelphia, Philadelphia, Pennsylvania, USA
[3] Perelman School of Medicine, University of Pennsylvania, Philadelphia, Pennsylvania, USA
[4] Department of Psychology, Hunter College, City University of New York, Manhattan, New York, USA
[5] Institute of Human Nutrition, Columbia College of Physicians and Surgeons, Columbia University, New York, New York, USA
[6] Emotional Brain Institute, Nathan Kline Institute, Orangeburg, New York, USA
[7] Child and Adolescent Psychiatry, New York University Langone Medical Center, New York, USA

Introduction

The infant's attachment to the caregiver is a profound and enduring emotional bond, ensuring that the infant remains in proximity to the caregiver to receive the caregiving necessary for survival (Bowlby, 1958; Bowlby, 1969). This infant attachment process is seen in altricial species widely distributed phylogenetically, including avian, mammalian, nonhuman primates, and humans (Hess, 1962; Harlow and Harlow, 1965; Salzen, 1970; Rajecki et al., 1978; Sanchez et al., 2001). As identified by Bowlby, this attachment has unique characteristics, including proximity seeking/maintenance behaviors, but also the paradoxical characteristic of attachment formation regardless of the quality of care received, including abusive relationships (Bowlby, 1969). A second function of attachment is cognitive and emotional programming of the infant brain, where the quality of maternal care received by the infant has dramatic and enduring effects on cognitive and emotional development (McEwen, 2003; Teicher et al., 2003; Gunnar et al., 2007; Toth and Cicchetti, 2011). Within a wide range of parenting styles, this programming interacts with genetics to define individual differences and adaptation to environments. However, abusive or neglectful parenting

Environmental Experience and Plasticity of the Developing Brain, First Edition.
Edited by Alessandro Sale.
© 2016 John Wiley & Sons, Inc. Published 2016 by John Wiley & Sons, Inc.

during attachment formation engages brain programming and initiates a pathway to pathology, including abnormal fear, stress regulation, and depressive behaviors.

This attachment learning and brain programing also occur within the dynamics of maturation. Indeed the developing organism is repeatedly presented with the daunting task of accommodating developmental transition and frequent behavioral reorganizing. That is, the infant is required to meet the demands of a changing environment and increasing skills enabling greater independence and self-regulation. Exactly how an organism reorganizes its behavior is not well defined, but is thought to include complex interactions between genes, experience, and learning. Furthermore, mechanisms of transitions and sensitive period windows that enable these rapid neurobehavioral transitions likely involve unique processes and can occur either rapidly or gradually. These periods of transitions, or reorganizations, have received more experimental attention in recent years (for reviews see Rice and Barone, 2000; Adriani and Laviola, 2004; Hensch, 2004; Crews et al., 2007; Sullivan and Holman, 2010), though researchers have long suggested the importance of these transitions and the critical role of proper reorganization for normal development (Levine, 1957; Denenberg, 1963). An understanding of the role of attachment in guiding these transitions and development has remained a challenge.

The importance of attachment and emotional well-being in humans was highlighted by Freud (Freud, 1938), expanded by Ainsworth (Ainsworth, 1973), and has continued to be further characterized by many others (e.g., Tottenham et al., 2010; Cicchetti et al., 2011; Bernard et al., 2013; Callaghan et al., 2014; Stellern et al., 2014). Mechanisms of causation have been highlighted by animal research that began in the 1950s, primarily using maternal separation in primates and rats (for recent reviews see Lyons et al., 2010; Stern et al., 2010; Branchi and Cirulli, 2014; Raineki et al., 2014). Here we review rodent work that has further documented attachment, the unique attachment learning circuitry, and behavioral outcomes associated with typical and atypical (abusive) attachment. It should be noted that animal studies cannot model all aspects of human attachment, especially as the child matures and more cognitive attributes, including a "mental representation" of the caregiver emerges. As reviewed here however, infant rodent studies have highlighted mechanisms of attachment and suggest that early attachment memories are formed within brain circuits that are different from those used for learning later in life. They also suggest that the circuitry involved in attachment learned with pain or abuse is mediated by an expanded brain circuit and hormonal facilitation. Comparisons of typical and atypical attachment circuits suggests similar behaviors in infancy expressed as prosocial behaviors, yet engage different neural substrates and epigenetic alterations that may lay the foundation for the enduring effects of early life trauma.

Infant attachment

One of life's first transitions occurs at birth as the newborn must reorganize their brain and behavior to adapt to the transition from an intrauterine to extrauterine environment. For altricial species, including humans, nonhuman primates, rodents and avian species, the first task is to learn to identify the caregiver and emit behaviors that produce proximity to the caregiver to ensure caregiver-infant bond formation. For many species, preference learning starts before birth as the young learn their caregivers' olfactory and auditory characteristics either through the mother's abdomen or through the egg's shell. These same stimuli are then preferred at birth. For example, newborn human infants will modify their sucking rate to hear their mother's voice (DeCasper and Fifer, 1980; Fifer and Moon, 1995) but also orient towards the odor of their mother's amniotic fluid and attempt to approach the breasts (Varendi et al., 1996). We know experience is important in these early life preferences because other voices (i.e., father) and food capable of scenting the amniotic fluid develop similar preferred status (Mennella et al., 1995; Schaal et al., 1995; Lecanuet and Schaal, 1996). It is also possible for the newborn to learn these rapidly through classical conditioning procedures delivered by scientists (Sullivan and Toubas, 1998). This early life attachment learning is phylogenetically widespread, and social behavior in rats, mice, sheep and rabbits has been repeatedly shown to be greatly influenced by this early life perinatal learning (Hofer et al., 1976; Teicher and Blass, 1977; Teicher et al., 1978; Blass and Teicher, 1980; Galef and Kaner, 1980; Hennessy et al., 1980; Hudson and Distel, 1983; Alberts and May, 1984; Distel and Hudson, 1985; Hudson, 1985; Risser and Slotnick, 1987; Leon, 1992; Coppola et al., 1994; Polan and Hofer, 1998; Moles et al., 2004; Armstrong et al., 2006; Logan et al., 2012; Roth et al., 2013; Stowers et al., 2013). The broad phylogenetically represented attachment system provides a strong foundation for use of animal models to explore the neurobiology of attachment since this circuit is inaccessible in infants and children.

The neurobiology of infant attachment has mostly been described using rodents. Olfaction has been the primary focus because immature pups can neither see nor hear until approaching the third week of life. Pups require their mother's odor for survival, as it is used for proximity seeking, nipple attachment, and social behavior. Indeed without the maternal odor pups frequently fail to nipple attach and anosmic pups rarely survive. Since a dam's odor is diet dependent and new food changes the maternal odor, a new maternal odor can be rapidly learned. For example, a novel odor (peppermint) placed either on or in the vicinity of the mother will readily take on the properties of maternal odor (Sullivan et al., 1990; Roth and Sullivan, 2005).

The attachment learning processes can be replicated outside the nest, where a novel odor paired with a stimulus that mimics maternal behavior supports rapid and robust olfactory learning. Indeed pairing an odor with either milk, warmth, or stroking to mimic maternal grooming and touching all produce a new maternal odor that is not just preferred, but can support nipple attachment and social behavior in the absence of the natural maternal odor (Sullivan et al., 1986; Roth and Sullivan, 2006; Roth et al., 2013).

Neurobiology of attachment learning

Infant behavioral results indicate attachment learning has unique properties, as the traditional framework for defining reward and storing information is not applicable and implicates a unique neural framework in the infant that is responsible for the olfactory-based attachment learning. Interestingly, a unique infant avian attachment circuit was defined in avian imprinting decades ago (for a recent review see Nakamori et al., 2013), and was critical in initiating the theoretical perspectives that humans must also have attachment learning circuits. We have worked to identify an attachment learning circuit in rodent pups, and as will be discussed here, this circuit does not involve the usual suspects known to mediate adult learning and memory processes, such as the amygdala, hippocampus and prefrontal cortex. We have also learned that pups have a sensitive period for attachment learning.

As illustrated in Figure 6.1, during the first 9 days of life pups readily learn a new maternal odor. The neurobiology of this learning is remarkably simple: learning-associated odor plasticity occurs within the olfactory bulb, which is the first relay station for olfactory processing and requires the pairing of the odor with copious amounts of norepinephrine (NE) (Sullivan et al., 1992; Sullivan et al., 2000a; Yuan et al., 2000). The infant locus coeruleus (LC) fails to habituate and show auto-inhibition, producing the large amounts of NE required for this attachment-related plasticity (Nakamura et al., 1987; Winzer-Serhan et al., 1996). The sensitive period ends when pups are around 10 days old as the LC becomes more adult-like and no longer supplies the required enhanced NE release. Once learned, the maternal odor produces enhanced olfactory bulb responding to the specific maternal odor as determined by a host of anatomical and physiological changes (Sullivan et al., 1990; Yuan et al., 2002; Roth et al., 2006; Raineki et al., 2009). The olfactory bulb axons (of mitral cells) project directly to the piriform cortex (Schwob and Price, 1984; Swanson and Petrovich, 1998; Haberly, 2001; Wilson and Stevenson, 2003), and the piriform cortex appears to have an important role in assigning the hedonic value to a learned odor. In particular, early life learned odor preferences engage the anterior piriform cortex (with no detectable activity in the posterior piriform), whereas learned odor aversions in older pups and adults engage posterior piriform cortical activity (Roth and Sullivan, 2005; Moriceau and Sullivan, 2006; Moriceau et al., 2006). Importantly, the same olfactory bulb learning-dependent responses occur to both the natural maternal odor and a learned artificial maternal odor (Roth and Sullivan, 2005; Raineki et al., 2010).

Neurobiology of abusive attachment learning

The paradox of attachment learning in humans is that strong attachments are formed to abusive caregivers. This can be modeled in other species and has enabled us to identify circuitry supporting this learning and to begin to understand how this experience initiates a pathway to pathology. Similar to typical (nurturing) attachment learning, abusive attachment learning is widely distributed phylogenetically. For example, shocking chicks during imprinting supports attachment learning (Hess, 1962; Salzen, 1970; Rajecki et al., 1978). Likewise, shocking an infant dog results in a strong attachment to the caregiver (Stanley, 1962). Perhaps the most striking demonstration, however, was Harlow's monkey's where abusive caregivers (the monkeys raised by the wire surrogate) severely abused their offspring, yet their infants demonstrated a profound preference for contact (Harlow and Harlow, 1965). More recent work has modeled abusive caregiving in nonhuman primates and again shows that infants retain strong motivation to remain with the abusive caregiver (Maestripieri et al., 1999; Sanchez et al., 2001; Suomi, 2003; O'Connor and Cameron, 2006). Together, these results show the strong proximity seeking behavior of abused offspring.

Rodent pups have also proven valuable in exploring the neurobiology of abuse-related attachment, including the short- and long-term consequences of abusive rearing on brain and behavioral development. In both rat and mouse pups, moderately painful stimuli paired with a novel odor support the learning of a new maternal odor. Specifically, pairing a novel odor with stimuli that mimic the mother stepping on pups or biting pups, such as a foot shock or tail pinch, are effective in supporting learning of a new maternal attachment odor (Spear, 1978; Haroutunian and Campbell, 1979; Sullivan et al., 1986; Camp and Rudy, 1988; Sullivan et al., 2000b; Roth and Sullivan, 2005; Moriceau and Sullivan, 2006; Moriceau et al., 2006; Roth et al., 2013). While behaviorally attachment formation with pain appears similar to typical attachment, as noted later, rearing with an abusive mother or odor-pain attachment learning alters brain development and behavioral outcomes.

Attachment learning from abusive attachment in the rodent is expressed as learned odor preferences, as indicated by pup orientation towards the odor and even the climbing of an obstacle to approach the odor (Camp and Rudy, 1988; Sullivan et al., 2000; Roth and Sullivan, 2001; Roth and Sullivan, 2005). Specifically, until pups reach postnatal day (PN) 10, pairing a novel odor with a painful stimulus, such as 0.5mA shock or tail pinch, results in pups approaching the odor when it is subsequently encountered (Spear, 1978; Sullivan et al., 1986; Camp and Rudy, 1988; Sullivan et al., 2000a; Roth and Sullivan, 2005; Moriceau

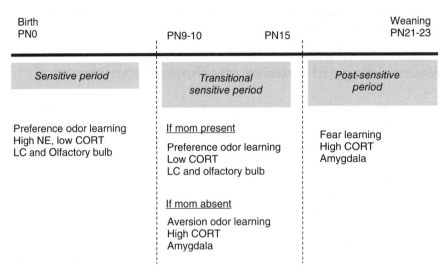

Figure 6.1 This schematic represents pups' transitions in attachment learning with odor-0.5 mA shock conditioning. Pups younger than PN10 have robust attachment learning during a sensitive period. Older pups readily learn fear, although maternal presence through social buffering enables the reinstatement of the sensitive period (PN, postnatal day; NE, norepinephrine; CORT, corticosterone; LC, locus coeruleus).

and Sullivan, 2006; Roth et al., 2013). After day 10, however, such conditioning results in learned odor aversions (this phenomenon is also illustrated in Figure 6.1). The inability of this Pavlovian conditioning procedure to produce fear learning is not due to pups' inability to detect the aversive stimulus. Noxious stimuli readily elicit pup escape responses and shock threshold does not appear to change as shock switches from supporting preference to supporting aversion learning (Stehouwer and Campbell, 1978; Collier and Bolles, 1980; Emerich et al., 1985; Barr, 1995). This suppressed aversion/fear learning's ecological significance may be due to the pup occasionally experiencing some pain from the mother and a learning system set up to prevent pups from learning aversions to the mother.

Using an infant animal model where the infant receives both abusive and positive caregiving offers another approach to understanding the neurobiology of abusive attachment and may more closely approximate abusive caregiving in children. A known stressor of rat mothers is resource deprivation (nesting material), and can be used to elicit aberrant caregiving behaviors. In a study we published in 2005, we utilized resource deprivation as a way to evoke aberrant caregiving, and explored whether pups learn a preference for a novel odor associated with the mother under these adverse conditions, similar to what we had shown with our odor-shock conditioning paradigm (Roth and Sullivan, 2005). Specifically, PN7-8 pups were placed in an apparatus with a lactating female who had not been given time to habituate to her new surroundings or provided adequate bedding to construct a nest (conditions that elicit maltreatment). A peppermint odor was also presented for the entire 30 min exposure session. Adverse caregiving behaviors displayed in the maltreatment condition included infant dragging, dropping, roughly handling, and active avoidance of the pups. Mothers within this condition also spent less time crouching over or nursing the pups and decreased amounts of licking and grooming behaviors. We observed that even though pups received multiple counts of maltreatment, they actively pursued contact with the mothers and later (memory test at 24 hours postconditioning) approached the peppermint odor that had been present in the caregiving environment.

We have partially documented the neurobiology for the paradoxical abuse attachment learning in the rodent. Brain areas involved in abuse attachment learning include the olfactory bulb and anterior piriform cortex, but not the amygdala (Sullivan et al., 2000b; Roth and Sullivan, 2005; Roth et al., 2006; Moriceau et al., 2009; Roth et al., 2013). It should be noted that pain information reaches the amygdala, yet the amygdala fails to exhibit plasticity normally associated with fear learning (Thompson et al., 2008; Barr et al., 2009). Our exploration of why the amygdala fails to be engaged in pups' fear learning revealed that it is not due to an immature amygdala per se, but rather due to pups' naturally low levels of the stress hormone corticosterone (CORT), a topic discussed further in the next section.

Maternal control of attachment

As illustrated in Figure 6.1, a sensitive period for attachment learning has been identified for infant rodents in which they are primed for odor learning to support acquisition of a maternal odor and proximity seeking of the caregiver. Termination of this sensitive period is largely due to decreasing levels of NE and the developmental functional emergence of the amygdala, though we have learned that the environment and CORT also have important control over when the sensitive period for attachment ends. Specifically, increasing CORT during the sensitive period either by systemic injections or by intra-amygdala infusions can prematurely end sensitive period learning, enabling the amygdala to become engaged with learning-related plasticity and allowing pups to learn fear and avoidance (Takahashi, 1994; Moriceau et al., 2004; Moriceau and Sullivan, 2004; Moriceau and Sullivan, 2006; Moriceau et al., 2009). In these same studies we have shown that decreasing CORT levels in older postsensitive period pups can reinstate sensitive period learning. As a side note here, disruption of endogenous opioids too alters sensitive period learning and transition (Roth and Sullivan, 2001; Roth et al., 2006; Roth and Sullivan, 2006).

An understanding of the effects of CORT in infants requires some understanding of their unique stress system. Specifically, CORT levels are quite low and stressful/painful events fail to mount a stress response in young pups: this is referred to as the "stress hyporesponsive period" (SHRP), and is in sharp contrast to the stress response exhibited by older pups and adults (Levine, 1962; Henning, 1978; Walker et al., 1986; Rosenfeld et al., 1992; Grino et al., 1994; Levine, 2001). Importantly, the age of SHRP termination begins around PN10. The environment has strong control over the SHRP: chronic early life stress (i.e., abusive rearing) is capable of precocious ending of the SHRP (Moriceau et al., 2006). Maternal presence can also reinstate the SHRP through a process referred to as "social buffering" where stressed pups fail to show a CORT increase (Stanton et al., 1987; Stanton and Levine, 1990; Suchecki et al., 1993). Maternal presence, through CORT reduction, blocks pups' fear learning, reinstating the attachment learning and preventing the participation of the amygdala in learning (Moriceau and Sullivan, 2006). After PN15, however, only fear will be learned during odor-shock conditioning regardless of maternal presence and CORT level (Upton and Sullivan, 2010).

To summarize, data indicate that during the attachment period, pups low CORT levels attenuate amygdala plasticity, which prevents infants from responding to fear/aversive stimuli and activates the attachment learning neural circuit. In pups older than PN9, there appears to be access to both the attachment and fear system. Specifically, if pups are alone and elicits a stress response, pups will learn fear. However, if the mother is present, and pups have their stress response buffered, pups will revert to sensitive period learning. This suggests that environmentally induced alterations of CORT levels and amygdala activity have the potential to disrupt the learning transition and attachment learning.

Although amygdala learning-related plasticity is suppressed during the sensitive period to facilitate attachment learning, there are long-term behavioral and epigenetic consequences after repeated odor-pain pairings or exposure to caregiver maltreatment. For example, such treatments increase CORT levels, alter engagement of the amygdala in response to maternal odor presentation, and induce later deficits in social and maternal behaviors (Roth et al., 2009; Raineki et al., 2010; Raineki et al., 2012). Unpaired presentations of the odor and shock stimuli (which do not produce learned odor preferences) are known to significantly alter gene expression patterns within the amygdala (Sarro et al., 2014), and exposure to caregiver maltreatment produces DNA methylation alterations that are present within the adult amygdala (Roth et al., 2014). These results suggest routes through which trauma within the attachment system (particularly at the level of the amygdala) could underlie many of the long-term behavioral effects associated with abuse, including vulnerability to the development of psychiatric disorders.

Attachment and epigenetic programming

Though the "programming" capacity of infant-caregiver experiences has long been recognized, it has only been within the last decade that studies have begun to provide empirical support for a mechanism whereby such experiences could

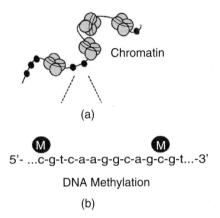

Chromatin

(a)

5'- ...c-g-t-c-a-a-g-g-c-a-g-c-g-t...-3'

DNA Methylation

(b)

Figure 6.2 DNA methylation. (a) DNA in the nucleus is wrapped around histone proteins, forming what is referred to as chromatin. (b) DNA methylation can occur at cytosine residues of cytosine-guanine (CG) dinucleotides that are clustered within gene regulatory regions. DNA methylation is an epigenetic mechanism typically associated with gene suppression, as methyl groups can either interfere with the binding of transcription factors necessary to promote gene transcription and/or recruit repressor proteins that promote a compact chromatin state not permissive to gene transcription.

render consequences for brain development and lifelong mental health. Studies that fall under the umbrella discipline of behavioral epigenetics have provided fascinating insight into biological factors that are extraordinarily sensitive to infant-caregiver interactions. In particular, DNA methylation, an epigenetic mechanism typically associated with gene silencing (Figure 6.2), has emerged as a leading candidate biological pathway capable of linking gene-environment interactions to long-term (and even multigenerational) trajectories in the development of behavior.

One way in which early life environmental events could render an individual with life-long altered stress responses and increased susceptibility to later-emergent stress- and mood-related psychiatric disorders is by epigenetic programming of hypothalamic-pituitary-adrenal (HPA) axis regulation. Many clinical studies have demonstrated that early life stress canalizes HPA axis function, as hypo- or hypercortisolism and the dysregulation of the circadian rhythm of cortisol production are common outcomes in children and adults with a history of maltreatment (Gunnar et al., 2007; Carpenter et al., 2009; Rogosch et al., 2011). HPA axis dysregulation is also a prominent symptom in adults with a history of child maltreatment and the diagnosis of major depressive disorder or post-traumatic stress disorder (De Bellis and Thomas, 2003; Bauer et al., 2010). Nonhuman primate models of early life adversity likewise demonstrate the negative impact of early life stress and maltreatment on the HPA axis, showing for example that separation of infants from their attachment figure can provoke increased activity of the HPA axis (Gunnar et al., 2007; Howell and Sanchez, 2011).

Early evidence that epigenetic changes could provide a route through which early life experiences influence HPA axis function came from a study demonstrating that methylation of DNA associated with the *glucocorticoid receptor* (*GR*) gene, a gene underlying stress-responsivity through its regulation of HPA activity, was directly associated with the type of caregiving experienced during the first postnatal week (Weaver et al., 2004). Adult male rats that had been reared by nurturing mothers that exhibited high levels of nurturing care (pup licking and grooming specifically) had low levels of methylation of DNA associated with the *GR* gene within their hippocampus, whereas adults who had been raised by less nurturing mothers exhibited hypermethylation of *GR* DNA. These observations were also consistent with *GR* gene expression patterns and anxiety-related behavior of the animals. Animals with low methylation had higher expression of the *GR* gene and exhibited less stress-responsivity and anxiety-like behavior (less fearful response to stimuli, decreased defensive response, and a more modest HPA response to a stress challenge), whereas animals with higher methylation had lower gene expression and increased anxiety-like behavior.

Since this seminal study, similar experience-induced alterations have been documented in humans at gene loci involved in stress regulation, and extended to other genomic sites involved in neural and behavioral plasticity and immune health and function. For example, investigators have found altered methylation states of many genes (including increased methylation of the human *GR* equivalent gene, *Nr3c1*) within the hippocampus of males suffering severe childhood abuse (McGowan et al., 2008; McGowan et al., 2009; Labonté et al., 2012). In buccal tissue or blood samples, DNA methylation alterations have been found present in children subjected to institutional care (Naumova et al., 2012), adults who experienced loss of a parent or maltreatment during their childhood years (Tyrka et al., 2012), and adults who experienced a disadvantaged socio-economic position during childhood (Borghol et al., 2012). Studies have also shown strong correlations between child abuse/life stressors, methylation states of immune- and synaptic plasticity-related genes, and the diagnosis of PTSD (Smith et al., 2011; Uddin et al., 2011). A recent study has even demonstrated that epigenetic marks in maltreated individuals can be changed through psychotherapeutic approaches (Perroud et al., 2013).

We have worked to provide a stronger empirical link between caregiver maltreatment, altered DNA methylation patterns, and aberrant behavioral outcomes (Roth et al., 2009; Blaze et al., 2013; Roth et al., 2014). To do this we have used a variation of the maltreatment paradigm described above (Roth and Sullivan, 2005). In our paradigm, rat pups are repeatedly exposed to maltreatment outside the homecage for 30 minutes each day beginning on PN1 and ending on PN7 (several within-litter control groups are also run at the same time). We have mainly focused on changes in methylation of DNA associated with the *Brain-derived neurotrophic factor* (*Bdnf*) gene as it codes for a protein that plays an essential role in the development and survival of neurons, as well as neural plasticity underlying life-long cognitive processes (Greenberg et al., 2009;

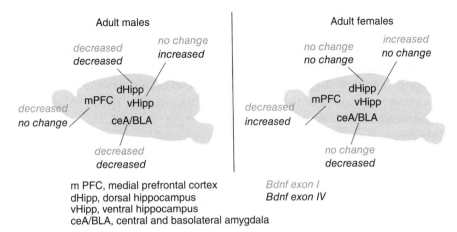

m PFC, medial prefrontal cortex
dHipp, dorsal hippocampus
vHipp, ventral hippocampus
ceA/BLA, central and basolateral amygdala

Bdnf exon I
Bdnf exon IV

Figure 6.3 Summary of maltreatment-induced DNA methylation alterations that we have observed in the brain of adult male (left panel) and female (right panel) rats (3 months removed from the infant experiences). *Increased, decreased,* or *no change* refers to methylation changes in maltreated rats in comparison to normal (nurturing) care controls. Changes in methylation are for DNA associated with important regulatory regions of the *Bdnf* gene (*Bdnf* I or IV). (Figure is recreated from data in Blaze et al., 2013 and Roth et al., 2009, 2014.)

Bath et al., 2012; Park and Poo, 2013). Further, there are ample data indicating that there are changes in *Bdnf* DNA methylation in response to a variety of environmental factors, especially stress (Lubin et al., 2008; Roth et al., 2011; Unternaehrer et al., 2012; Kundakovic et al., 2013), and many psychiatric disorders that are often associated with early life adversity have been linked to aberrant methylation of *Bdnf* DNA (Keller et al., 2010; Smith et al., 2011).

As summarized in Figure 6.3, we have shown that brief, but repeated, exposure to caregiver maltreatment (i.e., being stepped on, dropped, dragged, actively avoided, and roughly handled) produces DNA methylation alterations at *Bdnf* loci that are present in the adult brain (in the figure changes associated with exon I are represented by the lighter shaded text and those with exon IV are in black). Such data provide empirical support of the ability of caregiver maltreatment to produce DNA methylation alterations across behaviorally relevant brain networks known to support attachment and be affected by childhood maltreatment – the prefrontal cortex, hippocampus, and amygdala. They also provide insight of the ability of maltreatment to differentially affect brain regions at the molecular level and between sexes. Our observations of epigenetic alterations that differ between males and females parallel a similar phenomenon being increasingly reported by others (Mueller and Bale, 2008; Schwarz et al., 2010; Kundakovic et al., 2013; Kosten et al., 2014).

Another biological factor worth mentioning here is telomere biology. Telomere length, like DNA methylation, has recently emerged as an additional biomarker of the long-term impact of early life stress (Epel, 2009). Telomere length does appear to be epigenetically regulated (Gonzalo et al., 2006; Zhang et al., 2007), and the enzyme that replenishes telomere length, telomerase, can also directly influence the transcription of genes much like epigenetic factors do (Blasco, 2007; Zhang et al., 2007; Zhou et al., 2014). Telomeres are long stretches of TTAGGG nucleotide repeats that cap the ends of DNA (Blackburn, 2001). Telomere length plays a role in cellular aging with both biological and psychological environmental factors influencing the rate of their attrition in peripheral cells (von Zglinicki, 2002; Epel et al., 2004; Epel, 2009).

Emerging data indicate that telomere length is especially sensitive to variations in caregiving environments. For example, individuals exposed to chronic psychological stress during childhood (e.g., prolonged institutional care, maltreatment, exposure to violence) display accelerated telomere shortening in peripheral cells (i.e., buccal cells and leukocytes; Tyrka et al., 2010; Drury et al., 2012; Asok et al., 2013; Shalev et al., 2013). In a collaboration with Mary Dozier, we recently showed that high-quality responsive maternal care appears to protect telomeres from accelerated shortening in 4- to 6-year-old children living under chronically stressful conditions (Asok et al., 2013). Further, using our rodent model of caregiver maltreatment, we recently demonstrated that exposure to nurturing or aversive caregiving environments outside the homecage also results in long-term changes in telomere length within the brain (Asok et al., 2014). Together, these data suggest that future investigation of CNS epigenetic programming and telomere dynamics offers novel approaches for understanding the molecular and cellular effects of early life stress in relation to attachment and future physical and mental health.

Functional consequences

In a striking parallel to outcomes typically associated with abusive infant-caregiver relationships, we have shown long-term effects of pairing of cues with abuse during the sensitive period in rats. In one set of experiments, infants who had paired presentations of the odor and shock stimuli (which produce learned odor preferences) exhibited a depressive-like phenotype as adults (Sullivan et al., 2011; Rincón Cortés et al., 2015). This was accompanied by changes in genes involved in broad signaling pathways such as phospholipase C and ERK/MAPK paths, and atherosclerosis signaling, linked to inflammatory processes. Amazingly, re-exposure to the infant conditioned odor reversed the depression phenotype and reregulated gene expression, including changes in multiple paths representing cAMP and other G-protein coupled receptors that were not seen in the depression phenotype. Some pathways, such as those related to glucocorticoid receptor signaling were altered under both conditions.

Early life trauma and parental alcohol use are risk factors for adult alcohol abuse (see Enoch, 2012; Fenton et al., 2013 for recent reviews). We asked in our animal model of infant abuse whether early (postnatal day 8) pairing of ethanol odor with shock would alter ethanol intake in the adult. Using a two-bottle preference test, where the adult had access to increasingly concentrated alcohol solutions (1–7%) or water for 1 hour per day (Martinetti et al., 2000), the ethanol-shock paired infants took in more alcohol as adults than did the two control groups (1%; unpaired EtOH-shock > EtOH odor alone). After 9 days of access to alcohol (now at 7%), the paired animals maintained higher levels of intake over ethanol alone, but now the unpaired EtOH odor-shock animals also increased their intake to the same higher levels [Figure 6.4(a)]. Moreover, the percent of animals that preferred ethanol to water was greater than 90% in the

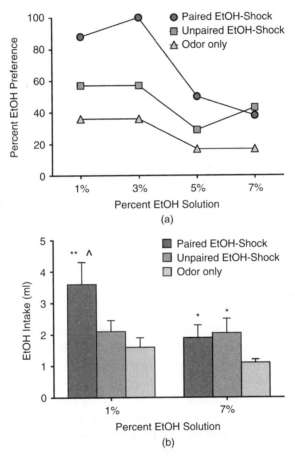

Figure 6.4 (a) Effects of pairing ethanol (EtOH) with shock at 8 days of age on adult EtOH preference (% preferring EtOH over water). Early odor-shock conditioning during the sensitive period had long-term consequences as determined in the two bottle preference test. Adults were given a choice of dilute EtOH (1% v/v) or water for 3 days and then the concentration was increased every 3 days (1%, 3%, 5%, 7%). The paired EtOH-shock animals showed a strong preference for alcohol over water when given free choice, upward of 85–99%. The unpaired shock-EtOH odor animals showed increased consumption compared to the odor-only animals but significantly less that the paired animals, except at the highest concentration. (b) These data are from the 3 days of testing. At the lowest concentration of EtOH (1%), the paired animals showed the greatest intake compared to unpaired odor-shock or EtOH alone. For the highest concentration, unpaired shock-odor as well as shocked paired with odor enhanced compared to controls. ** p < .01 from odor only; *p < .05 from odor only; ∧p < .05 from unpaired EtOH-shock.

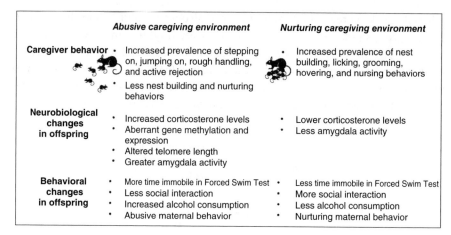

	Abusive caregiving environment	Nurturing caregiving environment
Caregiver behavior	• Increased prevalence of stepping on, jumping on, rough handling, and active rejection • Less nest building and nurturing behaviors	• Increased prevalence of nest building, licking, grooming, hovering, and nursing behaviors
Neurobiological changes in offspring	• Increased corticosterone levels • Aberrant gene methylation and expression • Altered telomere length • Greater amygdala activity	• Lower corticosterone levels • Less amygdala activity
Behavioral changes in offspring	• More time immobile in Forced Swim Test • Less social interaction • Increased alcohol consumption • Abusive maternal behavior	• Less time immobile in Forced Swim Test • More social interaction • Less alcohol consumption • Nurturing maternal behavior

Figure 6.5 Summary of outcomes associated with being raised in either abusive or nurturing caregiving environments.

paired EtOH shock group and remained elevated over all concentrations for the 12 day test [Figure 6.4(b)].

Thus, early life trauma and cues associated with it alter long-term behaviors and gene expression (particularly within the amygdala) that could underlie many of the enduring consequences of early abuse, including increased vulnerability to psychiatric disorders and increased risk for alcohol abuse.

Concluding remarks

Clinical data demonstrate that the lack of secure attachment to the caregiver, attributable to both environmental and biological factors, is associated with subsequent behavioral problems and psychopathologies. To contribute to the understanding of neurobiology underlying infant attachment, even in the context of aversive parenting, we have utilized several approaches in developing rodents. Our work (summarized in Figure 6.5) and that of others have shown that this early life attachment experience also programs brain and behavioral development, in part, mediated through gene expression and DNA methylation. Further elucidation of attachment circuitry and the regulatory role of epigenetics in typical and abusive attachment is certain to reveal substantial information regarding normal and abnormal brain and behavioral development and facilitate the development of treatments and interventions.

Acknowledgments

This work was supported by NIH grants HD33402 to RMS, MH80603 to GAB & RMS, and 1P20GM103653 to TLR.

References

Adriani W, Laviola G. (2004). Windows of vulnerability to psychopathology and therapeutic strategy in the adolescent rodent model. *Behav Pharmacol* 15(5–6):341–352.

Ainsworth M. (1973). The development of infant–mother attachment. In: *Review of Child Development Research*, B. Caldwell and H. Ricciuti, pp. 3:1–94. Chicago: University of Chicago Press.

Alberts JR, May B. (1984). Nonnutritive, thermotactile induction of filial huddling in rat pups. *Dev Psychobiol* 17(2):161–181.

Armstrong CM, DeVito LM, Cleland TA. (2006). One–trial associative odor learning in neonatal mice. *Chem Sens* 31(4):343–349.

Asok A, Bernard K, Roth TL, Rosen JB, Dozier M. (2013). Parental responsiveness moderates the association between early–life stress and reduced telomere length. *Dev Psychopathol* 25(3):577–585.

Asok A, Bernard K, Rosen JB, Dozier M, Roth TL. (2014). Infant–caregiver experiences alter telomere length in the brain. *PloS One* 9(7):e101437.

Barr GA. (1995). Ontogeny of nociception and antinociception. *NIDA Res Monogr* 158: 172–201.

Barr GA, Moriceau S, Shionoya K, Muzny K, Gao P, Wang S, Sullivan RM. (2009). Transitions in infant learning are modulated by dopamine in the amygdala. *Nat Neurosci* 12(11):1367–1369.

Bath KG, Akins MR, Lee FS. (2012). BDNF control of adult SVZ neurogenesis. *Dev Psychobiol* 54(6):578–589.

Bauer M, Wieck A, Lopes R, Teixeira A, Grassi–Oliveira R. (2010). Interplay between neuroimmunoendocrine systems during post–traumatic stress disorder: a minireview. *Neuroimmunomodulat* 17:192–195.

Bernard K, Meade E, Dozier M. (2013). Parental synchrony and nurturance as targets in an attachment based intervention: bulding upon Mary Ainsworth's insights about mother–infant interaction. *Attach Hum Dev* 15(5–6):507–523.

Blackburn EH. (2001). Switching and signaling at the telomere. *Cell* 106(6):661–673.

Blasco MA. (2007). The epigenetic regulation of mammalian telomeres. *Nat Rev Genet* 8(4):299–309.

Blass EM, Teicher MH. (1980). Suckling. *Sci* 210(4465):15–22.

Blaze J, Scheuing L, Roth TL. (2013). Differential methylation of genes in the medial prefrontal cortex of developing and adult rats following exposure to maltreatment or nurturing care during infancy. *Dev Neurosci* 35(4):306–316.

Borghol N, Suderman M, McArdle W, Racine A, Hallett M, Pembrey M, Hertzman C, Power C, Szyf M. (2012). Associations with early–life socio–economic position in adult DNA methylation. *Intl J Epidemiol* 41(1):62–74.

Bowlby J. (1958). The nature of the child's tie to his mother. *Intl J Psycho–Analysis* 39:350–373.

Bowlby J. (1969). Attachment. In: *Attachment and Loss*, Vol. 1. New York: Basic Books.

Branchi I, Cirulli F. (2014). Early experiences: building up the tools to face the challenges of adult life. *Dev Psychobiol* 56(8):1661–1674.

Callaghan BL, Sullivan RM, Howell B, Tottenham N. (2014). The International Society for Developmental Psychobiology Sackler Symposium: early adversity and the maturation of emotion circuits – a cross–species analysis. *Dev Psychobiol* 56(8):1635–1650.

Camp LL, Rudy JW. (1988). Changes in the categorization of appetitive and aversive events during postnatal development of the rat. *Dev Psychobiol* 21(1):25–42.

Carpenter LL, Tyrka AR, Ross NS, Khoury L, Anderson GM, Price LH. (2009). Effect of childhood emotional abuse and age on cortisol responsivity in adulthood. *Biol Psychiat* 66(1):69–75.

Cicchetti D, Rogosch FA, Toth SL, Sturge–Apple ML. (2011). Normalizing the development of cortisol regulation in maltreated infants through preventive interventions. *Dev Psychopathol* 23(3):789–800.

Collier A, Bolles R. (1980). The ontogensis of defensive reactions to shock in preweanling rats. *Dev Psychobiol* 13:141–150.

Coppola DM, Coltrane JA, Arsov I. (1994). Retronasal or internasal olfaction can mediate odor–guided behaviors in newborn mice. *Physiol Behav* 56(4):729–736.

Crews F, He J, Hodge C (2007). Adolescent cortical development: a critical period of vulnerability for addiction. *Pharmacology Biochem Behav* 86(2):189–199.

De Bellis MD, Thomas LA. (2003). Biologic findings of post–traumatic stress disorder and child maltreatment. *Curr Psychiatry Rep* 5:108–117.

DeCasper AJ, Fifer WP. (1980). Of human bonding: newborns prefer their mothers' voices. *Sci* 208(4448):1174–1176.

Denenberg V. (1963). Early experience and emotional development. *Sci Am* 208:138–146.

Distel H, Hudson R. (1985). The contribution of the olfactory and tactile modalities to the nipple–search behaviour of newborn rabbits. *J Comp Physiol A* 157(5):599–605.

Drury SS, Theall K, Gleason MM, Smyke AT, De Vivo I, Wong JY, et al. (2012). Telomere length and early severe social deprivation: linking early adversity and cellular aging. *Mol Psychiatry* 17(7):719–727.

Emerich D, Scalzo F, Enters E, Spear N, Spear L. (1985). Effects of 6–hydroxydopamine–induced catecholamine depletion on shock–precipitated wall climbing of infant rat pups. *Dev Psychobiol* 18(3):215–227.

Enoch MA. (2012). The influence of gene–environment interactions on the development of alcoholism and drug dependence. *Curr Psychiatry Rep* 14(2):150–158.

Epel ES. (2009). Psychological and metabolic stress: a recipe for accelerated cellular aging? *Hormones* 8(1):7–22.

Epel ES, Blackburn EH, Lin J, Dhabhar FS, Adler NE, et al. (2004). Accelerated telomere shortening in response to life stress. *Proc Natl Acad Sci USA* 101(49):17312–17315.

Fenton MC, Geier T, Keyes K, Skodol AE, Grant BF, Hasin DS. (2013). Combined role of childhood maltreatment, family history, and gender in the risk for alcohol dependence. *Psychol Med* 43(5):1045–1057.

Fifer W, Moon C. (1995). The effects of fetal experience with sound. In: *Fetal Development: A Psychobiological Perspective*, J. Lecanuet, W. Fifer, N. Krasnegor, and W. Smotherman, pp. 351–368. Hillsdale, NJ: Erlbaum.

Freud S. (1938). *An Outline of Psychoanalysis*. London: Hogarth.

Galef BG Jr., Kaner HC. (1980). Establishment and maintenance of preference for natural and artificial olfactory stimuli in juvenile rats. *J Comp Physiol Psychol* 94(4):588–595.

Gonzalo S, Jaco I, Fraga MF, Chen T, Li E, Esteller M, Blasco MA. (2006). DNA methyltransferases control telomere length and telomere recombination in mammalian cells. *Nat Cell Biol* 8(4):416–424.

Greenberg ME, Xu B, Lu B, Hempstead BL. (2009). New insights in the biology of BDNF synthesis and release: implications in CNS function. *J Neurosci* 29(41):12764–12767.

Grino M, Paulmyer–Lacroix O, Faudon M, Renard M, Anglade G. (1994). Blockade of alpha 2–adrenoceptors stimulates basal and stress–induced adrenocorticotropin secretion in the developing rat through a central mechanism independent from corticotropin–releasing factor and arginine vasopressin. *Endocrinol* 135(6):2549–2557.

Gunnar MR, Quevedo KM, Ronald De Kloet M. (2007). Early care experiences and HPA axis regulation in children: a mechanism for later trauma vulnerability. *Prog Brain Res* 167:137–149.

Haberly LB. (2001). Parallel–distributed processing in olfactory cortex: new insights from morphological and physiological analysis of neuronal circuitry. *Chem Sens* 26(5): 551–576.

Harlow H, Harlow M. (1965). The affectional systems. In: *Behavior of Nonhuman Primates*, A. Schrier, H. Harlow, and F. Stollnitz, pp. 2:287–334. New York: Academic Press.

Haroutunian, V, Campbell BA. (1979). Emergence of interoceptive and exteroceptive control of behavior in rats. *Sci* 205(4409):927–929.

Hennessy MB, Li J, Levine S. (1980). Infant responsiveness to maternal cues in mice of 2 inbred lines. *Dev Psychobiol* 13(1):77–84.

Henning SJ. (1978). Plasma concentrations of total and free corticosterone during development in the rat. *Am J Physiol* 235(5):E451–456.

Hensch TK. (2004). Critical period regulation. *Ann Rev Neurosci* 27(1):549–579.

Hess E. (1962). Ethology: an approach to the complete analysis of behavior. In: *New Directions in Psychology*, R. Brown, E. Galanter, E. Hess, and G. Mendler, pp. 159–199. New York: Holt, Rinehart and Winston.

Hofer MA, Shair H, Singh P. (1976). Evidence that maternal ventral skin substances promote suckling in infant rats. *Physiol Behav* 17(1):131–136.

Howell B, Sanchez M. (2011). Understanding behavioral effects of early life stress using the reactive scope and allostatic load models. *Dev Psychopathol* 23:1001–1016.

Hudson R. (1985). Do newborn rabbits learn the odor stimuli releasing nipple–search behavior? *Dev Psychobiol* 18(6):575–585.

Hudson R, Distel H. (1983). Nipple location by newborn rabbits: behavioral evidence for pheromonal guidance. *Behaviour* 85(260–275).

Keller S, Sarchiapone M, Zarrilli F, Videtic A, Ferraro A, et al. (2010). Increased BDNF promoter methylation in the Wernicke area of suicide subjects. *Arch Gen Psychiat* 67(3):258–267.

Kosten TA, Huang W, Nielsen DA. (2014). Sex and litter effects on anxiety and DNA methylation levels of stress and neurotrophin genes in adolescent rats. *Dev Psychobiol* 56(3):392–406.

Kundakovic M, Lim S, Gudsnuk K, Champagne FA. (2013). Sex–specific and strain–dependent effects of early life adversity on behavioral and epigenetic outcomes. *Front Psychiat* 4.

Labonté B, Suderman M, Maussion G, Navaro L, Yerko V, Mahar I, et al. (2012). Genome–wide epigenetic regulation by early–life trauma. *Arch General Psychiat* 69(7):722–731.

Lecanuet JP, Schaal B. (1996). Fetal sensory competencies. *Eur J Obstet Gyn R B* 68(1–2):1–23.

Leon M. (1992). The neurobiology of filial learning. *Ann Rev Psychol* 43:377–398.

Levine S. (1957). Infantile experience and resistance to physiological stress. *Sci* 126:405.

Levine S. (1962). Plasma–free corticosteroid response to electric shock in rats stimulated in infancy. *Sci* 135:795–796.

Levine S. (2001). Primary social relationships influence the development of the hypothalamic–pituitary–adrenal axis in the rat. *Physiol Behav* 73(3):255–260.

Logan DW, Brunet LJ, Webb WR, Cutforth T, Ngai J, Stowers L. (2012). Learned recognition of maternal signature odors mediates the first suckling episode in mice. *Curr Biol* 22(21):1998–2007.

Lubin FD, Roth TL, Sweatt JD. (2008). Epigenetic regulation of bdnf gene transcription in the consolidation of fear memory. *J Neurosci* 28(42):10576–10586.

Lyons DM, Parker KJ, Schatzberg AF. (2010). Animal models of early life stress: implications for understanding resilience. *Dev Psychobiol* 52(5):402–410.

Maestripieri D, Tomaszycki M, Carroll KA. (1999). Consistency and change in the behavior of rhesus macaque abusive mothers with successive infants. *Dev Psychobiol* 34(1):29–35.

Martinetti MP, Andrzejewski ME, Hineline PN, Lewis MJ. (2000). Ethanol consumption and the matching law: a choice analysis using a limited–access paradigm. *Exp and Clin Psychopharmacol* 8(3):395–403.

McEwen B. (2003). Early life influences on life–long patterns of behavior and health. *Ment Retard Dev D Research Rev* 9(3):149–154.

McGowan PO, Sasaki A, Huang TCT, et al. (2008). Promoter–wide hypermethylation of the ribosomal RNA gene promoter in the suicide brain. *PLoS ONE* 3(5):e2085.

McGowan PO, Sasaki A, D'Alessio AC, et al. (2009). Epigenetic regulation of the glucocorticoid receptor in human brain associates with childhood abuse. *Nat Neurosci* 12(3):342–348.

Mennella JA, Johnson A, Beauchamp GK. (1995). Garlic ingestion by pregnant women alters the odor of amniotic fluid. *Chem Sens* 20(2):207–209.

Moles A, Kieffer BL, D'Amato FR. (2004). Deficit in attachment behavior in mice lacking the mu–opioid receptor gene. *Sci* 304(5679):1983–1986.

Moriceau S, Sullivan RM (2004). Unique neural circuitry for neonatal olfactory learning. *J Neurosci* 24(5):1182–1189.

Moriceau S, Sullivan RM. (2006). Maternal presence serves as a switch between learning fear and attraction in infancy. *Nat Neurosci* 9(8):1004–1006.

Moriceau S, Roth TL, Okotoghaide T, Sullivan RM. (2004). Corticosterone controls the developmental emergence of fear and amygdala function to predator odors in infant rat pups. *Intl J Dev Neurosci* 22(5–6):415–422.

Moriceau S, Wilson DA, Levine S, Sullivan RM. (2006). Dual circuitry for odor–shock conditioning during infancy: corticosterone switches between fear and attraction via amygdala. *J Neurosci* 26(25):6737–6748.

Moriceau S, Shionoya K, Jakubs K, Sullivan RM. (2009). Early–life stress disrupts attachment learning: the role of amygdala corticosterone, locus coeruleus corticotropin releasing hormone, and olfactory bulb norepinephrine. *J Neurosci* 29(50):15745–15755.

Mueller BR, Bale TL. (2008). Sex–specific programming of offspring emotionality after stress early in pregnancy. *J Neurosci* 28(36):9055–9065.

Nakamori T, Maekawa F, Sato K, Tanaka K, Ohki–Hamazaki H. (2013). Neural basis of imprinting behavior in chicks. *Dev Growth Differ* 55(1):198–206.

Nakamura S, Kimura F, Sakaguchi T. (1987). Postnatal development of electrical activity in the locus ceruleus. *J Neurophysiol* 58(3):510–524.

Naumova OY, Lee M, Koposov R, Szyf M, Dozier M, Grigorenko EL. (2012). Differential patterns of whole–genome DNA methylation in institutionalized children and children raised by their biological parents. *Dev Psychopathol* 24(01):143–155.

O'Connor TG, Cameron JL. (2006). Translating research findings on early experience to prevention: animal and human evidence on early attachment relationships. *Am J Preve Med* 31(6 Suppl 1):S175–181.

Park H, Poo MM. (2013). Neurotrophin regulation of neural circuit development and function. *Nat Rev Neurosci* 14(1):7–23.

Perroud N, Salzmann A, Prada P, Nicastro R, et al. (2013). Response to psychotherapy in borderline personality disorder and methylation status of the BDNF gene. *Transl Psychiatry* 3:e207.

Polan HJ, Hofer MA. (1998). Olfactory preference for mother over home nest shavings by newborn rats. *Dev Psychobiol* 33(1):5–20.

Raineki C, Shionoya K, Sander K, Sullivan RM. (2009). Ontogeny of odor–LiCl vs. odor–shock learning: similar behaviors but divergent ages of functional amygdala emergence. *Learn Mem* 16(2):114–121.

Raineki C, Moriceau S, Sullivan RM. (2010). Developing a neurobehavioral animal model of infant attachment to an abusive caregiver. *Biol Psychiatry* 67(12):1137–1145.

Raineki C, Cortés MR, Belnoue L, Sullivan RM. (2012). Effects of early–life abuse differ across development: infant social behavior deficits are followed by adolescent depressive–like behaviors mediated by the amygdala. *J Neurosci* 32(22):7758–7765.

Raineki C, Lucion AB, Weinberg J. (2014). Neonatal handling: an overview of the positive and negative effects. *Dev Psychobiol* 56(8):1613–1625.

Rajecki D, Lamb M, Obmascher P. (1978). Towards a general theory of infantile attachment: a comparative review of aspects of the social bond. *Behav Brain Sci* 3:417–464.

Rice D, Barone S. (2000). Critical periods of vulnerability for the developing nervous system: evidence from humans and animal models. *Environ Health Persp* 108:511–533.

Rincón Cortés M, Barr GA, Mouly AM, Shionoya K, Nunez BS, Sullivan RM. (2015). Enduring good memories of infant trauma: rescue of adult neurobehavioral deficits via amygdala serotonin and corticosterone interaction. *Proc Natl Acad Sci USA* 112:881–886.

Risser JM, Slotnick BM. (1987). Nipple attachment and survival in neonatal olfactory bulbectomized rats. *Physiol Behav* 40(4):545–549.

Rogosch FA, Dackis MN, Cicchetti D. (2011). Child maltreatment and allostatic load: consequences for physical and mental health in children from low–income families. *Dev Psychopathol* 23(4):1107–1124.

Rosenfeld P, Suchecki D, Levine S. (1992). Multifactorial regulation of the hypothalamic pituitary–adrenal axis during development. *Neurosci Biohehav Rev* 16:553–568.

Roth TL, Sullivan RM. (2001). Endogenous opioids and their role in odor preference acquisition and consolidation following odor–shock conditioning in infant rats. *Dev Psychobiol* 39(3):188–198.

Roth TL, Sullivan RM. (2005). Memory of early maltreatment: neonatal behavioral and neural correlates of maternal maltreatment within the context of classical conditioning. *Biol Psychiatry* 57(8):823–831.

Roth TL, Sullivan RM. (2006). Examining the role of endogenous opioids in learned odor–stroke associations in infant rats. *Dev Psychobiol* 48(1):71–78.

Roth TL, Moriceau S, Sullivan RM. (2006). Opioid modulation of Fos protein expression and olfactory circuitry plays a pivotal role in what neonates remember. *Learn Mem* 13(5):590–598.

Roth TL, Lubin FD, Funk AJ, Sweatt JD. (2009). Lasting epigenetic influence of early–life adversity on the BDNF gene. *Biol Psychiatry* 65(9):760–769.

Roth TL, Zoladz PR, Sweatt JD, Diamond DM. (2011). Epigenetic modification of hippocampal Bdnf DNA in adult rats in an animal model of post–traumatic stress disorder. *J Psychiat Res* 45(7):919–926.

Roth TL, Raineki C, Salstein L, et al. (2013). Neurobiology of secure infant attachment and attachment despite adversity: a mouse model. *Genes Brain Behav* 12(7):673–680.

Roth TL, Matt S, Chen K, Blaze J. (2014). Bdnf DNA methylation modifications in the hippocampus and amygdala of male and female rats exposed to different caregiving environments outside the homecage. *Dev Psychobiol* 56(8):1755–1763.

Salzen E. (1970). Imprinting and environmental learning. In: *Development and Evolution of Behavior*, L. Aronson, E. Tobach, D. Lehrman, and J. Rosenblatt, pp. 158–178. San Francisco, W.H. Freeman.

Sanchez M, Ladd C, Plotsky P. (2001). Early adverse experience as a developmental risk factor for later psychopathology: evidence from rodent and primate models. *Dev Psychopathol* 13:419–449.

Sarro EC, Sullivan RM, Barr G. (2014). Unpredictable neonatal stress enhances adult anxiety and alters amygdala gene expression related to serotonin and GABA. *Neurosci* 258:147–161.

Schaal B, Marlier L, Soussignan R. (1995). Responsiveness to the odour of amniotic fluid in the human neonate. *Biol Neonate* 67(6):397–406.

Schwarz JM, Nugent BM, McCarthy MM. (2010). Developmental and hormone–induced epigenetic changes to estrogen and progesterone receptor genes in brain are dynamic across the life span. *Endocrinol* 151(10):4871–4881.

Schwob JE, Price, JL. (1984). The development of axonal connections in the central olfactory system of rats. *J Comp Neurol* 223(2):177–202.

Shalev I, Moffitt TE, Sugden K et al. (2013). Exposure to violence during childhood is associated with telomere erosion from 5 to 10 years of age: a longitudinal study. *Mol Psychiatry* 18(5):576–581.

Smith AK, Conneely KN, Kilaru V, et al. (2011). Differential immune system DNA methylation and cytokine regulation in post–traumatic stress disorder. *Am J Med Genets B* 156(6):700–708.

Spear N. (1978). *Processing Memories: Forgetting and Retention*. Hillsdale, NJ, Erlbaum.

Stanley W. (1962). Differential human handling as reinforcing events and as treatments influencing later social behavior in basenji puppies. *Psychol Rep* 10:775–788.

Stanton M, Levine S. (1990). Inhibition of infant glucocorticoid stress response: specific role of maternal cues. *Dev Psychobiol* 23(5):411–426.

Stanton ME, Wallstrom J, Levine S. (1987). Maternal contact inhibits pituitary-adrenal stress responses in preweanling rats. *Dev Psychobiol* 20(2):131–145.

Stehouwer D, Campbell B. (1978). Habituation of the forelimb-withdrawal response in neonatal rats. *J Exp Psychol Anim B* 4(2):104–119.

Stellern S, Esposito E, Mliner S, Pears K, Gunnar M. (2014). Increased freezing and decreased positive affect in postinstitutionalized children. *J Child Psychol Psychiat* 55(1):88–95.

Stern JM, Weinberg J, Hennessy MB. (2010). From freud to a modern understanding of behavioral, physiological, and brain development. *Dev Psychobiol* 52(7):609–615.

Stowers L, Cameron P, Keller JA. (2013). Ominous odors: olfactory control of instinctive fear and aggression in mice. *Curr Opin Neurobiol* 23(3):339–345.

Suchecki D, Rosenfeld P, Levine S. (1993). Maternal regulation of the hypothalamic–pituitary–adrenal axis in the infant rat: the roles of feeding and stroking. *Brain Res Dev Brain Res* 75(2):185–192.

Sullivan RM, Holman PJ. (2010). Transitions in sensitive period attachment learning in infancy: the role of corticosterone. *Neurosci Biobehav Rev* 34(6):835–844.

Sullivan RM, Toubas P. (1998). Clinical usefulness of maternal odor in newborns: soothing and feeding preparatory responses. *Biol Neonate* 74(6):402–408.

Sullivan RM, Hofer MA, Brake SC. (1986). Olfactory–guided orientation in neonatal rats is enhanced by a conditioned change in behavioral state. *Dev Psychobiol* 19(6):615–623.

Sullivan RM, Wilson DA, Wong R, Correa A, Leon M. (1990). Modified behavioral and olfactory bulb responses to maternal odors in preweanling rats. *Brain Res Dev Brain Res* 53(2):243–247.

Sullivan RM, Zyzak D, Skierkowski P, Wilson DA. (1992). The role of olfactory bulb norepinephrine in early olfactory learning. *Brain Res Dev Brain Res* 70(2):279–282.

Sullivan RM, Landers M, Yeaman B, Wilson DA. (2000a). Good memories of bad events in infancy. *Nat* 407(6800):38–39.

Sullivan RM, Stackenwalt G, Nasr F, Lemon C, Wilson DA. (2000b). Association of an odor with activation of olfactory bulb noradrenergic beta–receptors or locus coeruleus stimulation is sufficient to produce learned approach responses to that odor in neonatal rats. *Behav Neurosci* 114(5):957–962.

Sullivan RM, Raineki C, Barr GA. (2011). Enduring effects of infant attachment induced by odor–shock conditioning: adult depressive–like behaviors and amygdala gene expression normalized by infant odor. *Soc Neurosci Abstracts* 614.11.

Suomi SJ. (2003). Gene–environment interactions and the neurobiology of social conflict. *Ann NY Acad Sci* 1008(1):132–139.

Swanson LW, Petrovich GD. (1998). What is the amygdala? *Trends Neurosci* 21(8):323–331.

Takahashi LK. (1994). Organizing action of corticosterone on the development of behavioral inhibition in the preweanling rat. *Dev Brain Res* 81(1):121–127.

Teicher MH, Blass EM. (1977). First suckling response of the newborn albino rat: the roles of olfaction and amniotic fluid. *Sci* 198(4317):635–636.

Teicher MH, Flaum LE, Williams M, Eckhert SJ, Lumia AR. (1978). Survival, growth and suckling behavior of neonatally bulbectomized rats. *Physiol Behav* 21(4):553–561.

Teicher MH, Andersen SL, Polcari A, Anderson CM, Navalta CP, Kim DM. (2003). The neurobiological consequences of early stress and childhood maltreatment. *Neurosci Biobehav Rev* 27(1–2):33–44.

Thompson JV, Sullivan RM, Wilson DA. (2008). Developmental emergence of fear learning corresponds with changes in amygdala synaptic plasticity. *Brain Res* 1200C:58–65.

Toth SL, Cicchetti D. (2011). Frontiers in translational research on trauma. *Dev Psychopathol* 23(2):353–355.

Tottenham N, Hare TA, Quinn BT, et al. (2010). Prolonged institutional rearing is associated with atypically large amygdala volume and difficulties in emotion regulation. *Dev Sci* 13(1):46–61.

Tyrka AR, Price LH, Kao HT, Porton B, Marsella SA, Carpenter LL. (2010). Childhood maltreatment and telomere shortening: preliminary support for an effect of early stress on cellular aging. *Biol Psychiatry* 67(6):531–534.

Tyrka AR, Price LH, Marsit C, Walters OC, Carpenter LL. (2012). Childhood adversity and epigenetic modulation of the leukocyte glucocorticoid receptor: preliminary findings in healthy adults. *PloS One* 7(1):e30148.

Uddin M, Galea S, Chang SC, et al. (2011). Gene expression and methylation signatures of MAN2C1 are associated with PTSD. *Dis Markers* 30(2):111–121.

Unternaehrer E, Luers P, Mill J, et al. (2012). Dynamic changes in DNA methylation of stress–associated genes (OXTR, BDNF) after acute psychosocial stress. *Transl Psychiatry* 2:e150.

Upton KJ, Sullivan RM. (2010). Defining age limits of the sensitive period for attachment learning in rat pups. *Dev Psychobiol* 52(5):453–464.

Varendi H, Porter RH, Winberg J. (1996). Attractiveness of amniotic fluid odor: evidence of prenatal olfactory learning? *Acta Paediatr* 85(10):1223–1227.

von Zglinicki T. (2002). Oxidative stress shortens telomeres. *Trends Biochem Sci* 27(7):339–344.

Walker C, Sapolsky R, Meaney M, Vale W, Rivier C. (1986). Increased pituitary sensitivity to glucocorticoid feedback during the stress nonresponsive period in the neonatal rat. *Endocrinol* 119(4):1816–1821.

Weaver ICG, Cervoni N, Champagne FA, D'Alessio AC, Sharma S, Seckl JS, Dymov S, Szyf M, Meaney MJ. (2004). Epigenetic programming by maternal behavior. *Nat Neurosci* 7(8):847–854.

Wilson DA, Stevenson RJ. (2003). Olfactory perceptual learning: the critical role of memory in odor discrimination. *Neurosci Biobehav Rev* 27(4):307–328.

Winzer–Serhan UH, Raymon HK, Broide RS, Chen Y, Leslie FM. (1996). Expression of $\alpha 2$ adrenoceptors during rat brain development – II. $\alpha 2C$ messenger RNA expression and [3H]rauwolscine binding. *Neurosci* 76(1):261–272.

Yuan Q, Harley CW, Bruce JC, Darby–King A, McLean JH. (2000). Isoproterenol increases CREB phosphorylation and olfactory nerve–evoked potentials in normal and 5–HT–depleted olfactory bulbs in rat pups only at doses that produce odor prference learning. *Learn Mem* 7(6):413–421.

Yuan Q, Harley CW, McLean JH, Knöpfel T. (2002). Optical imaging of odor preference memory in the rat olfactory bulb. *J Neurophysiol* 87(6):3156–3159.

Zhang P, Dilley C, Mattson MP. (2007). DNA damage responses in neural cells: focus on the telomere. *Neurosci* 145(4):1439–1448.

Zhou J, Ding D, Wang M, Cong YS. (2014). Telomerase reverse transcriptase in the regulation of gene expression. *BMB Rep* 47:8–14.

CHAPTER 7

Early environmental manipulations and long-term effects on brain neurotrophin levels

Francesca Cirulli and Enrico Alleva

Section of Behavioral Neurosciences, Department of Cell Biology and Neurosciences, Istituto Superiore di Sanità, Rome, Italy

Introduction

The development of the mammalian brain involves a complex series of precisely timed events, directing the creation of the intricate neural circuitry that controls behavior. The pattern of connections present during prenatal development is only a rough approximation of the final wiring characterizing the adult brain. During development there is a continuous refinement of brain circuits through activity-dependent mechanisms that match the presynaptic neurons to their appropriate target cells. Indeed, the developing mammalian brain is "experience-sensitive" and "experience-dependent" and provided by high levels of plasticity allowing a fine-tuning of the external environment and the developing organism. While plasticity is certainly an advantageous characteristic, it can create a window of vulnerability for the developing nervous system. When adverse conditions occur, these can hinder brain maturation, leading to brain damage or susceptibility to psychiatric or neurodegenerative disorders (Cirulli et al., 2003).

One of the best examples of this concept comes from the study of the primary visual cortex, which has led to the collection of a wealth of information on brain plasticity and its regulation by experience (Wiesel and Hubel, 1963; Hensch, 2004). Studies addressing the timing, duration, and closure of these critical periods characterized by intense brain plasticity in the developing visual system have indicated that synaptic competition for the input from the eyes is able to shape cortical circuits (Hensch, 2004). A brief closure of one eye during such critical periods of visual system plasticity causes a pronounced shift of response preference of cortical neurons toward the open eye. This is one of the best-explained models of the importance of experience for the developing brain. Lack of input

Environmental Experience and Plasticity of the Developing Brain, First Edition.
Edited by Alessandro Sale.

from one eye – for example, following its closure – causes a permanent loss of visual acuity through the deprived eye (amblyopia), indicating the damaging effects of lack of sensory experience during developmental stages in which input is required for brain structuring (Berardi et al., 2000; Hensch, 2004).

Long-term effects of infantile stimulation on brain plasticity

It has been long recognized that early experiences can shape brain development. Seymour Levine has pioneered the field of studies of early experiences, producing an impressive amount of research clearly showing that stressful events can exert important long-term effects on brain development often lasting throughout the entire lifespan, influencing brain function and increasing the risk for depression and anxiety disorders (Levine, 1957). Studies performed in altricial rodents (e.g., mice and rats) have indicated that the mother–infant relationship is crucial for an adequate development of the offspring, representing the most relevant source of early stimulation: disrupting the maternal-infant relationship leads to long-term changes in the pattern of neuroendocrine and emotional/behavioral responses later in life (Levine, 1957). In his original work Levine has clearly shown that simple manipulations of the nest environment, such as removing rat pups from the mother and placing them in a novel compartment for up to 15 minutes until weaning (handling, H) has a profound effect on their stress physiology and their response to challenges in a way such that the ability of the adult organism to respond, cope, and adapt to novel and/or stressful stimuli is increased (Levine, 1957; Meaney et al., 1991). As a result of these early manipulations, immediately after the exposure to an electric shock, H rats (tested at adulthood) show a faster peak in the release of the stress hormones (glucocorticoids, GC), and a rapid return to basal levels when compared to nonhandled controls. The speed and short duration of the neuroendocrine response of H subjects is extremely adaptive preventing the organism from being exposed to high circulating GCs levels that can result, especially under chronic stressful conditions, in neurotoxicity through different mechanisms (Lupien et al., 1998). The long-term effects of the H procedure appear to depend upon changes in the phenotype of those neurons involved in the stress response (Meaney et al., 1996). As an example H subjects show an increased number of GR expression in the hippocampus, a brain region strongly implicated in GCs feedback regulation (Meaney et al., 1989). Longer periods of separation, however, result in decreased GR binding in both the hippocampus and the hypothalamus (Plotsky and Meaney, 1993).

Following up on these studies, many researchers have replicated these effects and showed that increasing the time pups spend away from the mother leads to opposite results compared to brief separations (Cirulli et al., 2003). It appears however that, as though handling always results in decreased emotionality at adulthood, longer intervals of separation of the pups, also known as "maternal separation" are not such a robust phenomenon and do not always lead to opposite effects. In one of our studies we compared these two paradigms and investigated the expression of the calcium binding proteins (CBPs) calretinin, calbindin and parvalbumin, which identify subpopulations of GABAergic neurons and serve important functional roles by buffering intracellular calcium levels, following brief (15 minute) and long (3 hour) periods of maternal separation, as compared to nonhandled controls (Giachino et al., 2007). CBP expressing neurons were analyzed in brain regions related to stress and anxiety. Emotionality was assessed in parallel using the social interaction test. Analyses were carried out at periadolescence, an important phase for the development of brain areas involved in stress responses. Our results indicate that density of CBP-immunoreactive neurons decreases in the paraventricular region of deprived rats but increases in the hippocampus and lateral amygdala of both early handled and deprived rats when compared to controls. Emotionality was reduced in both early handled and deprived animals. In conclusion, early handling and deprivation lead to neurochemical and behavioral changes linked to stress-sensitive brain regions. These data suggest that the effects of early experiences on CBP containing neurons might contribute to the functional changes of neuronal circuits involved in the emotional response, such as the GABAergic system (Giachino et al., 2007). This is apparently in contrast to several studies suggesting that brief versus long maternal separations result in different effects, respectively decreasing or increasing fear-related behavior and endocrine responses to stress (Francis and Meaney, 1999). It must be pointed out, that other reports have described that both handling and maternal deprivation have the same effects on the formation of neural circuits providing limbic and cortical control over autonomic emotional motor output. In addition, data in the literature suggest that both manipulations are able to stimulate maternal care to a similar degree (Pryce et al., 2001).

An important lesson that was learned from these studies – one that the former studies of Levine had already demonstrated – is that lack of any manipulation appears to be the most dramatic form of deprivation for the developing infant (Levine, 1957). A general chronic state of under-stimulation can induce neurochemical changes in the brain comparable to those induced by prenatal stress, resulting in increased stress responsiveness and emotionality at adulthood (Pryce and Feldon, 2003) (Figure 7.1).

Neurotrophins and brain plasticity

Neurotrophins (NTs) are involved in activity-dependent synaptic competition (Cellerino and Maffei, 1996). Originally, NTs were described as a family of growth factors promoting neuronal growth, differentiation, and survival. They

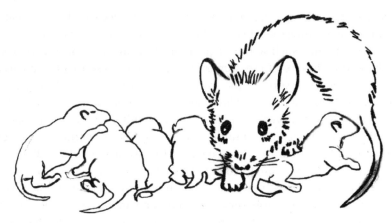

Figure 7.1 The mother–infant relationship is fundamental for brain and behavioral development of the offspring. The mother provides nourishment and produces a sensory-tactile stimulation that stimulates brain growth through maternal behaviors such as licking and grooming.

are clustered into families of structurally and functionally related molecules (Barde, 1990). The nerve growth factor (NGF) superfamily, for example, includes NGF, brain-derived neurotrophic factor (BDNF), neurotrophin-3 (NT-3), neurotrophin-4/5 (NT-4/5), and neurotrophin-6 (NT-6). NGF was discovered in the 1950s as a key player in target-mediated regulation of peripheral innervation (Levi–Montalcini, 1987). The concept of cell death was first formulated on the bases of the work performed by Victor Hamburger and Rita Levi-Montalcini investigating the role of the target tissue on the incoming innervation (Levi-Montalcini and Hamburger, 1951). The main concept arising from this work was that the nervous system shows an initial redundancy in the number of cells that are subsequently dealt with by the ensuing of a remarkable amount of neuronal death. Through a series of fascinating studies Rita Levi-Montalcini identified the target as key to the development of neuronal connections, the extent of innervation depending upon the supply of limited amounts of NTs. This mechanism allows the selection of those neurons capable to establish strong connections with the target. Subsequent studies have demonstrated that, during the development of the nervous system, NGF is released by the target tissue, taken up in responsive neurons and transported retrogradely to the cell body where it exerts its trophic/differentiative effects (Thoenen and Barde, 1980: Meakin and Shooter, 1992).

NGF has subsequently been one of the most thoroughly studied NTs, regulating the survival, development and trophism of specific neuronal populations in the peripheral and central nervous system (Levi-Montalcini and Angeletti, 1968). NGF, as all other NTs, binds with low affinity to a membrane spanning receptor molecule, known as the low-affinity NGF receptor that does not possess a cytoplasmatic kinase domain for signal transduction (p75NTR) (Meakin and

Shooter, 1992). The trophic effect of all neurotrophins, including NGF, requires binding to recognition molecules of the tyrosine kinase (Trk) family of receptors activated in response to neurotrophin binding, although Trk-independent signal transduction through p75NTR can also occur (Meakin and Shooter, 1992; Roux and Barker, 2002). NGF preferentially binds to TrkA, BDNF and NT-4/5 to TrkB and NT-3 to TrkC. Trk receptors display intracellular, transmembrane and extracellular domains, and transduce neurotrophin signaling through autophosphorylation, subsequently resulting in increased tyrosine phosphorylation of cellular proteins (Patapoutian and Reichardt, 2001). While the p75NTR can cause apoptosis in a variety of systems, when co-expressed with the appropriate Trk proteins, it can modify their ligand-binding activity, dose-responsiveness and kinase activity, leading to increased survival, neurite outgrowth and synaptic plasticity (Chao and Bothwell, 2002; Dechant and Barde, 2002). Some evidence indicates that NGF and BDNF may be secreted as pro-peptides, which often have biological effects opposite to those of mature neurotrophins, having a high affinity for p75NTR and inducing apoptosis in cultured neurons (Lee et al., 2001). This piece of data suggests that the balance between cell survival and cell death might depend upon the relative quantity of mature vs. pro-NTs available to cells expressing TRK and p75NTR receptors.

NGF acts as a trophic factor for cholinergic neurons since its administration in vivo increases the levels of choline acetyltransferase (Mobley et al., 1985). In addition, after transection of the septo-hippocampal pathways (a model of central cholinergic pathway) it rescues basal forebrain neurons from death (Korsching et al., 1986). BDNF, originally purified from pig brain (Barde et al., 1982) is more abundantly expressed and widely distributed than NGF in the CNS, acting as a trophic factor for dopaminergic neurons, in addition to cholinergic cells (Knusel et al., 1991). In addition to being retrogradely transported, BDNF is also anterogradely transported in the CNS and acts as both a target-derived neurotrophic factor and an autocrine/paracrine modulator. At the synapse BDNF has been shown to play an important role in long-term potentiation (LTP) (Kafitz et al., 1999; Lu and Chow, 1999; Pang et al., 2004). As an activity-dependent NT, with receptors densely distributed throughout the CNS, BDNF clearly has emerged as a major regulator of synaptic plasticity (Castren, 2004).

Neurotrophins as transducers of early experiences

NTs, such as NGF and BDNF, play a pivotal role in brain development and plasticity representing good candidates for mediating some of the effects triggered by early experiences on brain function.

It has been well demonstrated that, in the CNS, NTs are synthesized predominantly by neurons in an activity-dependent manner and that they are released upon neuronal depolarization. In vivo and in vitro studies have clearly shown that the activity-dependent regulation of NTs is mediated by classical neurotransmitters. Glutamate, via N-methyl-D-aspartate (NMDA) and non-NMDA receptors, as well as acetylcholine, via muscarinic receptors, can upregulate expression of neurotrophins (Zafra et al., 1990; Lindholm et al., 1994). While glutamate receptor stimulation increases NGF mRNA expression, gamma-aminobutyric acid (GABA) downregulates it. This regulation not only functions under extreme experimental conditions, such a kindling, but is also involved in the maintenance of physiological levels of NTs (Gall and Isackson, 1989). In addition, physiological stimuli, such as visual input, regulate neurotrophin mRNA levels in the rat visual cortex (Castren et al., 1992). Activity-dependent expression of BDNF has been shown to regulate cortical inhibition and duration of the critical period for visual cortical plasticity (Cellerino and Maffei, 1996). NTs effects on synaptic plasticity have been described as "very rapid local modes" since they do not require activation of gene transcription, being elicited within seconds from their application. There is evidence for short-term modulation of synaptic transmission by NTs as well as structural changes in axons and dendrites underlying plastic rearrangements in the nervous system (McAllister et al., 1999). Because of its action on neurite outgrowth, NGF seems especially well suited in determining structural changes in brain circuits, especially during early developmental periods when target innervation is still incomplete.

NTs are also able to control dendritic growth in a highly specific fashion (McAllister et al., 1999). Autocrine and paracrine roles for NTs have been described: if NTs can increase neuronal activity, this can, in turn, positively feed back on their production and release. Thus, positive loops between NTs and electrical activity could modify neuronal phenotype (Thoenen, 1995). NT receptor functions are also regulated in an activity-dependent manner. As an example, neuronal activity regulates the synthesis and the intracellular targeting of TrkB receptors (Lu, 2003). Therefore, both BDNF release and TrkB receptor expression must take place in a coordinated fashion at the relevant synaptic sites for an optimal synaptic response to occur. BDNF influences synaptic plasticity as a mature protein via the TrkB receptor signaling pathway; however, it needs to be mentioned here that proBDNF-p75NTR and the mature BDNF-TrkB signaling may exert opposite effects on spine density and morphology, although the physiological relevance of this effect of proBDNF has to be verified (Yang et al., 2009).

BDNF is capable of changing functional synaptic properties both in developing and in mature neurons. In addition, due to its effects on neurite outgrowth and differentiation of certain subtypes of neurons, BDNF has been implicated in numerous processes of functional and structural synaptic plasticity, such as sculpting the function and structure of synapses (Zagrebelsky and Korte, 2014). Synthesis and release of BDNF is induced by neuronal activity with

TrkB activation leading to the stabilization of axonal and dendritic branches and strengthening of active synaptic connections (Lu and Chow, 1999). In excitatory neurons of the mature CNS BDNF seems to be specifically involved in the fine-tuning of mature dendritic spine structure and possibly in the structural changes at spines upon activity-dependent plasticity (Zagrebelsky and Korte, 2014). This neurotrophin is most likely an instructive mediator of functional plasticity at synapses in the CNS. The evidence is especially good in the context of hippocampal LTP as BDNF increases neurotransmitter release and is able to change the excitation-inhibition balance by various means, for example, weakening GABAergic influence on excitatory neurons. In addition, while most of the data supporting a role for this trophic factor in modulating dendrite and dendritic spine morphology derive from experiments applying exogenous BDNF, data also suggest a role for endogenous BDNF in this context. Genetic approaches have indeed shown that homozygous as well as heterozygous BDNF knockout mice exhibit a marked reduction in LTP that can be rescued by adenovirus-mediated local overexpression of BDNF (Patterson, et al., 1996).

The effects of endogenous BDNF in modulating the structure of neurons seem to be extremely specific, depending on the developmental stage, the brain area as well as the cell-type. Indeed, there is ample evidence showing that BDNF controls the development of GABAergic neurons and the development of the neuronal structure of inhibitory neurons (Marty et al., 1996), a role especially important as it could well have long-term consequences on adult neuronal architecture. The analysis of hippocampal morphology in haploinsufficient BDNF mice (bdnf+/−) shows a significant decrease in total hippocampal volume associated to shorter and simplified CA3 apical dendritic trees suggestive for a role of BDNF in modulating neuronal architecture of hippocampal pyramidal neurons (Magarinos et al., 2011).

While BDNF is still a prime candidate for ensuring that changes in the form follow changes in the function of neurons as cellular correlates of learning and memory formation, more work is still needed to clarify which role endogenous BDNF exerts in a specific learning situation in vivo (Zagrebelsky and Korte, 2014).

Because of the fundamental role played by NTs in shaping brain function, impairments in any of the critical functions supported by neurotrophins are likely to contribute to a wide array of neurodevelopmental, neurodegenerative, and neuropsychiatric diseases (Li and Pozzo–Miller, 2014). As an example, much evidence has indicated a reduction in BDNF levels in MeCP2-based mouse models of Rett syndrome, the leading cause of intellectual disabilities in women world-wide, which becomes significant with the appearance of Rett-like features (Percy and Lane, 2005). Rett syndrome is a neurodevelopmental disorder that primarily affects girls, most of whom have mutations in the transcription regulatory gene MECP2. Conditional deletion of BDNF in postnatal forebrain excitatory neurons results in several phenotypes similar to those of Mecp2 knockout mice, such as hind limb clasping, decreased brain weight, and smaller olfactory and hippocampal neurons (Chang et al., 2006).

Overall, these data underline the importance of maintaining appropriate levels of NTs early during development for the correct development of the nervous system, strengthening the notion that any event affecting these regulations can have important long-term effects on brain function and on the susceptibility to psychiatric disorders.

Neurotrophins as transducers of stressful events

Early life stressful events, such as childhood trauma and neglect, could synergize with genetic susceptibility to create a long-term vulnerability for psychiatric disorders (Cirulli, 2001; Cirulli et al., 2003; Allcva and Francia, 2008; Cirulli and Alleva, 2009; Cirulli et al., 2009a). Many psychiatric disorders can be accounted for by a "two hit model" in which genetic and/or environmental factors disrupt early CNS development leading to vulnerability to a "second hit," in turn leading to the onset of psychiatric symptoms. This increased vulnerability is often associated to sustained changes in the hypothalamic-pituitary-adrenal (HPA) activity, producing enduring changes in stress physiology and emotional behavior. The signaling pathways activated by NTs and involved in cell survival and differentiation could be targets for a "first hit" during early development. These same pathways, responsible for brain plasticity, may be targets for a "second hit" in the adolescent or adult brain. Thus, if the same pathways in both the developing and the mature organism appear as targets of stress, we have a way of integrating genetic, developmental, and environmental factors that contribute to vulnerability and pathogenesis of psychopathology.

Since numerous data suggest that NT-mediated neuronal plasticity is a critical factor in mood disorders and in their therapy, alterations in neurotrophin levels as a result of exposure to stressful events at adulthood could interact synergistically with epigenetic changes caused by early stress, leading to greater susceptibility for stress-related psychiatric disorders (Duman and Monteggia, 2006; Castren et al., 2007; Alleva and Francia, 2008; Cirulli et al., 2009a).

Stress early in life may result in altered brain development and lead to a persistent sensitization of limbic circuits to even mild stress at adulthood, forming the basis for a greater susceptibility for mood and anxiety disorders. Numerous studies performed in rodents have indicated that NTs are sensitive to the stress of maternal separation and to changes in the rearing environment and that environmental stimulation can have both short- and long-term effects on NT levels (Pham et al., 1997; Cirulli et al., 1998; Cirulli et al., 2000; Cirulli, 2001; Cancedda et al., 2004; Roceri et al., 2004; Branchi et al., 2006; Cirulli et al., 2009a, 2009b).

Data from ours and other laboratories indicate that, while milder manipulations could promote neural plasticity, chronic stressful conditions could sensitize limbic circuits to stress, decreasing brain plasticity and leading to greater suscepti-bility to psychopathology (Cirulli, 2003; Cirulli and Alleva, 2009). As an example, separating mother and infant for brief periods of time leads to an increase in NGF expression in the hippocampus, cerebral cortex and hypothalamus in a time-dependent manner, an effect that might indicate a protective response to an adverse event (Cirulli et al., 1998; Cirulli et al., 2000). Longer periods of mater-nal separation (24 hours) result in increased rate of cell death in the neocortex, white matter, and granule cells of the dentate gyrus in 12-day-old rats (Zhang et al., 2002). Recent reports also indicate that at later life stages, such as postnatal day 30, responses to maternal separation lead to opposite effects, for example, a decrease in both NGF and BDNF in the ventral hippocampus (Dimatelis et al., 2014).

Communal nesting consists in more than one female building a common nest, a condition that, when reproduced in the laboratory, results in increased mater-nal behavior and increased interaction between peers (Branchi et al., 2013). Increased BDNF levels in association with reduced neurogenesis and increased depression-like behavior have been found following chronic communal nesting in CD-1 mice (Branchi et al., 2006), indicating that this neurotrophin is sen-sitive to an increase in social stimuli. A condition that is meant to reproduce a detrimental environment, such as daily maternal separations of 3 hours between mother and pups performed over the first 2 postnatal weeks, is also able to affect BDNF mRNA levels in limbic regions of rats (Roceri et al., 2004). Interestingly, different short- and long-term effects can be demonstrated with this manipu-lation: BDNF gene expression is increased shortly (on postnatal day 17) after maternal deprivation stress in the prefrontal cortex and hippocampus, while at adulthood a long-term depression in the expression of this neurotrophin in the prefrontal cortex can be found (Roceri et al., 2004). Although data on protein levels are not available, these changes in BDNF expression are also associated with impaired HPA axis responses to chronic swimming stress (Roceri et al., 2004). More recent data obtained in heterozygous null BDNF mice argue for an increased sensitivity to early environmental influences in mice with reduced BDNF function and support the important role of this neurotrophic factor in the developmental plasticity of brain circuits controlling anxiety (Carola and Gross, 2010).

We have been able to generalize these results to nonhuman primates show-ing that increased levels of NGF and BDNF in the circulation characterize sub-jects undergoing maternal deprivation from birth (Cirulli et al., 2009a). In line with the rodent model, BDNF levels measured in the peripheral circulation were increased in response to the stress provided by maternal deprivation. However, differently from rodents, changes in BDNF were found only in females, indepen-dently from HPA axis activity, and were accompanied by depressive-like behav-ior. This piece of data is especially interesting since, so far, only very few animal models have been sensitive enough to discriminate gender differences in the response to stress before puberty (Barr et al., 2004), and none reporting changes in BDNF, underlying the usefulness of this nonhuman primate model.

Haploinsufficiency of BDNF goes along with decreased peripheral BDNF levels as well as childhood-onset obesity (Han et al., 2008). Although this genetic variant is rare, as are several other coding region variants (Licinio et al., 2009), there is also a frequent nonsynonymous single-nucleotide polymorphism (SNP), which results in an aminoacid substitution in the pro-BDNF domain (rs6265, Val66Met). Met allele carriers have attenuated intracellular trafficking and secretion of BDNF and show comparatively lower hippocampal gray matter and poorer cognitive performance (Egan et al., 2003). Not surprisingly, this SNP has been tested for association with a wide range of psychiatric disorders. Rs6265 has been associated with substance abuse, eating disorders and schizophrenia (Verhagen et al., 2010). G×E interactions might add a further level of complexity, as it was shown that the Met allele interacts with severe life events thereby causing psychiatric symptoms (Kaufman et al., 2000; Savitz et al., 2007), also in interaction with serotonin transporter-linked polymorphic region (5-HTTLPR) (Kaufman et al., 2006; Wichers et al., 2008).

Taken together, there is thus ample evidence that rs6265 both predicts peripheral BDNF levels and interacts with life stress to increase the risk for depression, making this SNP a prime biomarker for susceptibility to psychopathology in humans, including depression. The precise interplay between rs6265 and life stress, however, cannot readily be tested in humans and strategies, such as variant BDNF mouse models (BDNF Met/Met), that reproduce phenotypic hallmarks characterizing humans with the variant allele (Chen et al., 2006), although of great advantage, bear the disadvantage of suboptimal behavioral repertoires that do not mirror well human psychopathology.

We have described for the first time a rhesus macaque single nucleotide polymorphism (SNP) that produces a Val to Met transition in the pro-BDNF domain. This polymorphism affects peripheral BDNF levels in a G×E manner, with Met allele carriers that were peer-reared displaying significantly lower peripheral levels of this neurotrophin as compared to Val allele carriers raised the same way (Cirulli et al., 2011). These data are in line with results from a variant BDNF mouse model in which the presence of the Met allele does not affect basal BDNF secretion but results in a 30% deficit in activity-dependent release of BDNF-Met from neurons (Chen et al., 2006). Since an increase in BDNF levels is an index of a coping response to stress, we believe that the presence of the Met allele might thwart such a response, thus endangering plasticity processes.

It is well established that alterations of the serotoninergic system may contribute to the pathophysiology of mood disorders. BDNF and serotonin (5-hydroxytryptamine, 5-HT) are two seemingly distinct signaling systems that play regulatory roles in many neuronal functions including survival, neurogenesis, and synaptic plasticity. A common feature of the two systems is their ability to regulate the development and plasticity of neural circuits involved in mood disorders, such as depression and anxiety. BDNF promotes the survival and differentiation of 5-HT neurons. Conversely, administration of antidepressant selective serotonin reuptake inhibitors (SSRIs) enhances BDNF gene expression. There is also evidence for a synergism between the two systems in affective behaviors and genetic epistasis between BDNF and the serotonin transporter genes (Martinowich and Lu, 2008). Accordingly, it has been demonstrated that genetic deletion of the serotonin transporter (SERT) in rodents leads to an anxious and depressive phenotype, which is also associated with reduced neuronal plasticity (Calabrese et al., 2013). In these studies, BDNF expression was reduced at birth and the magnitude of these changes became more pronounced starting from PND21, being sustained by epigenetic mechanisms as well as alterations in the expression of specific transcription factors. These results suggest that an impairment of SERT may affect BDNF expression throughout postnatal development. These early changes may increase stress susceptibility during critical windows of brain maturation, which may eventually lead to the heightened predisposition to mood disorders found in individual carrying genetic variants of the serotonin transporter (Calabrese et al., 2013).

Clinical studies also indicate a three-way interaction effect of 5-HTTLPR, BDNF Val66Met and childhood adversity on depression (Comasco et al., 2013). Family maltreatment, sexual abuse and depression were self-reported by an adolescent population-based cohort from Sweden. Neither 5-HTTLPR or BDNF genotypes separately, nor in interaction with each other, had any relation to depression, however in an environment-adjusted model a two-way interaction and a three-way interaction effect were found. Both 5-HTTLPR and BDNF Val66Met interacted with an unfavourable environment in relation to depressive symptoms. Depressive symptoms and depression were more common among carriers of either the ss/sl+Val/Val or the ll+Met genotypes in the presence of early life adversities, an effect more pronounced among girls.

Overall, increased levels of BDNF characterize acute responses to stressful events -including maternal separation- early during postnatal life, decreased expression being more reliably found at adulthood in response to a wide array of stressful stimuli. Although lower levels of BDNF characterize depressed patients, an increase in BDNF levels early on may modify the GABAergic system and contribute to the generation of individual differences in stress neurocircuitry, providing a substrate for altered vulnerability to depressive disorders at adulthood (Nair et al., 2007). Important interactions with the genetic background occur, which need to be taken into account to fully appreciate the effects of stressful conditions on both short- and long-term neural plasticity and susceptibility to psychiatric disorders. Ultimately, the timing, chronicity and environmental context of stressful stimuli in relationship with the genetic background are crucial variables in determining the effects on NTs and could help explain some controversial data found in the literature.

Windows of opportunity: environmental enrichment as a means to achieve a fine-tuning of brain plasticity and of social and emotional behavior

Recent studies on animal models and clinical trials have provided exciting evidence that intervention strategies boosting brain plasticity in adulthood may allow the reinstatement of brain plasticity (Castren, 2005).

Environmental enrichment (EE) has long been exploited to investigate the influence of the environment on brain structure and function. Robust morphological and functional effects elicited by EE at the neuronal level accompany improvements in cognitive performance. Recently, EE has been shown to accelerate the development of the visual system and to enhance visual-cortex plasticity in adulthood. These new findings highlight the potential of EE as a promising noninvasive strategy to ameliorate deficits in the maturation of the nervous system and to promote recovery of normal sensory functions in pathological conditions affecting the adult brain (Sale et al., 2009).

It has been suggested that differences in maternal behavior between enriched and nonenriched conditions could contribute to the earliest effects of enriched environment on brain development and that neurotrophins, particularly BDNF, might be involved indicating a positive effect of postnatal maternal care on brain development mediated through BDNF (Sale et al., 2004).

In agreement with these findings, active pup manipulations in the form of handling have been shown to favor behavioral and neural plasticity resulting in the maintenance of a high level of arousal and in increased neurotrophin levels in response to an acute manipulation (Cirulli et al., 2007). These studies clearly indicate that mild manipulations during the first 2 postnatal weeks have an effect opposite to that of stress, resulting in increased maternal behavior and increased hippocampal levels of NGF – this neurotrophin being potentially involved in the appraisal of subtle changes in the early social environment (Cirulli et al., 2007). Environmental enrichment during the peri-pubertal period has also been shown to completely reverse the effects of maternal separation on both HPA and behavioral responses to stress thus compensating the neural effects of early life adversity (Francis et al., 2002).

While pre- or postnatal stress can lead to impaired behavioral performance in learning and memory tasks in rats, pre- or postnatal enriched housing improves behavioral performance. These experience-dependent behavioral alterations are consistent with changes in 5-bromo-2'-deoxyuridine-labeled (BrdU) cell number in the granule cell layer of the hippocampus and in the expression level of synaptic markers, such as neuronal cell adhesion molecule, synaptophysin, and BDNF (Koo et al., 2003).

Communal nesting can be considered as another form of enrichment (Branchi et al., 2011a; Branchi et al., 2013): being reared in a CN affects adult behavior of CD-1 mice in a gender-dependent fashion, with reduced depression-like responses in females and increased anxiety-like behavior in males. Findings from these studies show that gender and early experiences interact in modulating adult behavior. In particular, early experiences modify developmental trajectories shaping adult endophenotypes of depression more markedly in females than in males (D'Andrea et al., 2010). At adulthood, CN-reared mice, compared to mice reared in standard nesting laboratory condition (SN), show an increase in BDNF protein levels and longer survival of BrdU-positive cells in the hippocampus. Open field and elevated plus maze results indicate that CN mice, although showing levels of exploratory and locomotor activity similar to those of SN mice, display increased anxiety-like behavior, performing more thigmotaxis in the open field and spending less time in the open arms of the plus maze. Furthermore, CN mice displayed higher levels of immobility behavior in the forced swim test. Overall, these findings show that CN, an highly stimulating early social environment, increases adult neuronal plasticity, as suggested by high BDNF levels and augmented number of newly generated cells in the hippocampus, which is associated to an increased anxiety- and depression-like behavior (Branchi et al., 2006). It is important to stress here that findings related to the forced swim test depend highly upon the specific protocol applied. In particular, it can be shown that when subjects are tested after acute antidepressant administration, both SN and CN mice decreased the immobility duration. This indicates that, when experimental subjects are tested according to the standardized protocol, both groups behave as expected (Branchi et al., 2010).

BDNF has a complex genomic structure rendering it an ideal target for multiple and complex transcriptional regulation (Lu, 2003). Multiple upstream promoters, each individually regulated, drive a short 50 exon that is alternatively spliced onto a common 30 exon, which encodes the pre-proBDNF protein. Evidence now indicates that the promoters of individual transcripts are regulated by diverse and varied physiological stimuli, and that these transcripts are distributed in different brain regions, different cell types and even different parts of the cell (e.g., soma vs. dendrites). Berry and coworkers found that prenatally stressed rats, at adolescence, showed not only a reduction in social interest and in affiliative behaviors, but also decreased hippocampal expression levels of BDNF (Cirulli and Alleva, 2009). These effects were also associated to a specific change in the hippocampal NKCC1/KCC2 ratio (two genes related to GABA signaling), suggesting an unbalance between neuronal inhibitory and excitatory mechanisms, possibly related to an immature GABA system (Hyde et al., 2011). Most intriguingly, the authors also provide evidence that, for a prenatally stressed rat, the interaction with a nonstressed control subject leads to an improvement in sociality suggesting that the social environment could be exploited for nonpharmacological therapeutic intervention.

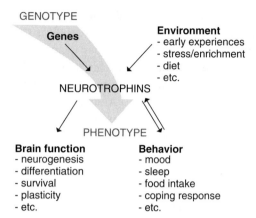

Figure 7.2 Stable changes in gene function might result from the interaction between the genotype and the environment leading to a specific phenotype. Neurotrophins are crucial effectors in changes in brain function deriving from external manipulations.

In addition to enriched living conditions, early pharmacological intervention to promote NTs levels in the brain has been attempted. Luoni and coworkers showed that early treatment with lurasidone, an atypical multireceptor antipsychotic, prevents the observed reduction in BDNF levels in prenatally stressed rats (Luoni et al., 2014) further suggesting that an early therapeutic intervention (environmental, pharmacological or, even better, a combination of the two) in vulnerable individuals, during critical developmental phases, has the potential to act on dynamic systems, enhancing the expression of neuroplastic molecules in key brain regions, leading to long-term beneficial effects on brain function, as well as enhanced resilience to stress-related disorders.

Although at the moment we have still limited knowledge of the neural basis of complex psychiatric conditions such as autism or depression and schizophrenia, there is good evidence that NTs act as important modulators of brain plasticity. It is possible to envision that, in the future, we may be able to exploit NTs – for example, through the use of environmental enrichment – to redirect brain development on the right track (see Figure 7.2).

Epigenetic changes as one mechanism linking early experiences and adult neurobehavioral profile

Epigenetics has been defined as the study of the effects of the environment operating over/above the level of the genetic code, leading to enduring changes in gene expression (Borrelli et al., 2008). Such a concept is perfectly suited to provide a mechanism underlying the effects of gene by environment interactions. The idea that a multitude of external or internal challenges can impact on the genome is particularly intriguing if considered in the context of the early perinatal phases. Thus, the earliest the occurrence of an environmental challenge, the

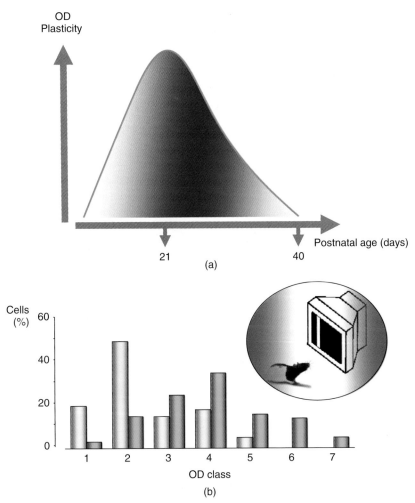

Figure 1.1 Critical period (CP) for ocular dominance plasticity in the rat visual cortex. (a) Schematic representation of the time course of CP for ocular dominance plasticity in the rat, which peaks around postnatal day (P) 21 and is definitively closed by the age of P45. (b) Single unit recordings from the primary visual cortex allow classification of neurons with respect to their ocular preferences: in a typical recording from a nondeprived animal (light cyan columns), cells in class 1 are activated exclusively by the contralateral eye, cells in class 7 are activated exclusively by the ipsilateral eye, neurons in classes 2–3 and 5–6 are activated to varying degrees by both eyes, and neurons in class 4 respond equally to both eyes. Following closure of the contralateral eye from 1 week during the CP, cells become much more responsive toward the ipsilateral open eye, at the expense of the deprived eye (dark cyan columns).

Environmental Experience and Plasticity of the Developing Brain, First Edition.
Edited by Alessandro Sale.
© 2016 John Wiley & Sons, Inc. Published 2016 by John Wiley & Sons, Inc.

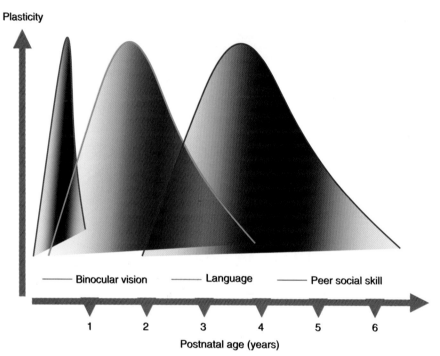

Figure 1.2 Critical periods across brain functions in humans. The picture represents a schematic of the critical period time course for acquisition of binocular vision, language learning, and adequate peer social skills in children. Different functions display different time courses, both in terms of total duration of the heightened sensitivity window and concerning the age of onset and closure of the potential for plasticity. In the three curves, levels of plasticity have been normalized to the peak.

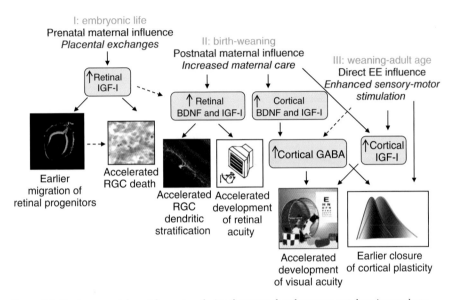

Figure 1.3 Environmental enrichment and visual system development acceleration: a three phases model. The figure depicts an interpretative framework of the data regarding EE effects on the developing visual system. Three consecutive temporal phases are differently controlled by the richness of the environment: (I) a prenatal phase in which the mother mediates the influence of the environment through placental exchanges with the fetus, leading to an accelerated anatomical retinal development that is mostly due to increased levels of IGF-1; (II) an early postnatal phase in which enhanced maternal care received by EE pups stimulates the expression of experience-dependent factors in the visual system, resulting in an early increase of BDNF and IGF-1 in the retina and the visual cortex; this guides the accelerated maturation of retinal ganglion cells (RGCs) observed in EE pups and, through an increased GABAergic inhibitory transmission, triggers a faster visual cortex development; and (III) a third and final phase in which the autonomous interaction of the developing pup with the enriched environment further increases cortical IGF-1, which promotes the maturation of the GABAergic system, also leading to an acceleration in visual acuity maturation. Continuous lines represent well-documented interactions between boxes; dashed lines indicate likely interactions in the context of visual cortex development requiring further experimental characterization.

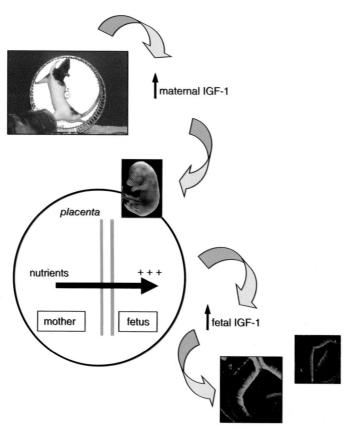

Figure 1.4 Prenatal enrichment modulates retinal development in the fetus. The figure shows a possible explicative model for the effects elicited by maternal enrichment during pregnancy on retinal development. Increased levels of physical exercise in gestating dams lead to higher amounts of circulating IGF-1 in the maternal blood stream, stimulating the supply of nutrients transferred to the fetus through the placental barrier. The enhancement in glucose and placental lactogens received by the fetus stimulates the autonomous production of IGF-1 in his tissues, with an increased expression detectable in the ganglion cell layer of the retina. IGF-1, in turn, stimulates the maturation of retinal circuitries. The photographs depict two examples of one enriched (left) and one nonenriched (right) retinal sections immunostained for double cortin, which labels migrating cells and is a good marker of the temporal and spatial distribution of neural progenitors during the early developmental stages of the rat retina. Reprinted from Sale et al., 2012.

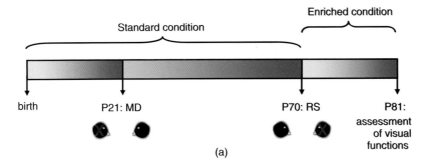

(a)

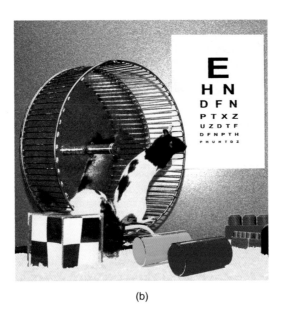

(b)

Figure 1.5 Exposure to enriched conditions promotes recovery of visual functions in adult amblyopic rats. (a) Experimental amblyopia is easily induced in juvenile rats by imposing an artificial closure of one eye through lid suture (monocular deprivation [MD]), started at the peak of the critical period (postnatal day 21) and maintained until the animals reach the adult age (around P70). Then, reverse suture (RS) is performed, consisting in the reopening of the long-term deprived eye and simultaneous closure of the fellow eye, in order to force the animals to use their lazy eye. After RS, the animals are divided in two groups, one left undisturbed under standard-rearing conditions, the other one being transferred to an enriched environment setting. (b) Rearing adult amblyopic rats in an enriched environment for 3 weeks leads to a complete recovery of visual functions, in terms of visual acuity, binocularity, and stereopsis.

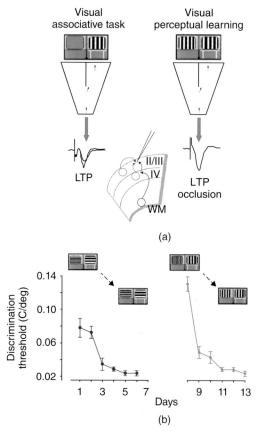

Figure 1.6 Visual perceptual learning induces long-term potentiation in the primary visual cortex. (a) A modified version of the visual water box task (Prusky et al., 2000; Cancedda et al., 2004) was used to induce visual perceptual learning in a group of adult rats that were first trained to distinguish a low 0.117 cycles per degree (c/deg) spatial frequency (SF) grating (reference grating) from a 0.712 c/deg SF grating (test grating) (right panel) and then learned to distinguish the two gratings when they became more and more similar to each other. A group of control animals was trained to distinguish the reference grating from a homogeneous gray (left panel). After training, LTP from layer II–III of V1 slices was occluded in PL animals compared to controls, at the level of both vertical (blue arrow) and horizontal (red arrow) connections. Sample traces from PL and control slices 5 minutes before (thin line) and 25 minutes after (thick line) induction of LTP are shown. (b) Visual perceptual learning is specific for stimulus orientation. The graphs show daily discrimination threshold values obtained in PL animals trained in discriminating first horizontal gratings and then tested with vertical. After the orientation change, the animals displayed a marked impairment in their discrimination abilities. Reprinted from Sale et al., 2012.

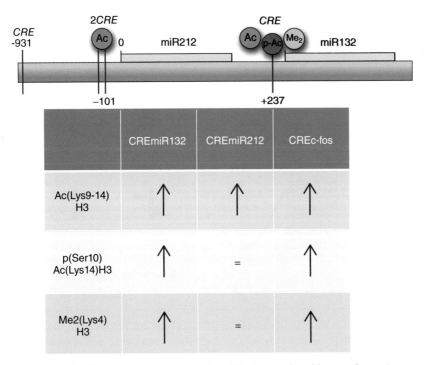

Figure 2.1 Sketch of histone post-translational modifications induced by visual experience on miR212/132 gene.

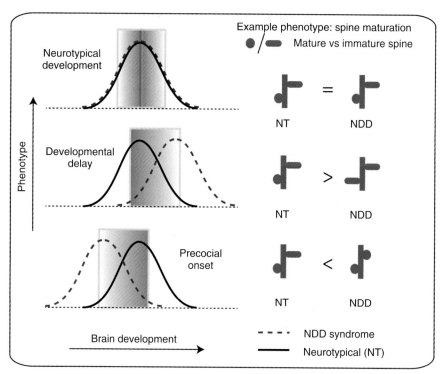

Figure 4.2 Regulation of developmental synaptic phenotypes and potential alteration in neurodevelopmental brain disorders (NDDs). (Left) Developmental profiles of synaptic phenotypes illustrating neurotypical development (top), developmental delay (middle), and precocial phenotypic onset (bottom). Gray bars indicate critical periods for phenotype plasticity. (Right) An example of a developmentally regulated synapse phenotype, spine morphology with longer, thinner filopodia-like spines observed in the immature state and shorter, stubbier spines in the mature state. Predicted phenotypic differences for developmental delay and precocial onset differences illustrated at phenotypic peak for neurotypical profile (black curves in lefthand panel). (Adapted from Meredith et al., 2012.)

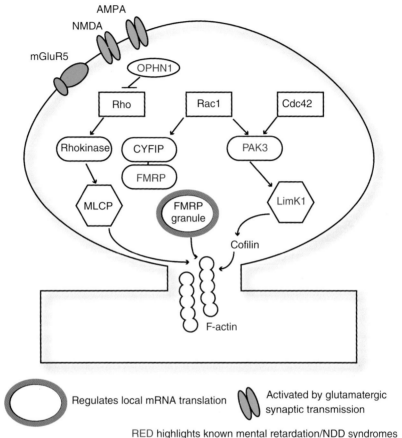

Figure 4.3 Many NDD-associated and linked genes function at the synapse to alter spine morphology. Many monogenic syndrome-associated genes (red) function at the synapse, illustrated here postsynaptically, to mediate changes in spine morphology via small GTPase-mediated signalling pathways and F-actin in response to synaptic activation (receptors highlighted in green). Abbreviations: AMPA, 2-amino-3-(3-hydroxy-5-methyl-isoxazol-4-yl) propanoic acid receptor; Cdc42, cell division cycle 42; CYFIP, cytoplasmic binding partner of Fragile X protein; FMRP, Fragile X Mental Retardation Protein; LimK1, LIM domain kinase 1; mGluR5 metabotropic glutamate receptor subunit 5; NMDA, N-Methyl-D-aspartic acid or N-Methyl-D-aspartate Receptor; OPHN1, oligophrenin-1; PAK, serine/threonine-protein kinase; Rac1, ras-related C3 botulinum toxin substrate; RhoA, ras homolog gene family, member A; MLCP, Myosin light-chain phosphatise. (Modified from Kroon et al., 2013.)

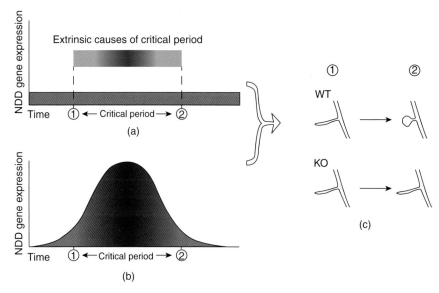

Figure 4.4 Illustrated hypothesis of how dysfunction of NDD-associated genes may dysregulate critical periods. A critical period is shown here as the timeframe between "1" and "2" (a). In this scenario, the critical period is caused by changing genetic expression (blue bar), such as expression of the GABA-synthesising enzyme, GAD65. Expression of the NDD gene (red bar) during neurotypical development is constant before, during, and after the critical period. Expression of genes that determine the dynamics of the critical period does not directly regulate the "NDD gene." Rather, the NDD gene role can indirectly regulate the critical period via its interaction with molecules that mediate synaptic changes during the critical period; for example, expression of GABAergic receptor subunits necessary to mediate synaptic inhibition. FMRP is able to interact with other 800 different mRNA targets in the adult brain, including many proteins with synaptic function and localization (Darnell et al., 2011). Hence dysfunction of the NDD gene can lead to an impaired critical period by indirect regulation. (b) Increased NDD gene expression changes during a restricted developmental stage (red curve) and directly regulates the occurrence of a critical period, independent of external factors. Such dynamic patterns of upregulated "NDD gene" expression, coincident with timing of thalamic and cortical critical periods, occur for many genes including Fmr1, neurofibromin (NF1), and ubiquitin-protein ligase E3A (UBE3A) (Figure 3 Kroon et al., 2013, Allen developing mouse brain atlas: http://developingmouse.brain-map.org). Therefore, dysfunction of the NDD gene causes the critical period to be absent completely. (c) In both scenarios, the NDD gene is ` necessary for the phenotypic change that takes place during the critical period ("WT" vs. "KO"), represented here by maturation of spine morphology. (Figure taken from Kroon et al., 2013.)

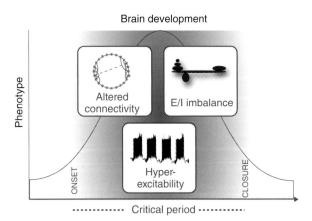

Figure 4.5 Framework of dysregulated critical periods and time windows during brain development as unifying theory for temporal aspects of mechanisms underlying many NDDs of ID and ASD, and prominently illustrated in this article with the Fmr1-KO mouse model for Fragile X syndrome. The three prominent hypotheses for the neurobiological bases of NDDs are shown, namely (1) altered connectivity at short- and long-range distances between neurons, (2) a relative imbalance between excitation (E) and inhibition (I) within brain circuitry, and (3) hyperexcitability of neurons with specific networks in the brain. Neuronal connectivity and both excitatory and inhibitory synaptic strength undergo heightened plasticity during early critical periods in the brain. It is likely that dysregulated phenotypes, such as an imbalance in the levels of synaptic excitation and inhibition, first arise during these critical periods in NDD models. Therefore, the use of known critical periods for cortical and hippocampal circuits may predict when these phenotypes first occur and how long they remain.

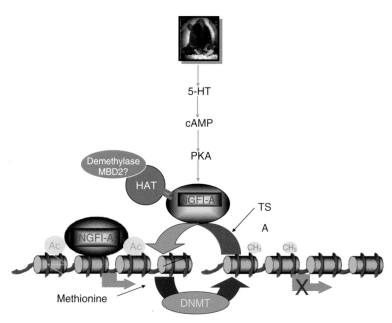

Figure 5.2 Epigenetic programming by maternal care. Maternal care causes activation of serotonin (5-HT) receptors, increases cAMP activation of protein kinase A followed by activation of NGFIA, which interacts with the *nr3c1* promoter and recruits chromatin modifying enzymes and MBD2/demethylase. Increased LG results in decreased methylation of DNA (CH3), increased histone acetylation (AC), and increased gene expression. The DNA methylation reaction is potentially reversible: histone deacetylase inhibitor TSA causes demethylation and activation of the gene, while methionine causes increased methylation and silencing of the gene.

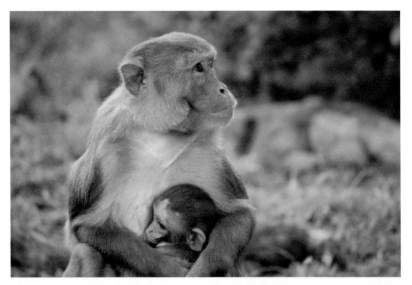

Figure 8.1 A rhesus macaque mother with her infant on Cayo Santiago, Puerto Rico. (Photo: Sean Coyne.)

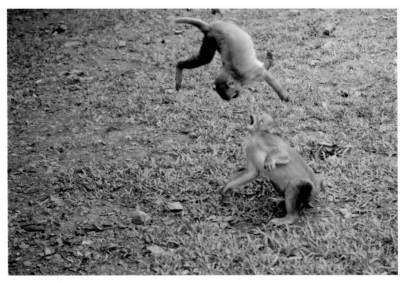

Figure 8.2 Social play (rough-and-tumble) between two rhesus macaque juveniles on Cayo Santiago, Puerto Rico. (Photo: Sean Coyne.)

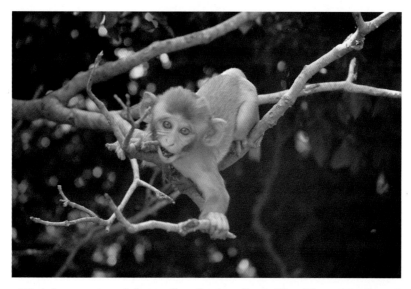
Figure 8.3 A rhesus macaque infant on Cayo Santiago, Puerto Rico. (Photo: Sean Coyne.)

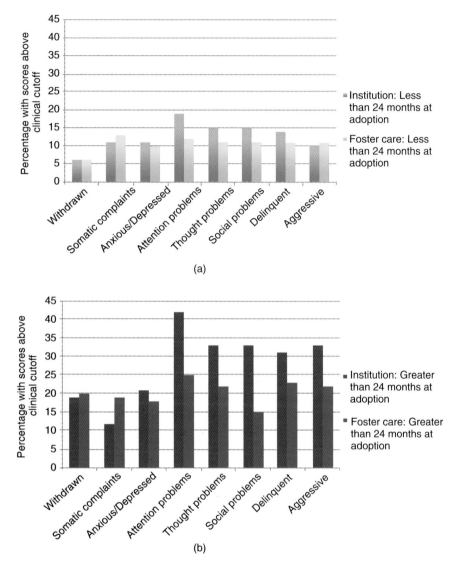

Figure 9.1 Percentage of children adopted from institutional or foster care with CBCL scores of >61 in each domain. (a) Children adopted before 24 months of age. (b) Children adopted after 24 months of age. Regardless of type of care, children adopted later were more likely to express elevated behavior problems. Main effects of institutional care were only noted for attention and social problems. Adapted from Gunnar & van Dulmen, 2007.

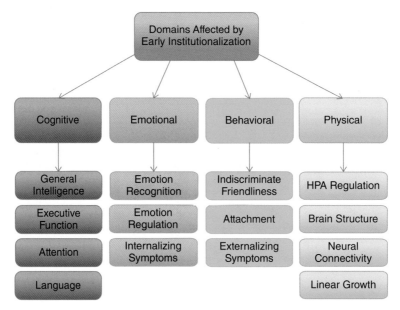

Figure 9.4 Potential effects of early institutional care. These effects are not specific to institutional care, as they may also follow other forms of early adversity. The duration of institutionalization increases the risk of these outcomes.

broader the potential to affect developmental trajectories by remodulating gene expression and, consequently, the availability of specific proteins, including NTs, playing a pivotal role during specific time windows (Boulle et al., 2012). In this sense, if the plasticity features of a developing organism are based on epigenetic mechanisms, health- or disease-related outcomes might result from disruption of such epigenetic processes prompted by internal or external challenges, during sensitive time periods.

A growing body of animal studies support the hypothesis that the early environment might shape brain function and behavior through epigenetic modulation (Tsankova et al., 2007; Zhang and Meaney, 2010). A striking example of this phenomenon is provided by the rat offspring of strains selected for low or high levels of maternal care that show a differential DNA methylation pattern, affecting chromatin structure and the levels of glucocorticoid receptor gene expression both at baseline and after stimulation (Weaver et al., 2004; McGowan and Szyf, 2010). Most intriguingly, these same authors provided also evidence that such early effects can be reversed by central infusion of methionine (a methyl donor) showing the dynamic nature of the epigenetic modifications leading to a potential reversibility later in life (Weaver et al., 2004; Szyf et al., 2005). Indeed, rat pups reared by abusive rat dams, an animal model of early life stress, are characterized by reduced levels of BDNF expression in the prefrontal cortex, which correlates with DNA hypermethylation in the activity-dependent promoter of exon IV (Roth et al., 2009). Interestingly, these same authors showed that epigenetic remodelling leads to long-term transgenerational effects that could be reversed by the infusion of the DNA methylation inhibitor zebularine (Roth et al., 2009). More recently, these researchers also provided evidence that different caregiving conditions (maltreatment or nurturing care) produce a complex array of DNA methylation that vary between developmental time points, sexes and gene loci (BDNF and REELIN). Thus, the alterations that can occur as a result of early experiences are quite complex, comprising both transient and later-emerging DNA methylation differences, which could shape developmental trajectories and underlie gender differences in outcomes (Blaze and Roth, 2013).

As far as early environment is concerned, not only social experiences within the mother–infant dyad, but also those occurring amidst peers can provide a main contribution to the epigenetic shaping of brain and behavior. In this regard, Branchi and coworkers, using the CN paradigm, have shown that mice reared in a CN are characterized by elaborate adult social competencies associated to a more active state of the BDNF gene (in the hippocampus) involving epigenetic remodelling (Branchi et al., 2011b). It is worth noting that such changes do not affect BDNF protein levels at baseline, but only following exposure to an environmental challenge, suggesting that the early social environment might result in a long-term impact on behavioral plasticity and coping-strategies involving epigenetic mechanisms (Branchi et al., 2011b).

So far, the above-mentioned examples refer to epigenetic modifications mediating the effects of the early postnatal environment. However, it is worth noting that such a mechanism is already in place during early prenatal development. Indeed prenatal stress is considered a risk factor for several neurodevelopmental disorders and preclinical studies have provided evidence that experimental paradigms such as restraint stress in both mice and rat dams carried out during the last third of pregnancy might result in specific epigenetic changes. As an example, a recent study from Boersma and colleagues has shown that prenatal stress in rats leads to a specific decrease in the expression of BDNF, possibly mediated by increased DNA methylation of BDNF exon IV (Boersma et al., 2014). More recently, Dong and colleagues found that exposure to stress during gestation leads to a schizophrenia-like behavioral phenotype in the adult offspring of prenatally stressed mice, including locomotor hyperactivity and impairment of sociability and these behavioral abnormalities were associated to a significant decrease in BDNF m-RNA variants accompanied by an enrichment of 5-methylcytosine and 5-hydroxymethylcytosine at BDNF gene regulatory regions (Dong et al., 2014).

Most of the above-mentioned studies have provided evidence for the hypothesis that epigenetic modifications occurring as a result of early life phases are potentially reversible also in predominantly postmitotic tissues, such as the adult brain (McGowan and Szyf, 2010). In particular, the DNA methylation pattern might be a consequence of a dynamic process involving methylation and demethylation reactions occurring as a result of physiological and environmental signals setting the ground for gene by environment interactions (Ramchandani et al., 1999). Thus, the dynamic nature of epigenetic modifications might provide a break-through towards reprogramming gene function in response to changes in life style and/or to pharmacological interventions. As an example, it has been shown that valproic acid, a well-known antiepileptic drug holding also mood stabilizing properties, might exert its function on mood by acting as a histone deacetylase inhibitor (HDACi) (Phiel et al., 2001). Although the effects of HDACi have been characterized in the brain, the mechanisms underlying specificity in the gene targeted by these compounds, which are fundamental for an effective use in mental illnesses, are still being actively investigated.

Overall, identifying epigenetic changes accounting for behavioral pathological traits as a result of adverse early experiences, might have important therapeutic values because these mechanisms are potentially reversible (McGowan and Szyf, 2010). In this regard, future studies aimed at building an epigenomic map of brain NTs, comparing and contrasting mental illnesses, also in relation to gene by environment interactions, might be an appealing strategy.

Conclusion

Overall, in this chapter we have described experimental evidence clearly indicating that the development of the mammalian brain results from the combination of multiple internal and external inputs, ultimately modifying expression levels of NTs, shaping the nervous system. The continuous refinement of brain circuits through activity-dependent mechanisms allows for external manipulations (e.g., environmental enrichment) to sculpt and refine connections in the brain, offering potential for therapeutic intervention when a derangement in plasticity might occur.

References

Alleva E, Francia N. (2008). Psychiatric vulnerability: suggestions from animal models and role of neurotrophins. *Neurosci Biobehav Rev* (in press).

Barde YA. (1990). The nerve growth factor family. *Prog Growth Factor Res* 2(4):237–248.

Barde YA, Edgar D, Thoenen H. (1982). Purification of a new neurotrophic factor from mammalian brain. *Embo J* 1(5):549–553.

Barr CS, Newman TK, Shannon C, et al. (2004). Rearing condition and rh5–HTTLPR interact to influence limbic–hypothalamic–pituitary–adrenal axis response to stress in infant macaques. *Biol Psychiatry* 55(7):733–738.

Berardi N, Pizzorusso T, Maffei L. (2000). Critical periods during sensory development. *Curr Opin Neurobiol* 10(1):138–145.

Blaze J, Roth TL. (2013). Exposure to caregiver maltreatment alters expression levels of epigenetic regulators in the medial prefrontal cortex. *Int J Dev Neurosci* 31(8):804–810.

Boersma GJ, Lee RS, Cordner ZA, Ewald ER, Purcell RH, Moghadam AA, Tamashiro KL. (2014). Prenatal stress decreases Bdnf expression and increases methylation of Bdnf exon IV in rats. *Epigenetics* 9(3):437–447.

Borrelli E, Nestler EJ, Allis CD, Sassone–Corsi P. (2008). Decoding the epigenetic language of neuronal plasticity. *Neuron* 60(6):961–974.

Boulle F, van den Hove DL, Jakob SB, et al. (2012). Epigenetic regulation of the BDNF gene: implications for psychiatric disorders. *Mol Psychiatry* 17(6):584–596.

Branchi I, D'Andrea I, Sietzema J, Fiore M, Di Fausto V, Aloe L, Alleva E. (2006). Early social enrichment augments adult hippocampal BDNF levels and survival of BrdU–positive cells while increasing anxiety– and depression–like behavior. *J Neurosci Res* 83(6):965–973.

Branchi I, D'Andrea I, Cirulli F, Lipp HP, Alleva E. (2010). Shaping brain development: mouse communal nesting blunts adult neuroendocrine and behavioral response to social stress and modifies chronic antidepressant treatment outcome. *Psychoneuroendocrinology* 35(5):743–751.

Branchi I, D'Andrea I, Santarelli S, Bonsignore LT, Alleva E. (2011a). The richness of social stimuli shapes developmental trajectories: are laboratory mouse pups impoverished? *Prog Neuropsychopharmacol Biol Psychiatry* 35(6):1452–1460.

Branchi I, Karpova NN, D'Andrea I, Castren E, Alleva E. (2011b). Epigenetic modifications induced by early enrichment are associated with changes in timing of induction of BDNF expression. *Neurosci Lett* 495(3):168–172.

Branchi I, Curley JP, D'Andrea I, Cirulli F, Champagne FA, Alleva E. (2013). Early interactions with mother and peers independently build adult social skills and shape BDNF and oxytocin receptor brain levels. *Psychoneuroendocrinology* 38(4):522–532.

Calabrese F, Guidotti G, Middelman A, Racagni G, Homberg J, Riva MA. (2013). Lack of serotonin transporter alters BDNF expression in the rat brain during early postnatal development. *Mol Neurobiol* 48(1):244–256.

Cancedda L, Putignano E, Sale A, Viegi A, Berardi N, Maffei L. (2004). Acceleration of visual system development by environmental enrichment. *J Neurosci* 24(20):4840–4848.

Carola V, Gross C. (2010). BDNF moderates early environmental risk factors for anxiety in mouse. *Genes Brain Behav* 9(4):379–389.

Castren E. (2004). Neurotrophins as mediators of drug effects on mood, addiction, and neuroprotection. *Mol Neurobiol* 29(3):289–302.

Castren E. (2005). Is mood chemistry? *Nat Rev Neurosci* 6(3):241–246.

Castren E, Zafra F, Thoenen H, Lindholm D. (1992). Light regulates expression of brain–derived neurotrophic factor mRNA in rat visual cortex. *Proc Natl Acad Sci USA* 89(20): 9444–9448.

Castren E, Voikar V, Rantamaki T. (2007). Role of neurotrophic factors in depression. *Curr Opin Pharmacol* 7(1):18–21.

Cellerino A, Maffei L. (1996). The action of neurotrophins in the development and plasticity of the visual cortex. *Prog Neurobiol* 49(1):53–71.

Chang Q, Khare G, Dani V, Nelson S, Jaenisch R. (2006). The disease progression of Mecp2 mutant mice is affected by the level of BDNF expression. *Neuron* 49(3):341–348.

Chao MV, Bothwell M. (2002). Neurotrophins: to cleave or not to cleave. *Neuron* 33(1): 9–12.

Chen ZY, Jing D, Bath KG, et al. (2006). Genetic variant BDNF (Val66Met) polymorphism alters anxiety–related behavior. *Science* 314(5796):140–143.

Cirulli F. (2001). Role of environmental factors on brain development and nerve growth factor expression. *Physiol Behav* 73(3):321–330.

Cirulli F, Alleva E. (2009). The NGF saga: from animal models of psychosocial stress to stress–related psychopathology. *Front Neuroendocrinol* 30(3):379–395.

Cirulli F, Micera A, Alleva E, Aloe L. (1998). Early maternal separation increases NGF expression in the developing rat hippocampus. *Pharmacol Biochem Behav* 59(4):853–858.

Cirulli F, Alleva E, Antonelli A, Aloe L. (2000). NGF expression in the developing rat brain: effects of maternal separation. *Brain Res Dev Brain Res* 123:129–134.

Cirulli F, Berry A, Alleva E. (2003). Early disruption of the mother–infant relationship: effects on brain plasticity and implications for psychopathology. *Neurosci Biobehav Rev* 27(1–2): 73–82.

Cirulli F, Capone F, Bonsignore LT, Aloe L, Alleva E. (2007). Early behavioural enrichment in the form of handling renders mouse pups unresponsive to anxiolytic drugs and increases NGF levels in the hippocampus. *Behav Brain Res* 178(2):208–215.

Cirulli F, Francia N, Berry A, Aloe L, Alleva E, Suomi SJ. (2009a). Early life stress as a risk factor for mental health: role of neurotrophins from rodents to non–human primates. *Neurosci Biobehav Rev* 33(4):573–585.

Cirulli F, Francia N, Branchi I, Antonucci MT, Aloe L, Suomi SJ, Alleva E. (2009b). Changes in plasma levels of BDNF and NGF reveal a gender–selective vulnerability to early adversity in rhesus macaques. *Psychoneuroendocrinology* 34(2):172–180.

Cirulli F, Reif A, Herterich S, Lesch KP, Berry A, Francia N, Aloe L, Barr CS, Suomi SJ, Alleva E. (2011). A novel BDNF polymorphism affects plasma protein levels in interaction with early adversity in rhesus macaques. *Psychoneuroendocrinology* 36(3):372–379.

Comasco E, Aslund C, Oreland L, Nilsson KW. (2013). Three–way interaction effect of 5–HTTLPR, BDNF Val66Met, and childhood adversity on depression: a replication study. *Eur Neuropsychopharmacol* 23(10):1300–1306.

D'Andrea I, Gracci F, Alleva E, Branchi I. (2010). Early social enrichment provided by communal nest increases resilience to depression–like behavior more in female than in male mice. *Behav Brain Res.*

Dechant G, Barde YA. (2002). The neurotrophin receptor p75(NTR): novel functions and implications for diseases of the nervous system. *Nat Neurosci* 5(11):1131–1136.

Dimatelis JJ, Russell VA, Stein DJ, Daniels WM. (2014). Methamphetamine reversed maternal separation–induced decrease in nerve growth factor in the ventral hippocampus. *Metab Brain Dis* 29(2):433–439.

Dong E, Dzitoyeva SG, Matrisciano F, Tueting P, Grayson DR, Guidotti A. (2014). Brain–Derived Neurotrophic Factor Epigenetic Modifications Associated with Schizophrenia–like Phenotype Induced by Prenatal Stress in Mice. *Biological Psychiatry.*

Duman RS, Monteggia LM. (2006). A neurotrophic model for stress–related mood disorders. *Biol Psychiatry* 59(12):1116–1127.

Egan MF, Kojima M, Callicott JH, et al. (2003). The BDNF val66met polymorphism affects activity–dependent secretion of BDNF and human memory and hippocampal function. *Cell* 112(2):257–269.

Francis DD, Meaney MJ. (1999). Maternal care and the development of stress responses. *Curr Opin Neurobiol* 9:128–134.

Francis DD, Diorio J, Plotsky PM, Meaney MJ. (2002). Environmental enrichment reverses the effects of maternal separation on stress reactivity. *J Neurosci* 22(18):7840–7843.

Gall CM, Isackson PJ (1989). Limbic seizures increase neuronal production of messenger RNA for nerve growth factor. *Science* 245(4919):758–761.

Giachino C, Canalia N, Capone F, et al. (2007). Maternal deprivation and early handling affect density of calcium binding protein–containing neurons in selected brain regions and emotional behavior in periadolescent rats. *Neuroscience* 145(2):568–578.

Han JC, Liu QR, Jones M, et al. (2008). Brain–derived neurotrophic factor and obesity in the WAGR syndrome. *N Engl J Med* 359(9):918–927.

Hensch TK. (2004). Critical period regulation. *Annu Rev Neurosci* 27:549–579.

Hyde TM, Lipska BK, Ali T, et al. (2011). Expression of GABA signaling molecules KCC2, NKCC1, and GAD1 in cortical development and schizophrenia. *J Neurosci* 31(30): 11088–11095.

Kafitz KW, Rose CR, Thoenen H, Konnerth A. (1999). Neurotrophin–evoked rapid excitation through TrkB receptors. *Nature* 401(6756):918–921.

Kaufman J, Plotsky PM, Nemeroff CB, Charney DS. (2000). Effects of early adverse experiences on brain structure and function: clinical implications. *Biol Psychiatry* 48(8):778–790.

Kaufman J, Yang BZ, Douglas–Palumberi H, Grasso D, Lipschitz D, Houshyar S, Krystal JH, Gelernter J. (2006). Brain–derived neurotrophic factor–5–HTTLPR gene interactions and environmental modifiers of depression in children. *Biol Psychiatry* 59(8):673–680.

Knusel B, Winslow JW, Rosenthal A, Burton LE, Seid DP, Nikolics K, Hefti K. (1991). Promotion of central cholinergic and dopaminergic neuron differentiation by brain–derived neurotrophic factor but not neurotrophin 3. *Proc Natl Acad Sci USA* 88(3):961–965.

Koo JW, Park CH, Choi SH, et al. (2003). The postnatal environment can counteract prenatal effects on cognitive ability, cell proliferation, and synaptic protein expression. *FASEB J* 17(11):1556–1558.

Korsching S, Heumann R, Thoenen H, Hefti F. (1986). Cholinergic denervation of the rat hippocampus by fimbrial transection leads to a transient accumulation of nerve growth factor (NGF) without change in mRNANGF content. *Neurosci Lett* 66(2):175–180.

Lee R, Kermani P, Teng KK, Hempstead BL. (2001). Regulation of cell survival by secreted proneurotrophins. *Science* 294(5548):1945–1948.

Levi–Montalcini R. (1987). The nerve growth factor 35 years later. *Science* 237(4819):1154–1162.

Levi–Montalcini R, Angeletti PU. (1968). Nerve growth factor. *Physiol Rev* 48(3):534–569.

Levi–Montalcini R, Hamburger V. (1951). Selective growth stimulating effects of mouse sarcoma on the sensory and sympathetic nervous system of the chick embryo. *J Exp Zool* 116(2):321–361.

Levine S. (1957). Infantile experience and resistance to physiological stress. *Science* 126:405.

Li W, Pozzo–Miller L. (2014). BDNF deregulation in Rett syndrome. *Neuropharmacology* 76 Pt C:737–746.

Licinio J, Dong C, Wong ML. (2009). Novel sequence variations in the brain–derived neurotrophic factor gene and association with major depression and antidepressant treatment response. *Arch Gen Psychiatry* 66(5):488–497.

Lindholm D, Castren E, Berzaghi M, Blochl A, Thoenen H. (1994). Activity–dependent and hormonal regulation of neurotrophin mRNA levels in the brain—implications for neuronal plasticity. *J Neurobiol* 25(11):1362–1372.

Lu B. (2003). BDNF and activity–dependent synaptic modulation. *Learn Mem* 10(2):86–98.

Lu B, Chow A. (1999). Neurotrophins and hippocampal synaptic transmission and plasticity. *J Neurosci Res* 58(1):76–87.

Luoni A, Berry A, Calabrese F, et al. (2014). Delayed BDNF alterations in the prefrontal cortex of rats exposed to prenatal stress: preventive effect of lurasidone treatment during adolescence. *Eur Neuropsychopharmacol* 24(6):986–995.

Lupien SJ, de Leon M, de Santi S, et al. (1998). Cortisol levels during human aging predict hippocampal atrophy and memory deficits. *Nat Neurosci* 1(1):69–73.

Magarinos AM, Li CJ, Gal Toth J, et al. (2011). Effect of brain–derived neurotrophic factor haploinsufficiency on stress–induced remodeling of hippocampal neurons. *Hippocampus* 21(3):253–264.

Martinowich K, Lu B. (2008). Interaction between BDNF and serotonin: role in mood disorders. *Neuropsychopharmacology* 33(1):73–83.

Marty S, Carroll P, Cellerino A, et al. (1996). Brain–derived neurotrophic factor promotes the differentiation of various hippocampal nonpyramidal neurons, including Cajal–Retzius cells, in organotypic slice cultures. *J Neurosci* 16(2):675–687.

McAllister AK, Katz LC, Lo DC. (1999). Neurotrophins and synaptic plasticity. *Annu Rev Neurosci* 22:295–318.

McGowan PO, Szyf M. (2010). The epigenetics of social adversity in early life: implications for mental health outcomes. *Neurobiol Dis* 39(1):66–72.

Meakin SO, Shooter EM. (1992). The nerve growth factor family of receptors. *Trends Neurosci* 15(9):323–331.

Meaney MJ, Aitken DH, Viau V, Sharma S, Sarrieau A. (1989). Neonatal handling alters adreno-cortical negative feedback sensitivity and hippocampal type II glucocorticoid receptor binding in the rat. *Neuroendocrinology* 50(5):597–604.

Meaney MJ, Diorio J, Francis D, et al. (1996). Early environmental regulation of forebrain glu-cocorticoid receptor gene expression: implications for adrenocortical responses to stress. *Dev Neurosci* 18(1–2):49–72.

Meaney MJ, Mitchell JB, Aitken DH, et al. (1991). The effects of neonatal handling on the development of the adrenocortical response to stress: implications for neuropathology and cognitive deficits in later life. *Psychoneuroendocrinology* 16(1–3):85–103.

Mobley WC, Rutkowski JL, Tennekoon GI, Buchanan K, Johnston MV. (1985). Choline acetyl-transferase activity in striatum of neonatal rats increased by nerve growth factor. *Science* 229(4710):284–287.

Nair A, Vadodaria KC, Banerjee SB, et al. (2007). Stressor–specific regulation of distinct brain–derived neurotrophic factor transcripts and cyclic AMP response element–binding protein expression in the postnatal and adult rat hippocampus. *Neuropsychopharmacology* 32(7):1504–1519.

Pang PT, Teng HK, Zaitsev E, et al. (2004). Cleavage of proBDNF by tPA/plasmin is essential for long–term hippocampal plasticity. *Science* 306(5695):487–491.

Patapoutian A, Reichardt LF. (2001). Trk receptors: mediators of neurotrophin action. *Curr Opin Neurobiol* 11(3):272–280.

Patterson SL, Abel T, Deuel TA, Martin KC, Rose JC, Kandel ER. (1996). Recombinant BDNF rescues deficits in basal synaptic transmission and hippocampal LTP in BDNF knockout mice. *Neuron* 16(6):1137–1145.

Percy AK, Lane JB. (2005). Rett syndrome: model of neurodevelopmental disorders. *J Child Neurol* 20(9):718–721.

Pham TM, Soderstrom S, Henriksson BG, Mohammed AH. (1997). Effects of neonatal stimulation on later cognitive function and hippocampal nerve growth factor. *Behav Brain Res* 86(1):113–120.

Phiel CJ, Zhang F, Huang EY, Guenther MG, Lazar MA, Klein PS. (2001). Histone deacetylase is a direct target of valproic acid, a potent anticonvulsant, mood stabilizer, and teratogen. *J Biol Chem* 276(39):36734–36741.

Plotsky PM, Meaney MJ. (1993). Early, postnatal experience alters hypothalamic corticotropin-releasing factor (CRF) mRNA, median eminence CRF content and stress–induced release in adult rats. *Brain Res Mol Brain Res* 18:195–200.

Pryce CR, Feldon J. (2003). Long–term neurobehavioural impact of the postnatal environment in rats: manipulations, effects and mediating mechanisms. *Neurosci Biobehav Rev* 27(1–2):57–71.

Pryce CR, Bettschen D, Bahr NI, Feldon J. (2001). Comparison of the effects of infant handling, isolation, and nonhandling on acoustic startle, prepulse inhibition, locomotion, and HPA activity in the adult rat. *Behav Neurosci* 115(1):71–83.

Ramchandani S, Bhattacharya SK, Cervoni N, Szyf M. (1999). DNA methylation is a reversible biological signal. *Proc Natl Acad Sci USA* 96(11):6107–6112.

Roceri M, Cirulli F, Pessina C, Peretto P, Racagni G, Riva MA. (2004). Post–natal repeated maternal deprivation produces age–dependent changes of brain–derived neurotrophic factor expression in selected rat brain regions. *Biol Psychiatry* 55(7):708–714.

Roth TL, Lubin FD, Funk AJ, Sweatt JD. (2009). Lasting epigenetic influence of early–life adversity on the BDNF gene. *Biol Psychiatry* 65(9):760–769.

Roux PP, Barker PA. (2002). Neurotrophin signaling through the p75 neurotrophin receptor. *Prog Neurobiol* 67(3):203–233.

Sale A, Putignano E, Cancedda L, Landi S, Cirulli F, Berardi N, Maffei L. (2004). Enriched environment and acceleration of visual system development. *Neuropharmacology* 47(5):649–660.

Sale A, Berardi N, Maffei L. (2009). Enrich the environment to empower the brain. *Trends Neurosci* 32(4):233–239.

Savitz J, van der Merwe L, Stein DJ, Solms M, Ramesar R. (2007). Genotype and childhood sexual trauma moderate neurocognitive performance: a possible role for brain–derived neurotrophic factor and apolipoprotein E variants. *Biol Psychiatry* 62(5):391–399.

Szyf M, Weaver IC, Champagne FA, Diorio J, Meaney MJ. (2005). Maternal programming of steroid receptor expression and phenotype through DNA methylation in the rat. *Front Neuroendocrinol* 26(3–4):139–162.

Thoenen H. (1995). Neurotrophins and neuronal plasticity. *Science* 270(5236):593–598.

Thoenen H, Barde YA. (1980). Physiology of nerve growth factor. *Physiol Rev* 60(4):1284–1335.

Tsankova N, Renthal W, Kumar A, Nestler EJ. (2007). Epigenetic regulation in psychiatric disorders. *Nat Rev Neurosci* 8(5):355–367.

Verhagen M, van der Meij A, van Deurzen PA, et al. (2010). Meta–analysis of the BDNF Val66Met polymorphism in major depressive disorder: effects of gender and ethnicity. *Mol Psychiatry* 15(3):260–271.

Weaver IC, Cervoni N, Champagne FA, et al. (2004). Epigenetic programming by maternal behavior. *Nat Neurosci* 7(8):847–854.

Wichers M, Kenis G, Jacobs N, et al. (2008). The BDNF Val(66)Met x 5–HTTLPR x child adversity interaction and depressive symptoms: an attempt at replication. *Am J Med Genet B Neuropsychiatr Genet* 147B(1):120–123.

Wiesel TN, Hubel DH. (1963). Effects of Visual Deprivation on Morphology and Physiology of Cells in the Cats Lateral Geniculate Body. *J Neurophysiol* 26:978–993.

Yang J, Siao CJ, Nagappan G, et al. (2009). Neuronal release of proBDNF. *Nat Neurosci* 12(2):113–115.

Zafra F, Hengerer B, Leibrock J, Thoenen H, Lindholm D. (1990). Activity dependent regulation of BDNF and NGF mRNAs in the rat hippocampus is mediated by non–NMDA glutamate receptors. *Embo J* 9(11):3545–3550.

Zagrebelsky M, Korte M. (2014). Form follows function: BDNF and its involvement in sculpting the function and structure of synapses. *Neuropharmacology* 76 Pt C:628–638.

Zhang LX, Levine S, Dent G, et al. (2002). Maternal deprivation increases cell death in the infant rat brain. *Brain Res Dev Brain Res* 133(1):1–11.

Zhang TY, Meaney MJ. (2010). Epigenetics and the environmental regulation of the genome and its function. *Annu Rev Psychol* 61:439–466, C431–433.

CHAPTER 8

Effects of genes and early experience on the development of primate behavior and stress reactivity

Sean P. Coyne and Dario Maestripieri

Department of Comparative Human Development, The University of Chicago, Chicago, Illinois, USA

Introduction

Among the over 300 species in the Primate order there is great variability in social systems (Mitani et al., 2012). Very few species have a solitary lifestyle, while all the others are characterized by permanent associations between two or more adults and their young. Pair-living, however, is relatively rare, while over 90% of primate species live in groups with one adult male and several reproductively active females (harems), groups with multiple adult males and females and their young, or groups that fluctuate between the one-male and the multimale structure (Mitani et al., 2012). Paternal care is rare in primates and limited to species in which adults live in pairs or in small family groups. All primate infants are reared by their mothers and, with the exception of some species of prosimians in which infants are parked in a nest for brief periods of time, mothers carry their infants on their chest or on their back on an almost continuous basis for weeks, months, or even years. After infants have acquired their locomotor independence, they travel close to their mothers for long periods of time, and in some cases throughout their lives. Given how much time they spend in contact or in proximity with their infants, mothers represent the most important aspects of the infants' social environment during infancy, juvenility, and adolescence. In solitary species or species that live in small family groups, infants' interactions with individuals other than their mother are limited to those with one older sibling or one adult. In species that live in groups with multiple females (with either one male or multiple males), infants have the opportunity to interact with other females' infants, with other immatures, and with adults.

Early behavioral development in nonhuman primates has been studied in the wild, in semi-naturalistic captivity conditions, and in the lab (e.g., Hinde and Spencer-Booth, 1967; Rosenblum and Kaufman, 1967; Fossey, 1979; Altmann, 1980; Plooij, 1984; Nakamichi, 1989; Maestripieri, 1994). Behavioral studies conducted in the wild or in semi-naturalistic conditions have typically involved infants reared by their mothers and living in species-typical social groupings. Behavioral studies in the lab have often involved individuals housed in small cages and in atypical social environments (e.g., a single mother-infant pair or a small peer group). In addition to documenting age-related changes in infant behavior with longitudinal or cross-sectional approaches, developmental studies have also often addressed infant behavioral and physiological reactivity to various types of environmental and psychosocial stress (see Parker and Maestripieri, 2011). The most systematic studies of the development of behavior and reactivity to stress have been conducted with some species of prosimians and New World monkeys (e.g., ring-tailed lemurs, capuchin monkeys, squirrel monkeys, marmosets, and tamarins), cercopithecine monkeys such as macaques or baboons, and all the great apes (chimpanzees, bonobos, gorillas, and orangutans). In addition to differences in the patterns and trajectories of behavioral development across different species, studies have uncovered also a great deal of within-species variation in social development and in behavioral and physiological reactivity to stress (e.g., Hinde and Spencer-Booth, 1967; 1971).

The mother's own behavior toward the infant, namely her parenting style, has emerged as a major source of variation in both behavioral development and reactivity to stress (e.g., Fairbanks, 1996). Variation in artificial-rearing conditions in the laboratory (e.g., rearing infants with or without their mothers, with peers, and under various conditions of social deprivation or social enrichment) can also affect the development of behavior and reactivity to stress. The extent to which behavioral development and reactivity to stress are influenced by variation in the quality of social relationships between infants and other individuals in the wild or in semi-naturalistic environments has not been systematically investigated. Finally, in addition to influences of environment and early experience, there is evidence that variation in infant behavior and physiology is the result of inherited genetic variation or of gene-environment interactions.

In this chapter we summarize and discuss our knowledge of the role of genes and early experience in the development of behavior and reactivity to stress in nonhuman primates, with particular focus on species that have been well-studied in different environmental settings. In terms of variable early experience, we focus on variability in maternal behavior and do not to address variability in artificial-rearing environments in the lab (e.g., isolation-reared or peer-reared monkeys; see Parker and Maestripieri, 2011; Kinnally, 2012 for recent reviews and discussion of these studies). Genetic influences will be examined with particular emphasis on evidence of main effects of genetic polymorphisms on infant behavior or reactivity to stress in the wild, in semi-naturalistic environments, or in the lab. Gene-environment interactions will be addressed when they have been demonstrated in normal social environments and in mother-reared infants; laboratory studies of isolation-reared or peer-reared monkeys will not be systematically reviewed (see Kinnally, 2012 for a recent review).

Assessment of infant behavior and stress reactivity

Observational studies of early behavioral development in nonhuman primates in which infants are studied with their mothers, and often in the context of their social group, generally report data on the acquisition of infant independence. This is quantified by measuring the frequency with which infants break ventro-ventral contact (or any bodily contact) with their mothers or walk away from them beyond their arm's reach (e.g., Hinde and Spencer-Booth, 1967; Maestripieri, 1994). Duration of time spent out of contact or out of close proximity to the mother can also be used as a measure of infant independence. More independent infants break contact more often, leave the mother's proximity more often, and generally spend less time in contact and in proximity with their mother than less independent infants. Observational studies of behavior also quantify the infant exploratory behavior and both solitary and social play. More rarely, observations are made of the infant's tendency to approach novel objects or older and potentially dangerous conspecifics (see Fairbanks, 1996).

Observational studies of infant behavior generally report remarkable inter-individual variation in the acquisition of locomotor and social independence from the mother. Some infants are more active, or more active earlier in life, than others and appear more comfortable spending time away from their mother and interacting with other individuals. Variation is also reported in the tendency to explore a novel environment, and approach novel objects or unfamiliar individuals. Individual differences in social and exploratory behavior may be accompanied by differences in the expressions of behavioral indicators of anxiety such as displacement activities or self-directed behaviors (SDBs). SDBs include such activities as scratching, yawning, self-grooming, or shaking. Not only do these displacement activities tend to occur in situations of psychosocial stress, their occurrence is affected by both anxiogenic and anxiolytic drugs (Maestripieri et al., 1992). Developmental differences in reactivity to novel stimuli or responsiveness to other individuals are likely to be accompanied by differences in neurochemical and neuroendocrine substrates regulating emotional and social processes. Neuropeptides and hormones of the HPA axis such CRF, ACTH, and cortisol, along with the brain monoamine neurotransmitters norepinephrine, serotonin, and dopamine would be likely candidates, as these substances play an important role in the regulation of emotional and behavioral processes and their concentrations can be relatively stable over long periods of time.

While measuring stress reactivity and other stress-related behaviors during typical social interactions among free-living primates can be enlightening, often differences are more easily detected through direct experimentation. There are several available paradigms to assess stress reactivity in primates. One such paradigm is the Free Play task in which the subject is removed from its home cage/environment and social group and placed in a novel environment, typically with novel enrichment in order to assess how the individual reacts to novel stimuli free of social influence. A simplification of the Free Play task is the Novel Object task in which a novel object is presented to the subject in its home cage/enclosure. Another common test is the human intruder task, in which the subjects are confined to an area either in their home enclosures, or a novel environment and allowed to habituate to that area, which is followed by the introduction a novel human experimenter. The experimenter enters, stands next to the subject's cage and stares at the subject with a threatening expression. Finally, another test used with infant primates is the maternal separation task. In maternal separation tasks, the mother-infant pair is typically trapped together, then mother and infant are separated and the infant is housed alone in a cage, either in the same room as the cage with the mother, or in a different room, for variable amounts of time (usually a half hour or 1 hour).

In the above-described tasks, many different aspects of infant behavior can be observed and quantified. For example, in free play/novel object tests, behavioral measures usually include latency to approach the novel objects, latency to leave the home/transport cage, and how much movement the animal makes around the novel environment, with the underlying assumption that more stressed/less bold animals will have longer latencies to leave the home cage and approach novel objects, as well as move around the novel environment less. Standard measures for the human intruder task include fear behaviors, such as freezing or fear grimacing, as well as aggressive behaviors (typically threats) and total amount of movement during the task. Some studies use a variation of this task in which rather than using a human as an intruder they instead use a novel conspecific. Typically the novel conspecific is placed in a smaller cage in the subjects' home enclosure. Finally, in maternal separation tasks, measures often include distress vocalizations, stereotypic behaviors, and amount of locomotion.

In controlled laboratory experiments, many physiological measures can be obtained as well. Typically, experimenters can obtain blood samples for both pretest conditions and post-test conditions to assess the effects of the experimental manipulation on stress physiology by measuring the difference in hormone levels between the two time points. The process of stress response includes the activation of multiple central nervous system and peripheral pathways, including neurotransmitters (e.g., serotonin, dopamine, norepinephrine) and hormones (cortisol, vasopressin, neuropeptide Y, epinephrine). The physiological stress response includes the coordination of the autonomic nervous system with the hypothalamic-pituitary-adrenal (HPA) axis (Sapolsky et al., 2000).

The coordination of these two systems to maintain homeostasis in the presence of a challenge enables the individual to mobilize energetic resources needed and conserving those that are not needed. The autonomic nervous system enables a fast response to stress, increasing heart rate and decreasing metabolism and stimulating epinephrine release from the adrenal medulla. The HPA axis responds to stress by regulating the level of cortisol that is released into the bloodstream. Corticotropin-releasing hormone (CRH) is released from the hypothalamus in response to stressful stimuli. This response activates the release of adrenocorticotropic hormone (ACTH) from the pituitary gland, which in turn activates the release of glucocorticoids (i.e, cortisol) from the adrenal cortex. Cortisol negatively feeds back to multiple sites in the brain to shut down cortisol output. Plasma levels of ACTH and cortisol indicate the amount of activity in the HPA axis and can give insight into the overall physiological stress response of the animal.

Influence of naturally occurring variation in maternal style on offspring behavior and stress reactivity

In Old World monkeys, mothers show marked individual differences in maternal style along the two orthogonal dimensions of maternal Protectiveness and Rejection (e.g., Hinde and Spencer-Booth, 1971; Maestripieri, 1998a; Tanaka, 1989; Schino et al., 1995; Fairbanks, 1996). The dimension of maternal Protectiveness includes variation in the degree to which the mother physically restrains infant exploration, initiates contact and proximity and cradles or grooms her infant. The dimension of maternal Rejection includes the degree to which the mother limits the timing, frequency, and duration of suckling, carrying, and contact. These dimensions combine to make four parenting style types: mothers who are high on both dimensions are classified as Controlling; mothers low on both dimensions are classified as Laissez-Faire; mothers high on one dimension and low on the other are classified as Protective or Rejecting. Longitudinal studies have demonstrated that parenting style tends to be consistent over time and across infants of the same mother (Berman, 1990; Fairbanks, 1989; Maestripieri et al., 1999). See Figure 8.1.

Studies of macaques and vervet monkeys have examined how exposure to variable levels of maternal protectiveness and maternal rejection experienced in early infancy affects variation in offspring independence from the mother and infants' tendency to explore the environment or respond to challenges at various ages. An early study by Simpson (1985) showed that exposure to high levels of maternal rejection in the first few months of life was associated with reduced infant's exploration at the end of the first year. Subsequent studies, however, showed that infants reared by highly rejecting (or less responsive mothers) mothers generally develop independence at an earlier age (e.g., spend more

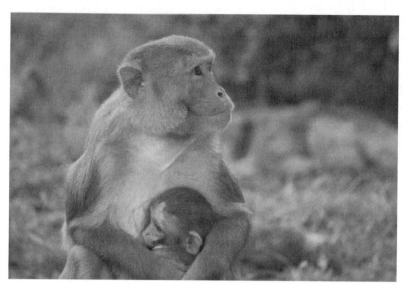

Figure 8.1 A rhesus macaque mother with her infant on Cayo Santiago, Puerto Rico. (Photo: Sean Coyne.) (See insert for color representation of this figure.)

time out of contact with their mothers, explore the environment more, and play more with their peers) than infants reared by mothers with low rejection levels (Bardi and Huffman, 2006; Simpson et al., 1989; Simpson and Datta, 1990). In contrast, infants reared by more protective mothers appear to be delayed in the acquisition of their independence and are relatively fearful and cautious when faced with challenging situations (Fairbanks and McGuire, 1988; 1993). Similar findings were also obtained in studies in which maternal protectiveness was experimentally enhanced through manipulations of the environment (Fairbanks and McGuire, 1987; Vochteloo et al., 1993). For example, Fairbanks and McGuire (1987) showed that following the introduction of new males, vervet monkey mothers became more protective of their infants, presumably because of the increased risk of infanticide, or male aggression, or simply the social instability resulting from this manipulation. The offspring of mothers who became more protective showed increased anxiety/fearfulness and lower tendency to explore when tested for responsiveness to novelty months or years later (Fairbanks and McGuire, 1987; 1988). Effects of maternal style and other aspects of the infant's early social environment have also been documented with regard to responsiveness to negative visual stimuli. Mandalaywala et al. (2014) have shown that 9-month-old infants reared by more protective mothers (in the first 2–3 months of life) and those reared by high-ranking mothers (protectiveness and rank were not correlated in this study) exhibited a stronger attentional bias toward faces with threatening expressions, as opposed to faces

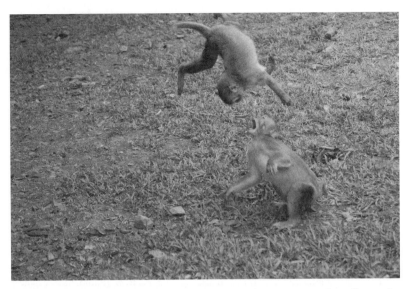

Figure 8.2 Social play (rough-and-tumble) between two rhesus macaque juveniles on Cayo Santiago, Puerto Rico. (Photo: Sean Coyne.) (See insert for color representation of this figure.)

with neutral expressions, when compared to infants reared by less protective mothers and those reared by lower-ranking mothers. See Figure 8.2.

The issue of whether these effects of early experience on offspring reactivity to the environment also persist into later stages of development and adulthood has been addressed by a few studies. In vervet monkeys, juveniles who were exposed to greater maternal protectiveness in infancy had a higher latency to enter a new enclosure and to approach novel food containers (Fairbanks and McGuire, 1988; 1993), whereas adolescent males reared by highly rejecting mothers were more willing to approach and challenge a strange adult male (Fairbanks, 1996). Schino et al. (2001) found no significant association between variation in maternal protectiveness or rejection early in life and the offspring's behavior several years later in Japanese macaques. However, they did report a relationship between early maternal rejection and offspring responsiveness to stressful situations. Specifically, individuals that were rejected more by their mothers early in life were less likely to respond with submissive signals or with avoidance to an approach from another individual and exhibited lower rates of scratching in the 5-minute period following the receipt of aggression. Finally, Maestripieri et al. (2006b) showed that rhesus macaques that were rejected more by their mothers in the first 6 months of life engaged more in solitary play and greater avoidance of other individuals in the second year. In this study, the association between maternal behavior and offspring behaviors later in life was also reported in females that were

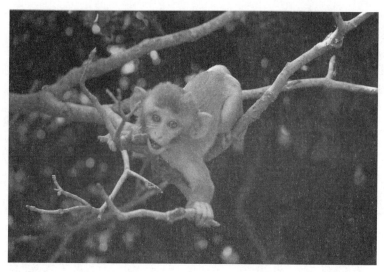

Figure 8.3 A rhesus macaque infant on Cayo Santiago, Puerto Rico. (Photo: Sean Coyne.) (See insert for color representation of this figure.)

cross-fostered at birth and reared by unrelated adult females, thus excluding the possibility of inherited temperamental similarities between mothers and offspring. See Figure 8.3.

Only a few data are available about the relationship between variable maternal care and offspring hormonal measures in nonhuman primates (e.g., Bardi et al., 2005). Maestripieri et al. (2006a; 2006b) reported that offspring reared by mothers with higher levels of maternal rejection exhibited lower CSF levels of 5-Hydroxyindoleacetic acid (5-HIAA), 3 methoxy-4-hydroxyphenylglycol (MHPG), and Homovanillic acid (HVA) in the first 3 years of life than offspring reared by mothers with lower levels of rejection. This difference was observed in both nonfostered and cross-fostered infants, suggesting that exposure to variable parenting style early in life interacts with genetically inherited propensities in determining CSF monoamine metabolite levels (Rogers et al., 2004). Furthermore, CSF MHPG levels in the second year of life were negatively correlated with solitary play and avoidance of other individuals, while CSF 5-HIAA levels were negatively correlated with scratching rates, suggesting that individuals with low CSF 5-HIAA had higher anxiety (Maestripieri et al., 1992). In contrast, variation in maternal protectiveness early in life did not predict later variation in CSF monoamine metabolite levels or offspring behavior (Maestripieri et al., 2006a). Taken together, the studies by Maestripieri et al. (2006a; 2006b) suggest that exposure to maternal rejection early in life may affect the development of different neural circuits underlying emotion regulation, ranging from fear to anxiety to impulse control.

It is very likely that the effects of variable maternal protectiveness and rejection on behavioral and neuroendocrine development result from different mechanisms. Maternal rejection is a physically and psychologically stressful experience for a primate infant. Mothers often reject their infants by hitting them or biting them, which appears to cause pain and distress in the infant. Being denied bodily contact and access to nipple, even in the absence of physical punishment, also causes significant distress in infants, which is expressed in loud screams and geckers, and temper tantrums (Maestripieri, 2002). Frequently rejected infants also show behavioral signs of depression. Therefore, exposure of different rates of maternal rejection early in life is directly comparable to exposure to a stressor with different levels of intensity. In rhesus macaques, the average infant begins being rejected in the 3rd or 4th week of life at the rate of 1 episode every 2 hours, or less (Maestripieri, 1998b). The rate of rejection gradually increases as infants grow older and peaks at 6 months of age, when mothers resume their mating activities. Some infants do not experience rejection at all, however, while others are rejected at the rate of 3–4 episodes per hour, or higher, as early as in their first week of life (Maestripieri, 1998b). When the behavioral and physiological effects of rejection are considered together, they support the resilience model of stress development, which assumes a J-shaped relationship between early stress intensity and the development of stress vulnerability and rejection (Lyons et al., 1999; Parker et al., 2006; Parker and Maestripieri, 2011). In fact, the data reviewed above suggest that infants that experience little or no rejection become fearful and behaviorally inhibited later in life, whereas those exposed to extremely high rates of rejection become highly anxious and impulsive.

Unlike rejection, maternal protectiveness in itself is not stressful and exposure to different levels of protectiveness is not expected to directly affect the development of stress-sensitive physiological systems such as the HPA axis or the serotonergic system. Different levels of maternal protectiveness, however, provide infants with different opportunities to independently explore the environment and develop behavioral and physiological coping strategies to deal with stress. Again, the data reviewed above suggest that moderate levels of protectiveness may provide infants with opportunities to master environmental challenges with their mothers' supervision and support, and therefore foster resilience, while too little or too much protectiveness may hamper the developing individual's ability to effectively cope with challenges. More behavioral and physiological data are needed to demonstrate the developmental effects of variation in maternal protectiveness, as well as to investigate the interactive effects of simultaneous variation in protectiveness and rejection.

That variation in maternal style, at least in the maternal rejection dimension, has long-lasting consequences for development is also demonstrated by intergenerational effects. Maestripieri et al. (2007) found significant similarities in maternal rejection rates between mothers and daughters for both nonfostered and cross-fostered rhesus females (see also Berman, 1990), suggesting that the daughters' behavior was affected by exposure to their mothers' rejection in their first 6 months of life. Both nonfostered and cross-fostered rhesus females reared by mothers with high rates of maternal rejection had significantly lower CSF concentrations of 5-HIAA in their first 3 years of life than females reared by mothers with lower (below the median) rates of maternal rejection, and low CSF 5-HIAA was associated with high rejection rates when the daughters produced and reared their first offspring (Maestripieri et al., 2006a; 2007).

Long-term changes in the offspring serotonergic system and concomitant changes in anxiety and impulsivity resulting from early exposure to variable maternal rejection may be responsible not only for the intergenerational transmission of maternal rejection rates, but also for the transmission of infant abuse. The natural occurrence of infant abuse in monkeys provides the opportunity to study the developmental consequences of an early adverse experience that is within the range of experience of the species and shares many similarities with child maltreatment (Maestripieri and Carroll, 1998a; 1998b; Maestripieri et al., 1997). Among rhesus macaques and other cercopithecine monkeys living in large captive groups, 5–10% of all infants born in a given year are physically abused by their mothers (Maestripieri and Carroll, 1998a; 1998b; Maestripieri et al., 1997). In rhesus macaques, abusive mothers may drag their infants by their tail or leg, or throw them in the air. Abuse bouts last only a few seconds, and the rest of the time abusive mothers show competent patterns of maternal behavior. Abuse is most frequent in the first month of infant life and rare or nonexistent after the third month, when infants are more independent from their mothers (Maestripieri, 1998b; McCormack et al., 2006). Although monkey infants who survive early maternal abuse appear to be far less behaviorally and physically traumatized than socially deprived monkeys, abuse perpetrated by the infant's biological mother probably entails a psychological trauma with profound negative consequences. Moreover, even if abuse is limited to the first months of infant life, continuous coexistence with the abusive mother and observation of abuse being repeated with younger siblings could contribute to reinforce and perpetuate the traumatic effects of abuse into adulthood. Cross-fostering experiments demonstrated that early experience plays an important role in the intergenerational transmission of infant abuse (Maestripieri, 2005a). Approximately half of cross-fostered and non-cross-fostered females abused early in life exhibit abusive parenting with their first-born offspring (Maestripieri, 2005a), and those who do so have lower CSF concentrations of 5-HIAA than those who do not (Maestripieri et al., 2006a; 2007).

Observations of social and behavioral development have suggested that abused infants may be delayed in the acquisition of independence from their mothers and in the development of peer relations in the first year of life (Maestripieri and Carroll, 1998c). In rhesus macaques, the stressful (both physically and psychologically) experience of being abused early in life results in both acute and long-term alterations in HPA axis function.

In a recent study, basal morning levels of cortisol in 10 abused and 10 control infants were measured at 1, 3 and 6 months of age, and ACTH and cortisol responses to stress were measured in month 6 (McCormack et al., 2009). In addition, infants were genotyped for the serotonin transporter gene (*5-HTTLPR*) and individuals carrying one or two copies of the short allele of this gene were compared to those carrying two copies of the long "protective" allele (function of *5-HTTLPR* discussed in greater detail below). During the first month, when physical abuse rates were the highest, abused infants had elevated basal morning cortisol levels compared to controls and showed greater distress responses to handling. In this month, in addition to a main effect of abuse on basal cortisol levels, there was also a significant interaction between early experience and *5-HTTLPR* genotype such that the effects of abuse on basal cortisol levels were especially strong in infants carrying the short *5-HTTLPR* allele. After the first month, abused infants' basal HPA axis function recovered to levels similar to controls. Despite the normalization of basal activity, there were group by sex effects on the HPA axis stress response in month 6, such that abused males showed significantly higher ACTH stress responses than control males when exposed to novelty stress in the absence of the mother. The higher ACTH stress responses were associated with higher levels of anxious behaviors at that age. Thus, abused exhibited both increased HPA axis activity and increased emotional reactivity in the period of time while abuse occurred for a few months following abuse.

In a larger study comparing the development of 21 abused and 21 nonabused rhesus monkey infants, the infants who were physically abused by their mothers in the first 3 months of life showed significantly different responses to CRF challenges performed at 6-month intervals during their first 3 years of life when compared to nonabused infants (Sanchez et al., 2010). Specifically, the administration of exogenous CRF resulted in a greater increase in plasma cortisol concentrations in abused than in nonabused infants, both males and females, when these were 6, 12, 18, 24, 30 and 36 months old. The abused infants also showed a blunted plasma ACTH response to CRF, but this difference was observed only at 6 months of age. Finally, a subset of abused females, but not males, also showed greater plasma cortisol responses to stress test (a 20-minute novel environment test) than nonabused females during their first 3 years of life (Maestripieri, 2005b). Taken together, these results suggest that early maternal abuse results in greater adrenocortical, and possibly also pituitary, responsiveness to challenges later in life. The greater cortisol levels (basal, in response to stress, and in response to CRF) observed in the abused subjects are consistent with the results of many animal and human studies showing that individuals who are exposed to traumatic stress early in life exhibit later HPA hyperreactivity to challenges (see Gunnar and Quevedo, 2007 for a review).

All of the above-reviewed research on the developmental effects of maternal abuse in macaques has been conducted with infants exposed to relatively low rates of abuse, whose life was not in jeopardy and which, in many cases, suffered only minor bruises and scratches that did not require an intervention. Although maternal abuse invariably begins in the 1st or 2nd week of life, peaks in frequency later in the first month, and gradually decreases until it ends by the end of the 3rd month (Maestripieri, 1998b), there are stable differences among abusive mothers in the rate with which they exhibit abuse. Essentially, abuse that occurs at a rate of one or more episodes per hour in the 1st or 2nd week of life can potentially jeopardize the infant's life (some rhesus monkey mothers that exhibit such high rates of abuse end up killing all of their infants, year after year; Maestripieri and Carroll, 1998b), whereas abuse rates lower than 1 episode per hour are associated with good chances of infant survival. Since no data are available on the behavioral and neuroendocrine development of infants exposed to very different levels of abuse, the effects of variation in the intensity of this stressor on the development of stress vulnerability vs. resilience are not well understood (see Parker and Maestripieri, 2011). The data reviewed above concerning infants exposed to low/moderate levels of abuse suggest that these infants exhibit increased vulnerability to stress later in life, rather than resilience. This effect, however, may be the result of the high rates of maternal rejection that typically accompany maternal abuse, regardless of its frequency, rather than the result of abuse alone. Further research is needed to examine the effects of different rates of abuse on development as well as to disentangle the effects of high maternal rejection and abuse when they co-occur.

Main genetic effects on the development of infant behavior and stress reactivity

Heritability, broadly defined, is the proportion of phenotypic variance that is attributable to genotypic variance (H^2). A more useful tool, however, is narrow-sense heritability, which is the proportion of phenotypic variation that is explained by additive variance, given by the formula $h^2 = V_A/V_P$ (Blomquist, 2012; Blomquist and Brent, 2014). While the denominator (V_P) includes all observed variation, it typically excludes factors that are known to affect variation in a fixed way, such as sex, age, or birth cohort. Further, the numerator (V_A) is the sum of the average effects of the parents' alleles (Visscher et al., 2008). It is important to note that traditionally many studies of heritability, both in humans and nonhuman primates, are done with adult individuals, and rarely include infants or juveniles. However, in more recent studies in nonhuman primates there is an increasing trend to use infants and adolescents as subjects. This trend is important as we know that the heritability of traits may change over time (i.e, genetic and environmental factors exert differing influences at different life stages).

Studies of genotyped primate populations and studies of cross-fostered individuals have provided evidence for moderate to strong heritability of CSF concentrations of 5-HIAA and other monoamine metabolites (Higley et al., 1993; Rogers et al., 2004). Little is known about the heritability of stress hormones (e.g., baseline cortisol or stress cortisol levels), while there have been several studies that have investigated the heritability of various stress-related behaviors. For example, a study by Fairbanks and colleagues (2004) investigated the impulsive and aggressive behaviors of vervet monkeys. The investigators tested both adolescents and adults on an intruder challenge task. In this version of the task, 3–4 subjects at a time were tested in their home enclosure with a sex-matched adult intruder. The behavioral measure was a Social Impulsivity Index that the authors created combining the following behaviors: latency to approach the intruder, standing or sitting within 1 meter of the intruder, and touching, sniffing, displaying to, or threatening the intruder. Results indicate that the heritability of the Social Impulsivity Index was $h^2 = 0.35$ [0.11], which is similar to the heritability of human personality traits (Fairbanks et al., 2004). In another study involving infant rhesus macaques, the subjects were assessed in both a free play task and a human intruder task (Fawcett et al., 2014). However, in this free play task the infants were brought into a novel environment with their anesthetized mother, in order to allow for the relative calming effect of her presence without the direct social influence she would exert while awake. The investigators measured the latency to leave the mother (if at all) during the free play task, as well as exploratory behavior and attempted escape behavior during the human intruder task. Results indicate that both latency to leave the mother during free play (estimated $h^2 = 0.263$ [0.003]) and attempted escapes during the intruder change (estimated $h^2 = 0.295$ [0.007]) are heritable. In these examples, it is clear that various measures of behavioral responses to stressful tasks are heritable traits and most likely have identifiable molecular genetic influences.

One potential source of variation in genetic influences on behavior is polymorphisms, or population variation in the structure of the DNA. Polymorphisms may be at a single nucleotide (single nucleotide polymorphism, or SNP) at a particular genomic locus or may include longer, often repeated, strings of sequences (variable tandem number of repeats, or VTNR). Polymorphisms in genes involved in emotion regulation such as brain neurotransmitter genes are likely to be particularly important in influencing variation in behavioral development and reactivity to stress. We here focus on the influence of several specific genes that have been extensively studied in regard to stress reactivity and emotional behavior: the serotonin transporter gene (*5HTT*) the *μ*-opioid receptor gene (*OPRM1*), and the dopamine D4 receptor gene (*DRD4*). Other genetic polymorphisms that have been investigated in nonhuman primates, which may also have an influence on stress reactivity, include the serotonin receptor 1A (*5-HT1A*) gene, the tryptophan hydroxylase 2 (*TPH2*) gene, the monoamine oxidase A (*MAO-A*) gene, the dopamine receptor 1 (*DRD1*) gene, the glucocorticoid receptor (*GR*) gene, the corticotropin-releasing hormone (*CRH*) gene, and genes involved in neuropeptide Y (*NPY*) and in the brain-derived neurotrophic factor (*BDNF*). Work with these other gene polymorphisms will not be systematically reviewed but they will be briefly discussed where appropriate.

Gene polymorphisms can potentially moderate the effects of early experience, so that such effects will be greater or smaller in individuals carrying particular alleles. Epigenetic regulation of the expression of these genes can also be a mechanism through which early experience can influence behavior or stress reactivity. Epigenetic regulation may involve changes in histone modification or DNA methylation patterns (DNA methylation is the addition of a methyl group to cytosine-guanine [CpG] dinucleotides). When it occurs within gene regulatory regions, DNA methylation typically inhibits gene expression, which we discuss further below.

Serotonin transporter gene (*5HTT*) and its linked polymorphic region (*5-HTTLPR*)

Serotonin is a monoaminergic neurotransmitter that serves many functions in the body, but most importantly here, plays a crucial role in modulating emotional behavior in the brain. Heritability of variation in serotonergic function could arise from any genes whose products participate in serotonin's synthesis, release, reuptake, or metabolism, or in genes that encode serotonin receptors (Manuck et al., 2006). In both humans and in rhesus macaques, there is an orthologous (i.e, similar to, but not inherited from a common ancestor) mutation in the promoter region of the serotonin transporter (*5-HTT*) gene referred to as the serotonin transporter linked polymorphic region (*5-HTTLPR*). The gene has two alleles referred to as "short" or *s* and "long" or *l*. The short allele confers lower transcriptional efficiency to the serotonin transporter gene (Bennett et al., 2002) and is associated with reduced serotonin reuptake into the presynaptic neuron and reduced serotonergic responsivity to neuroendocrine challenges (Manuck et al., 2006). Human studies have shown that individuals with one or two copies of the short allele have greater neuroticism and anxiety (Greenberg et al., 2000) and greater amygdala neuronal activation in response to faces with threatening expressions (Hariri et al., 2002; Skuse, 2006).

In rhesus macaques, the *5-HTTLPR* polymorphism is generally unrelated to CSF concentrations of 5-HIAA (Bennett et al., 2002; see also Maestripieri et al., 2006a). Nevertheless, individuals who carry the short allele for *5-HTTLPR* appear to share some behavioral traits with individuals with low CSF 5-HIAA, including higher aggressiveness and earlier age of male emigration from the group (Trefilov et al., 2000). Some evidence exists that the *5-HTTLPR* can influence early behavioral development and reactivity to the environment in rhesus macaques. In a recent study, 6-month-old infants were separated from their mothers for 4 days and returned to them for 3 days, before being separated again over a total of four weeks (Spinelli et al., 2012). Results indicate that individuals carrying a short allele exhibited greater rates of environmental exploration and locomotion than homozygous long individuals. Further, there was an interaction effect such that short-allele individuals increased their SDBs compared to long-allele individuals over the course of multiple separations. In a study of similar design (i.e, 4 days of maternal separation followed by 3 days of reunion repeated four times; Spinelli et al., 2007), there was a main effect of genotype such that individuals with a short allele showed lower levels of behavioral acute despair (measured as distress vocalization, SDBs, and behavioral withdrawal), higher stereotypic behavior, and lower environmental exploration.

Another study assessed differences in behavior of infant and juvenile rhesus macaques across four testing paradigms: a free play test, a remote-controlled car test (a type of novel object test, only here the novel object is mobile), a human intruder test, and a novel fruit test (Bethea et al., 2004). In addition to being genotyped for the *5-HTTLPR* and given the above behavioral tests, a small subset of the subjects was tested postpuberty for differences in neuroendocrine serotonergic function via a fenfluramine challenge. In a fenfluramine challenge, an anesthetized animal is injected with fenfluramine and prolactin levels are measured regularly post injection. Prolactin responses to fenfluramine are an indicator for overall central serotonin function, and the short allele of the *5-HTTLPR* has been demonstrated to confer an attenuated prolactin response to a fenfluramine challenge in humans (Reist et al., 2001). Individuals homozygous for the short allele were behaviorally inhibited in the free play test, engaged in more fear behaviors in the remote-controlled car test, and threatened the intruder more in the human intruder test. There was no difference between genotypes of either sex in the prolactin response to fenfluramine. Therefore, individuals homozygous for the short allele demonstrate greater anxiety across domains, and this increased anxiety is independent of a global neurohormonal challenge. Further, in a study of the physiological effects of *5-HTTLPR*, Barr and colleagues (2004) employed a maternal separation test and showed that individuals carrying the short allele had higher ACTH levels than those with two copies of the long allele. Finally, in a study of the effects of maternal abuse of infants, investigators examined the *5-HTTLPR* in both abused and nonabused infants and the reaction of those infants to a novel environment test (McCormack et al., 2009). Infants with the short allele were more behaviorally stressed by human handling (e.g., resistant to being handled, unable to be consoled, and produced more tantrums). Infants with the short allele also displayed higher cortisol and ACTH levels compared to peers homozygous for the long allele. Furthermore, infants with the short allele who were separated from their mothers at birth or physically abused by them were more likely to show anxiety and fear in response to novelty and dysregulated HPA axis responses to stress than individuals with the same early experience who were homozygous for the long allele.

The *5-HTTLPR* polymorphism has recently been the subject of studies examining the possible epigenetic mechanisms through which early experience affects primate behavioral development. In one study by Kinnally and colleagues (2010a), infant rhesus macaques (age 90–120 days old) were genotyped for the

5-HTTLPR as well as sampled for methylation at a promoter region, an 800 base pair long "island" approximately 200bp downstream from the *5-HTTLPR*, and then given a maternal separation test. Results indicate that methylation of the *5-HTT* promoter region (i.e, lowered *5-HTT* function) was greater in individuals with a short allele of the *5-HTTLPR* than those with the long alleles. Further, only the methylation patterns and not *5-HTTLPR* genotype predicted variation in two measures of stress reactivity: activity (measured by proportion of time spent in locomotion, proportion of time in the hang position, rate of environmental exploration and whether the animal displayed eating, drinking or crouching) and emotionality (measured by distress vocalizations, SDBs, and aggressive behaviors). Another study of DNA methylation in a different promoter region (*H3K4me3*) of the *5-HTT* gene also showed greater methylation (i.e, lowered gene function) for individuals carrying the short *5-HTTLPR* allele (Lindell et al., 2012).

In another related investigation of the integrated nature of the *5-HTTLPR* gene, one study looked at the function of both the *5-HTTLPR* and the *MAOA-LPR* (Kinnally et al., 2010b). Monoamine Oxidase A (MAOA) is an enzyme that oxidates and inactivates monoaminergic compounds, such as serotonin (Sabol et al., 1998). The *MAOA-LPR* gene (which is present in both humans and NHPs, displays a variable tandem number of repeats, VTNR, and is located in a promoter region) affects the production of MAOA, with certain repeats conferring "high" transcription efficiency while others confer "low" transcription efficiency (e.g., in rhesus macaques, 5 or 6 repeats confer high-functioning gene activity, while 7 repeats confers low-functioning gene activity). These transcription efficiencies functionally affect the levels of available serotonin. In order to detect the effects of *5-HTTLPR* and *MAOA-LPR*, Kinnally and colleagues (2010b) employed a maternal separation test and a human intruder test. The infant rhesus macaques were 90–120 days old, placed in social isolation for 25-hours and then tested on the human intruder task. The investigators measured stress reactivity on two dimensions: behavioral reactivity (e.g., locomotion, crouching, environmental exploration) and emotional reactivity (e.g., distress vocalizations, SDBs, threatening signals). There were no main effect of either single gene on behavior, but there was an interaction effect between the genes. Individuals with both high-function genotypes were less behaviorally reactive to the human intruder test than individuals with at least one low-functioning gene. Further, infants with one high-functional allele and one low-functional allele of the two different genes (i.e, a high-function *5-HTTLPR* and low-function *MAOA-LPR* or low-function *5-HTTLPR* and high-function *MAOA-LPR*) were less emotionally reactive than other infants (i.e, two high-functioning genes or two low-functioning genes). In a study solely investigating the effects of *MAOA-LPR*, infant rhesus macaques that carried the low-activity *rhMAOA-LPR* genotype and were reared in small social groups were at higher risk for expression of aggressive behaviors during a stressful situation, while those reared by mothers alone in a restricted environment exhibited greater rates of behavior thought to reflect anxiety (Karere et al., 2009).

The mechanisms by which *5-HTTLPR* and other polymorphisms interact with early experience in affecting behavioral development and reactivity to stress are still largely unknown. If early stress exerts long-term effects on *5-HTT* expression and behavior, we would expect to observe *5-HTT* dysregulation soon after the experience of an early stressor. Lower poststressor *5-HTT* expression in peripheral blood mononuclear cells (white blood cells) has been observed in infant rhesus macaques that experience early life stress (maternal deprivation or aggression, Kinnally et al., 2008) and was associated with behavioral disinhibition during stress at an early stage in development (Kinnally et al., 2008). These findings suggest that *5-HTT* impairment, when induced by stress at a critical period in development, may lead to emotion dysregulation that may be long lasting.

The *μ*-opioid receptor gene (*OPRM1*)

Both humans and nonhuman primates have a single nucleotide polymorphism, albeit at different locations, of the *μ*-opioid receptor (*OPRM1)* gene. In nonhuman primates, two alleles for this gene have been reported (C and G), with the homozygous C/C being the most common genotype. Endogenous opioids have been implicated in the formation and maintenance of social bonds, including mother-infant bonds, in nonhuman primates and other animals (Nelson and Panksepp, 1998). For example, *β*-endorphins, which preferentially bind to the *μ*-opioid receptors, are released after grooming behavior in monkeys (Keverne et al., 1989). Consistent with the opioid hypothesis of attachment, there is now some evidence that the *OPRM1* gene polymorphism is associated with variation both in maternal attachment and in infant responses to separation from the mother. In terms of maternal attachment, one study of free-ranging rhesus macaques showed that mothers with a G allele displayed greater restraining behavior (i.e, preventing the infant from breaking contact and leaving the mother) as well as higher CSF oxytocin levels during lactation compared to individuals with the C allele (Higham et al., 2011). Two studies have investigated behavioral and physiological responses of 6-month old rhesus macaque infants to separation from their mothers in relation to the *OPRM1* polymorphism. Barr et al. (2008) conducted a 4-day mother-infant separation, followed by a 3-day reunion; separation and reunion were repeated for a total of four times. Prior to separation test (i.e, under natural, nonexperimental conditions), G allele infants showed the highest maternal attachment rates. During the separation test, C allele infants decreased their distress vocalization over time but individuals with the G allele persisted in calling throughout the test. Further, upon reunion with the mother, infants with the G allele spent increasing amounts of social contact with their mother and less with other social group members while C allele infants interacted equally with their mother and other group mates, as well as solitary exploration. In another study from the same research group, it was shown that rhesus infants with the G allele had lower ACTH and cortisol responses to the stress of maternal separation than C allele individuals (Schwandt et al., 2011). Miller et al. (2004) proposed that in individuals carrying different *OPRM1* alleles, β-endorphins have differential affinity to the receptors. β-endorphins have an inhibitory effect on μ-opioid function and such inhibition affects ACTH production, which in turn modulates the release of cortisol. Therefore, the observed effects of the *OPRM1* polymorphism on infant responses to separation stress may be an expression of a more general relationship between the endogenous opioid system and HPA axis reactivity to stress.

Dopamine receptor D4 (*DRD4*) and other reward-related genes

In the central nervous system, dopamine serves as a neurotransmitter that is primarily associated with reward-motivated behavior, but is also important for motor control. Like *OPRM1*, *DRD4* displays a polymorphism with a VNTR, in both humans and NHPs, and has certain repeats that confer a high functioning of the receptor and other repeats that confer low function. In nonhuman primates, the *DRD4* polymorphism has been investigated in relation to personality traits such as novelty seeking, which are expected to influence behaviors such as exploration, assertiveness, aggressiveness, and dominance. In one study of juvenile vervet monkeys, individuals with the low-functioning 5-repeat (5R) allele showed significantly shorter latencies to approach a potentially threatening novel object that was in their home enclosure than those who carried the high-functioning 6R allele (Bailey et al., 2007). In another study of juvenile vervets that used a conspecific intruder challenge, groups of 3–5 juveniles were presented with a novel adult male in their home enclosure (Fairbanks et al., 2012). The investigators measured what they called the Social Impulsivity Index, which combines latency to approach the intruder with risky, assertive, and aggressive behaviors, all of which are validated reactions to the stress inducing intruder challenge. Individuals with the low-functioning copy of *DRD4* showed higher rates of social impulsivity, which included shorter latencies to approach the intruder, touch the intruder, and direct behavioral displays toward the intruder (Fairbanks et al., 2012). Research in our lab has investigated the role of *DRD4* on several behaviors of juvenile rhesus macaques in a free-ranging population. Of interest here, we examined how individuals allocated the time spent within or away from social proximity of their mother, an attempt at a naturalistic (albeit self-imposed) measure of maternal separation, as well as preventative submissive behaviors (i.e, submissive signals directed at individuals without any aggressive provocation), a potential measure of social anxiety. Our results indicate that individuals with low-functioning *DRD4* alleles spend significantly less time within proximity of their mother, but engage in more preventative submissive behaviors (Coyne et al., 2015).

Another single nucleotide polymorphism in the promoter of the gene that encodes the dopamine receptor type 1 (*DRD1*), which is thought to be involved with the experience of reward, is linked with higher alcohol consumption in macaques (Newman et al., 2009) and may also influence infant behavioral development and stress reactivity. Additionally, two other SNPs, one in the promoter of the CRH gene and one in the neuropeptide Y (*NPY*) gene promoter, have also each been linked with an increased stress response (HPA and behavioral activation during a stressful social separation) as well as greater propensity for alcohol consumption in macaques (*CRH*: Barr et al., 2009, *NPY*: Lindell et al., 2010).

The above studies indicate that *DRD4*, *DRD1*, and other reward-related or emotion-related genes may play important roles in regulating behavioral development and stress reactivity in nonhuman primates. Most, if not all of these studies, however, have been conducted with rhesus macaques and only a few behavioral responses have been examined. Genetic variation in dopaminergic function and its influence on behavioral development and stress reactivity need to be further investigated in species other than rhesus macaques and using experimental paradigms involving more diverse measures of behavior and reactivity to the environment. Moreover, further research is needed to elucidate the physiological mechanisms through which genetic variation in dopaminergic function affects behavior and stress reactivity. Finally, the effects of early experience on the development of the brain dopamine system, and how these effects interact with genetic variation, should be addressed in future primate research.

Summary and conclusions

Variation in early experience can have major long-lasting consequences for behavioral development and stress reactivity in nonhuman primates. In particular, many studies have shown that variable maternal style along the dimensions of protectiveness and rejection can influence many aspects of infant social development as well as behavioral and physiological reactivity to the environment. These effects, in many cases, are mediated by experience-induced alterations in neural and neuroendocrine systems involved in emotion regulation such as the brain serotonin system and the HPA axis. Variation in neurotransmitter or endocrine function can also be the result of inherited genetic variation, and both early experience and genetic inheritance contribute to the maintenance of individual differences in behavior and reactivity to the environment across generations.

Although the study of genetic influences on behavioral development and stress reactivity in nonhuman primates is a relatively new area of research, a growing body of evidence has already accumulated about the importance of gene polymorphisms involved in emotion regulation, and in particular, of *5-HTTLPR*, *OPRM1*, and *DRD4*. The effects of these polymorphisms often interact with each other and with early experience, such as exposure to stress in the first few months of life. The mechanisms underlying main genetic effects on behavior or gene-environment interactions are still poorly understood but research on epigenetics appears to be particularly promising.

Although systematic research on the effects of genes and early experience in primates has been conducted with a very limited number of species such as rhesus macaques and vervet monkeys, it is highly likely that the results of this research are generalizable to other nonhuman primate species and also to humans. Nonhuman primate research has contributed in the past to our understanding of many fundamental aspects of early human behavioral development (e.g., the discovery of the attachment system and its role in mother-child relationships and in the acquisition of independence) and, in the future, has the potential to enhance our knowledge of brain-behavior relationships early in life and how these relationships are affected by genes and environment.

References

Altmann J. (1980). *Baboon Mothers and Infants*. Cambridge, MA: Harvard University Press.

Bailey JN, Breidenthal SE, Jorgensen MJ, Mccracken JT, Fairbanks LA. (2007). The association of DRD4 and novelty seeking is found in a nonhuman primate model. *Psychiatric Genetics* 17:23–27.

Bardi M, Huffman MA. (2006). Maternal behavior and maternal stress are associated with infant behavioral development in macaques. *Developmental Psychobiology* 48:1–9.

Bardi M, Bode AE, Ramirez SM, Brent LY. (2005). Maternal care and the development of the stress response. *Am J Primatology* 66:263–278.

Barr CS, Newman TK, Shannon C, et al. (2004). Rearing condition and rh5–HTTLPR interact to influence limbic–hypothalamic–pituitary–adrenal axis response to stress in infant macaques. *Biological Psychiatry* 55:733–738.

Barr CS, Schwandt ML, Lindell SG, et al. (2008). Variation at the mu–opioid receptor gene (OPRM1) influences attachment behavior in infant primates. *Proc Natl Acad Sci USA* 105:5277–5281.

Barr CS, Dvoskin RL, Gupte M, et al. (2009). Functional CRH variation increases stress–induced alcohol consumption in primates. *Proc Natl Acad Sci USA* 106:14593–14598.

Bennett AJ, Lesch KP, Heils A, Long JC, Lorenz JG, Shoaf SE, Champoux M, Suomi SJ, Linnoila M, Higley JD. (2002). Early experience and serotonin transporter gene variation interact to influence primate CNS function. *Molecular Psychiatry* 7:118–122.

Berman CM. (1990). Intergenerational transmission of maternal rejection rates among free–ranging rhesus monkeys. *Animal Behaviour* 39:329–337.

Bethea CL, Streicher JM, Coleman K, Pau FKY, Moessner R, Cameron JL. (2004). Anxious behavior and fenfluramine–induced prolactin secretion in young rhesus macaques with different alleles of the serotonin reuptake transporter polymorphism (5HTTLPR). *Behavior Genetics* 34:295–307.

Bird AP. (1986). CpG–rich islands and the function of DNA methylation. *Nature* 321: 209–213.

Blomquist GE. (2012). Female age of first reproduction at Cayo Santiago: Heritability and shared environments. In: *Bones, Genetics, and Behavior of Rhesus Macaques*, ed. S. Wang. Berlin: Springer.

Blomquist GE, Brent LJN. (2014). Applying quantitative genetic methods to primate social behavior. *International J Primatology* 35:108–128.

Coyne SP, Lindell SG, Clemente J, Barr CS, Parker KJ, Maestripieri D. (2015). Dopamine D4 receptor genotype variation in free-ranging rhesus macaques and its association with juvenile behavior. *Behav Brain Res*, 292:50–55.

Fairbanks LA. (1989). Early experience and cross–generational continuity of mother–infant contact in vervet monkeys. *Developmental Psychobiology* 22:669–681.

Fairbanks LA. (1996). Individual differences in maternal style: causes and consequences for mothers and offspring. *Adv Study Behavior* 25:579–611.

Fairbanks LA, Mcguire MT. (1987). Mother–infant Relationships in vervet monkeys: Response to new adult males. *International J Primatology* 8:351–366.

Fairbanks LA, Mcguire MT. (1988). Long–term effects of early mothering behavior on responsiveness to the environment in vervet monkeys. *Developmental Psychobiology* 21:711–724.

Fairbanks LA, Mcguire MT. (1993). Maternal protectiveness and response to the unfamiliar in vervet monkeys. *Am J Primatology* 30:119–129.

Fairbanks LA, Newman TK, Bailey JN, et al. (2004). Genetic contributions to social impulsivity and aggressiveness in vervet monkeys. *Biological Psychiatry* 55:642–647.

Fairbanks LA, Way BM, Breidenthal SE, Bailey JN, Jorgensen MJ. (2012). Maternal and offspring dopamine D4 receptor genotypes interact to influence juvenile impulsivity in vervet monkeys. *Psychological Sci* 23:1099–1104.

Fawcett GL, Dettmer AM, Kay D, Raveendran M, Higley JD, Ryan ND, Cameron JL, Rogers J. (2014). Quantitative genetics of response to novelty and other stimuli by infant rhesus macaques (Macaca mulatta) across three behavioral assessments. *International J Primatology* 35:325–339.

Fossey D. (1979). Development of the mountain gorilla (Gorilla gorilla beringei): The first thirty–six months. In: *The Great Apes*, ed. D.A. Hamburg and E.R. McCrown, pp. 139–184. Menlo Park, CA: Benjamin Cummings.

Greenberg BD, Li Q, Lucas FR, Hu S, Sirota LA, Benjamin J, Lesch KP, Hamer D, Murphy DL. (2000). Association between the serotonin transporter promoter polymorphism and personality traits in a primarily female population sample. *Am J Medical Genetics* 96:202–216.

Gunnar M, Quevedo K. (2007). The neurobiology of stress and development. *Annu Rev Psychology* 58:145–173.

Hariri AR, Tessitore A, Mattay VS, Fera F, Weinberger DR. (2002). The amygdala response to emotional stimuli: a comparison of faces and scenes. *Neuroimage* 17:317–323.

Higham JP, Barr CS, Hoffman CL, Mandalaywala TM, Parker KJ, Maestripieri D. (2011). Mu–opioid receptor (OPRM1) variation, oxytocin levels and maternal attachment in free–ranging rhesus macaques Macaca mulatta. *Behavioral Neurosci* 125:131–136.

Higley JD, Thompson WW, Champoux M, et al. (1993). Paternal and maternal genetic and environmental contributions to cerebrospinal–fluid monoamine metabolites in rhesus monkeys (Macaca mulatta). *Archives General Psychiatry* 50:615–623.

Hinde RA, Spencer–Booth Y. (1967). The behaviour of socially living rhesus monkeys in their first two and a half years. *Animal Behaviour* 15:169–196.

Hinde RA, Spencer–Booth Y. (1971). Effects of brief separation from mother on rhesus monkeys. *Science* 173:111–118.

Karere GM, Kinnally EL, Sanchez JN, Famula TR, Lyons LA, Capitanio JP. (2009). What is an "adverse" environment? Interactions of rearing experiences and MAOA genotype in rhesus monkeys. *Biological Psychiatry* 65:770–777.

Keverne EB, Martensz ND, Tuite B. (1989). Beta–endorphin concentrations in cerebrospinal fluid of monkeys are influenced by grooming relationships. *Psychoneuroendocrinology* 14:155–161.

Kinnally EL. (2012). Gene–environment coordination in neurobehavioral development. In: *Building Babies: Primate Development in Proximate and Ultimate Perspectives*, ed. K. Clancy, K. Hinde, and J.N. Rutherford. New York: Springer.

Kinnally EL, Lyons LA, Abel K, Mendoza S, Capitanio JP. (2008). Effects of early experience and genotype on serotonin transporter regulation in infant rhesus macaques. *Genes Brain Behav* 4:481–486.

Kinnally EL, Capitanio JP, Leibel R, Deng L, Ledue C, Haghighi F, Mann JJ. (2010a). Epigenetic regulation of serotonin transporter expression and behavior in infant rhesus macaques. *Genes, Brain Behavior* 9:575–582.

Kinnally EL, Karere GM, Lyons LA, Mendoza SP, Mason WA, Capitanio JP. (2010b). Serotonin pathway gene–gene and gene–environment interactions influence behavioral stress response in infant rhesus macaques. *Development Psychopathology* 22:35–44.

Lesch KP, Bengel D, Heils A, Sabol SZ, Greenberg BD, Petri S, Benjamin J, Muller CR, Hamer DH, Murphy DL. (1996). Association of anxiety–related traits with a polymorphism in the serotonin transporter gene regulatory region. *Science* 274:1527–1531.

Lindell SG, Schwandt ML, Sun H, Sparenborg JD, Bjork K, Kasckow JW, Sommer WH, Goldman D, Higley JD, Suomi SJ, Heilig M, Barr CS. (2010). Functional NPY variation as a factor in stress resilience and alcohol consumption in rhesus macaques. *Archives General Psychiatry* 67:423–431.

Lindell SG, Yuan QP, Zhou ZF, Goldman D, Thompson RC, Lopez JF, Suomi SJ, Higley JD, Barr CS. (2012). The serotonin transporter gene is a substrate for age and stress dependent epigenetic regulation in rhesus macaque brain: potential roles in genetic selection and Gene x Environment interactions. *Development Psychopathology* 24:1391–1400.

Lyons DM, Martel FL, Levine S, Risch NJ, Schatzberg AF. (1999). Postnatal experiences and genetic effects on squirrel monkey social affinities and emotional distress. *Hormones Behavior* 36:266–275.

Maestripieri D. (1994). Mother–infant relationships in three species of macaques (Macaca mulatta, M. nemestrina, M. arctoides). I. Development of the mother–infant relationship in the first three months. *Behaviour* 131:75–96.

Maestripieri D. (1998a). Social and demographic influences on mothering style in pigtail macaques. *Ethology* 104:379–385.

Maestripieri D. (1998b). Parenting styles of abusive mothers in group–living rhesus macaques. *Animal Behaviour* 55:1–11.

Maestripieri D. (2002). Parent–offspring conflict in primates. *International J of Primatology*, 23, 923–951.

Maestripieri D. (2005a). Early experience affects the intergenerational transmission of infant abuse in rhesus monkeys. *Proc Natl Acad Sci USA* 102:9726–9729.

Maestripieri D. (2005b). Effects of early experience on female behavioural and reproductive development in rhesus macaques. *Proc Royal Society London B* 272:1243–1248.

Maestripieri D, Carroll KA. (1998a). Behavioral and environmental correlates of infant abuse in group–living pigtail macaques. *Infant Behavior Development* 21:603–612.

Maestripieri D, Carroll KA. (1998b). Risk factors for infant abuse and neglect in group–living rhesus monkeys. *Psychological Sci* 9:143–145.

Maestripieri D, Carroll KA. (1998c). Child abuse and neglect: Usefulness of the animal data. *Psychological Bulletin* 123:211–223.

Maestripieri D, Schino G, Aureli F, Troisi A. (1992). A modest proposal: Displacement activities as an indicator of emotions in primates. *Animal Behaviour* 44:967–979.

Maestripieri D, Wallen K, Carroll KA. (1997). Infant abuse runs in families of group–living pigtail macaques. *Child Abuse Neglect* 21:465–471.

Maestripieri D, Tomaszycki M, Carroll KA. (1999). Consistency and change in the behavior of rhesus macaque abusive mothers with successive infants. *Developmental Psychobiology* 34:29–35.

Maestripieri D, McCormack K, Lindell SG, Higley JD, Sanchez MM. (2006a). Influence of parenting style on the offspring's behaviour and CSF monoamine metabolite levels in crossfostered and noncrossfostered female rhesus macaques. *Behavioural Brain Research* 175:90–95.

Maestripieri D, Higley JD, Lindell SG, Newman TK, Mccormack KM, Sanchez MM. (2006b). Early maternal rejection affects the development of monoaminergic systems and adult abusive parenting in rhesus macaques (Macaca mulatta). *Behavioral Neurosci* 120:1017–1024.

Maestripieri D, Lindell SG, Higley JD. (2007). Intergenerational transmission of maternal behavior in rhesus macaques and its underlying mechanisms. *Developmental Psychobiology* 49:165–171.

Mandalaywala TM, Parker KJ, Maestripieri D. (2014). Early experience affects the strength of vigilance for threat in rhesus monkey infants. *Psychological Sci* 25:1893–1902.

Manuck SB, Kaplan JR, Lotrich FE. (2006). Brain serotonin and aggressive disposition in humans and nonhuman primates. In: *Biology of Aggression*, ed. R.J. Nelson, pp. 65–113. Oxford: Oxford University Press.

McCormack K, Sanchez MM, Bardi M, Maestripieri D. (2006). Maternal care patterns and behavioral development of rhesus macaque abused infants in the first 6 months of life. *Dev Psychobiol* 48:537–50.

McCormack K, Newman TK, Higley JD, Maestripieri D, Sanchez MM. (2009). Serotonin transporter gene variation, infant abuse, and responsiveness to stress in rhesus macaque mothers and infants. *Hormones Behavior* 55:538–547.

Miller GM, Bendor J, Tiefenbacher S, Yang H, Novak MA, Madras BK. (2004). A mu–opioid receptor single nucleotide polymorphism in rhesus monkey: association with stress response and aggression. *Molecular Psychiatry* 9:99–108.

Mitani J, Call J, Kappeler P, Palombit R, Silk J. (2012). *The Evolution of Primate Societies*. Chicago: University of Chicago Press.

Nakamichi M. (1989). Sex differences in social development during the first 4 years in a free–ranging group of Japanese monkeys, Macaca fuscata. *Animal Behaviour* 38:737–748.

Nelson EE, Panksepp J. (1998). Brain substrates of infant–mother attachment: contributions of opioids, oxytocin, and norepinephrine. *Neurosci Biobehavioral Rev* 22:437–452.

Newman TK, Parker CC, Suomi SJ, Goldman D, Barr CS, Higley JD. (2009). DRD1 5′ UTR variation, sex and early infant stress influence ethanol consumption in rhesus macaques. *Genes, Brain Behavior* 8:626–630.

Parker KJ, Maestripieri D. (2011). Identifying key features of early stressful experiences that produce stress vulnerability and resilience in primates. *Neurosci Biobehavioral Rev* 35:1466–1483.

Parker KJ, Buckmaster CL, Sundlass K, Schatzberg AF, Lyons DM. (2006). Maternal mediation, stress inoculation, and the development of neuroendocrine stress resistance in primates. *Proc Natl Acad Sci USA* 103:3000–3005.

Plooij FX. (1984). *The Behavioral Development of Free–Living Chimpanzee Babies and Infants*. Amsterdam: Ablex Publishing.

Reist C, Mazzanti C, Vu R, Tran D, Goldman D. (2001). Serotonin transporter promoter polymorphism is associated with attenuated prolactin response to fenfluramine. *Am J Medical Genetics* 105:363–368.

Rogers J, Martin LJ, Comuzzie AG, Mann JJ, Manuck SB, Leland M, Kaplan JR. (2004). Genetics of monoamine metabolites in baboons: overlapping sets of genes influence levels of 5–hydroxyindolacetic acid, 3–hydroxy–4–methoxyphenylglycol, and homovanillic acid. *Biological Psychiatry* 55:739–744.

Rosenblum LA, Kaufman IC. (1967). Laboratory observations of early mother–infant relations in pigtail and bonnet macaques. In: *Social Communication among Primates*, ed. S.A. Altmann, pp. 33–41. Chicago: University of Chicago Press.

Sabol S, Hu S, Hamer D. (1998). A functional polymorphism in the Monoamine Oxidase A gene promoter. *Human Genetics* 103:273–279.

Sanchez MM, Mccormack K, Grand AP, Fulks R, Graff A, Maestripieri D. (2010). Effects of sex and early maternal abuse on adrenocorticotropin hormone and cortisol responses to the corticotropin–releasing hormone challenge during the first 3 years of life in group–living rhesus monkeys. *Development Psychopathology* 22:45–53.

Sapolsky RM, Romero LM, Munck AU. (2000). How do glucocorticoids influence stress responses? Integrating permissive, suppressive, stimulatory, and preparative actions. *Endocrine Rev* 21:55–89.

Schino G, D'Amato FR, Troisi A. (1995). Mother–infant relationships in Japanese macaques: sources of interindividual variation. *Animal Behaviour* 49:151–158.

Schino G, Speranza L, Troisi A. (2001). Early maternal rejection and later social anxiety in juvenile and adult Japanese macaques. *Developmental Psychobiology* 38:186–190.

Schwandt ML, Lindell SG, Higley JD, Suomi SJ, Heilig M, Barr CS. (2011). OPRM1 gene variation influences hypothalamic–pituitary–adrenal axis function in response to a variety of stressors in rhesus macaques. *Psychoneuroendocrinology* 36:1303–1311.

Simpson MJA. (1985). Effects of early experience on the behaviour of yearling rhesus monkeys (Macaca mulatta) in the presence of a strange object: classification and correlation approaches. *Primates* 26:57–72.

Simpson MJA, Datta SB. (1990). Predicting infant enterprise from early relationships in rhesus macaques. *Behaviour* 116:42–62.

Simpson MJA, Gore MA, Janus M, Rayment FDG. (1989). Prior experience of risk and individual differences in enterprise shown by rhesus monkey infants in the second half of their first year. *Primates* 30:493–509.

Skuse D. (2006). Genetic influences on the neural basis of social cognition. *Philosophical Transactions Royal Society London B* 361:2129–2141.

Spinelli S, Schwandt ML, Lindell SG, Newman TK, Heilig M, Suomi SJ, Higley JD, Goldman D, Barr CS. (2007). Association between the recombinant human serotonin transporter linked promoter region polymorphism and behavior in rhesus macaques during a separation paradigm. *Development Psychopathology* 19:977–987.

Spinelli S, Schwandt ML, Lindell SG, Heilig M, Suomi SJ, Higley JD, Goldman D, Barr CS. (2012). The serotonin transporter gene linked polymorphic region is associated with the behavioral response to repeated stress exposure in infant rhesus macaques. *Development Psychopathology* 24:157–165.

Tanaka I. (1989). Variability in the development of mother–infant relationships among free–ranging Japanese macaques. *Primates* 30:477–491.

Trefilov A, Berard J, Krawczak M, Schmidtke J. (2000). Natal dispersal in rhesus macaques is related to serotonin transporter gene promoter variation. *Behavior Genetics* 30:295–301.

Visscher PM, Hill WG, Wray NR. (2008). Heritability in the genomics era: concepts and misconceptions. *Nature Rev Genetics* 9:255–266.

Vochteloo JD, Timmermans PJA, Duijghuisen JAH, Vossen JMH. (1993). Effects of reducing the mother's radius of action on the development of mother–infant relationships in longtailed macaques. *Animal Behaviour* 45:603–612.

CHAPTER 9

Institutional deprivation and neurobehavioral development in infancy

Jenalee R. Doom and Megan R. Gunnar

Institute of Child Development, University of Minnesota, Minneapolis, Minnesota, USA

Introduction

Institutional care during infancy often deprives children of the social interaction, environmental experiences, and the nutrients needed to promote healthy development. Prolonged institutionalization is associated with deficits across cognitive, socioemotional, and physical domains. However, the poor levels of functioning observed while children are in institutional care are not permanent. Research has demonstrated that removal from depriving environments, especially early in life, is associated with a remarkable rebound in many domains. As such, it is impossible to discuss the impact of institutional care in infancy without also focusing on neural plasticity and the capacity of young children to rebound if their conditions improve. On the other hand, there is evidence for sensitive periods for development in some domains, such that despite improvements following removal from deprived conditions, impairments and delays continue to be observed for years postinstitutionalization. Thus, children who were placed in more enriched environments following institutional care serve as models of the potential and limitations of plasticity in early childhood.

Before discussing evidence for sensitive periods and plasticity following early institutional care, several principles of development that are pertinent to this research must be discussed. First, longer periods of deprivation are related to poorer outcomes, and earlier removal from the depriving environment is generally related to better long-term outcomes and greater plasticity. This principle likely has to do with the timing of brain development, which is protracted across childhood with sensory and primary association areas developing first followed by areas that govern higher order abilities. Thus, longer durations of institutional care likely coincide with the rapid development of a greater number of neural

Environmental Experience and Plasticity of the Developing Brain, First Edition.
Edited by Alessandro Sale.
© 2016 John Wiley & Sons, Inc. Published 2016 by John Wiley & Sons, Inc.

systems than a shorter period in an institution. Likewise, earlier placement into an enriched environment increases the likelihood that rapidly developing systems will be positively stimulated by necessary environmental inputs.

Second, it has so far not been possible to isolate what aspects of institutional care are responsible for certain outcomes, and it is likely that multiple factors, including physical, chemical, social, and nutritional factors, are interacting to produce the phenotype. While it may be tempting to ascribe certain behavioral traits to a particular cause, it is impossible to tease apart the effects of so many interacting influences in the institutional environment. We have previously noted, however, that cognitive and language development proceeded on pace in institutions that served as model, training institutions in Britain over a half century ago (Tizard and Joseph 1970). These institutions provided children with excellent nutrition, high levels of stimulation, adult:child ratios about 1:3 or 1:4, multi-aged small groups that were more family like, and lots of social interaction with adults and children. Yet, staff turnover was high as nurses came to be trained and left for permanent jobs, and emotional development and behavior problems emerged and were persistent long after the children were placed in families (Hodges and Tizard, 1989). Thus, we concluded that nutrition and stimulation seem to be critical for cognitive and language development, but that emotional development is more strongly influenced by the presence and availability of relationships with a consistently available, supportive adult (Gunnar, 2001).

Third, individual differences in functioning often result even after experiencing similar environments. Although some children are quite sensitive to harsh early environments, others are resilient and either adapt successfully in the face of adversity or rebound more effectively once conditions improve. Differences in genetics may partially explain individual differences, but there are also a number of psychosocial factors involving how other people respond to the child and chance factors (e.g, a caretaker takes a particular shine to a child and provides them with more stimulation) that contribute to risk and resilience. Additionally, in studies of internationally adopted children who come from many different institutions, measuring the quality of preadoption conditions is difficult and of unknown reliability as it is based on parent report of what they were allowed to see.

Fourth, the particular stages of brain development that are underway during periods of institutional care must be considered when trying to understand sensitive periods of development and what functions may be most affected. Additionally, disruptions in functioning associated with early institutionalization should be studied together with the underlying brain regions and neural networks that map onto each particular domain. It must be noted that institutional care may have direct and/or indirect effects on each region of the brain and social/cognitive domain. The prefrontal cortex is a prime example of a brain region affected by institutional care both directly and indirectly as it develops rapidly early in life when institutionalization is most likely to occur, making it more susceptible to environmental perturbations. The prefrontal cortex is also a "hub-region" for coordinating information across the brain (Gao et al., 2009), meaning that it may be particularly at risk for indirect effects of institutional care on associated brain regions. For example, during the first year of life, the putamen shows the fastest growth rate in comparison to all other areas of the brain (Choe et al., 2012). As the putamen scaffolds the initiation of voluntary movement and environmental learning, and shares expansive connections with the prefrontal cortex, any damage to the putamen sustained during early life may negatively affect the development of the prefrontal cortex. In addition, larger effects could unfold over time in regions that are quickly developing during the period of deprivation (Nishida et al., 2006). On the other hand, the more we learn about the development of regions like the prefrontal cortex, the more we realize that these regions, while once thought of as late developing, are active and serve important functions during infancy. Thus, there may be more direct influences of stimulus deprivation on what were once thought of as only "late developing" regions (Kolb et al., 2012).

There is increasing evidence for sensitive periods of development, during which the experience of institutional care or placement into an enriched environment has lasting effects on functioning. Nonetheless, while it would be very helpful to be able to differentiate duration of deprivation from the timing of deprivation, because most children arrive in institutional care at birth or shortly thereafter, timing and duration are typically too highly correlated to disentangle. This complicates sensitive period analyses, leaving the field with suggestive but far from conclusive evidence.

Fifth, unlike a deprived environment, which promotes plasticity that may reduce the potential for positive development, an enriched environment promotes plasticity that supports positive development by stimulating the brain with necessary social and sensory inputs. Although catch-up in certain domains may not be complete, the vast majority of research indicates that children who have been placed into adoptive or foster care homes outperform those who still live in institutions (van IJzendoorn and Juffer, 2006). Thus, relieving conditions of deprivation in order to support healthier development is the direction of policy advice, while whether or not this means removal from institutions depends on the availability of an infrastructure that supports the availability of safe, supportive family care arrangements (McCall, 2011).

Unfortunately, institutions that provide care for orphaned or abandoned children are unlikely to disappear in the near future, so research and interventions targeting institutions around the world are necessary to aid children's development despite unfavorable circumstances. In addition to improving children's outcomes, attention to within-institution interventions, can provide insight into the factors that promote psychosocial and neurobiological recovery in institutionalized children, which contributes valuable information about the nature of human development and necessary factors for healthy functioning.

The current review will cover cognitive, emotional, and behavioral systems impacted by early institutional care as well as neural systems, as evidenced by the use of imaging technology and electrophysiology. Impacts on stress-mediating systems such as the hypothalamic-pituitary-adrenal (HPA) axis and relatively recent research on genetic moderation of outcomes and epigenetics will be discussed as these are expected to relate to physical and mental health outcomes. Finally, we will discuss sensitive periods of development, postinstitutional factors affecting outcomes (e.g, parenting and attachment), and the plasticity of brain and behavioral systems following early intervention. Implications of studying children within institutions, children placed into foster care or adopted into families, and those undergoing psychosocial or nutritional interventions will be discussed in relation to what these groups can tell us about institutionalization and the human condition. Comparisons to children experiencing other forms of adversity will be discussed in order to understand the specific sequelae of institutional care and how research on children who have experienced institutionalization can be applied to other groups facing adversity.

Cognition

General intelligence and higher order cognitive skills (executive function) are negatively impacted by time spent in institutional care, and recovery following institutional care varies by the cognitive domain affected and the brain regions rapidly developing during the period of institutionalization. A meta-analysis of 75 studies reported an effect size of $d = 0.74$ for the effect of institutionalization on IQ between children living in orphanages versus those raised in their families, which is on average a 20 point IQ difference (Van IJzendoorn et al., 2008). The Bucharest Early Intervention Project (BEIP) has provided valuable insight into the effect of institutional care on cognitive function. The BEIP followed institutionalized children randomized into foster care or care as usual, which initially meant continued institutional care. Among other measures, the BEIP assessed cognitive outcomes. At 54 months of age, children who were placed in project-supported foster care or who were never institutionalized performed better on cognitive tasks than the "care as usual" children (Nelson et al., 2007). Additionally, those children who were the youngest at foster care placement showed the greatest improvement in cognitive functioning, suggesting a sensitive period for the development of general intellectual abilities and that early placement out of institutions aids plasticity following adversity (Nelson et al., 2007). These effects remained constant through 8 years of age and IQ recovery was particularly evident for children who remained with their original project-supported foster care families (Fox et al.,). The latter finding suggests that stability following early institutional care may enhance plasticity following removal from the institution. Finally, for the most impaired, general cognitive abilities may continue to improve long after placement in an enriching home. Rutter and his colleagues noted continued, gradual improvement in IQ into the adolescent years for postinstitutionalized Romanian children whose Denver developmental quotients averaged around 50 at adoption (Rutter et al., 2010).

Executive function skills are particularly affected by institutionalization, likely reflecting the sensitivity of the prefrontal cortex to early experiences (e.g. Kolb et al., 2012). As early as 1 year after adoption, after controlling for IQ, postinstitutionalized children show deficits in several aspects of executive function (EF), including working memory, cognitive flexibility, and inhibitory control (Hostinar et al., 2012). Lower quality of institutional care and less time spent with the birth family before institutional placement predict poorer EF performance (Hostinar et al., 2012), which supports the hypothesis that greater severity and duration of deprivation are related to altered or impaired neurodevelopment. Evidence from the Minnesota and Wisconsin International Adoption Studies (Pollak et al., 2010) and BEIP studies (Bos et al., 2009) indicates that children who experienced a period of early life institutional care continued to perform more poorly for years after removal from institutional care on executive function and visual memory tasks than family reared children. However, after controlling for confounding factors such as birth weight, head circumference, and length of institutional care, children randomized into the foster care group in the BEIP study performed better compared to children in the care as usual group (Bos et al., 2009). Evidence that those randomly assigned to living in families perform better than those randomized to care as usual may highlight the potential for plasticity in executive functions following early deprivation. Alternatively, improved care after deprivation may only prevent children from further declines in functioning in certain domains.

All executive functions may not be equally affected by early institutional care. While children experiencing early institutionalization perform poorly on many executive function tasks, they do remarkably well on planning and sequencing tasks such as Tower of London (Bos et al., 2009; Pollak et al., 2010). Alternatively, declarative memory, especially recall following a delay, appears to be impaired in postinstitutionalized children compared to never institutionalized children (Kroupina et al., 2010). These findings suggest that precise neural circuits underlying executive functions are affected or are less capable of recovery/compensation once the child is removed from deprivation rather than all circuitry supporting functioning on EF tasks. Given problems with executive functions, it is no surprise that children who spend their early years in institutional care are at high risk of being diagnosed with attention deficit, hyper-activity disorder (ADHD; Walshaw et al., 2010). Indeed, the aspects of EF affected in postinstitutionalized children overlap extensively with both the aspects that differ for children with ADHD (i.e, inhibitory control and working memory), while those spared (planning and set-shifting, see Pollak et al., 2010) also seem to be spared in ADHD (Walshaw et al., 2010).

Early nutritional status is also related to attentional outcomes in postinstitutionalized children. Greater ADHD symptoms in postinstitutionalized children 2.5–5 years postadoption are related to more severe iron deficiency at adoption and longer duration of institutional care (Doom et al., 2015). Unfortunately, postinstitutionalized children do not show reductions in ADHD symptoms over time (Doom et al., 2015). This finding suggests that while IQ in postinstitutionalized children generally improves over time, attentional problems do not show the same pattern of recovery postadoption.

Language is another cognitive domain that is affected by early institutional care but shows significant recovery following improvements in the environment. There may be a sensitive period, however. Work by the BEIP group revealed that children placed in families before the major spurt in word learning (i.e, before 15 months) exhibited the same expressive and receptive language scores as never institutionalized children in Romania at 30 and 42 months (Windsor et al., 2011). However, those placed later remained delayed. Followed up at 8 years of age, a similar pattern emerged with a cut-point at before and after age 2 years on measures of word identification and nonword repetition, an index of phonological memory (Windsor et al., 2013). Notably, several studies have shown that the rate of language learning in children old enough to learn language is a sensitive early indicator of which children will recover in cognitive abilities more rapidly and which will continue to struggle years after adoption (Croft et al., 2007). Thus, language skills and areas of the brain that support language show resilience if the child is placed in a language-rich setting before age two and preferably before the burst in word learning that occurs around 15 to 18 months of age (Windsor et al., 2011).

Deficits in theory of mind have been reported in postinstitutionalized children. Children who spent part of their lives in an institution performed worse on a false belief task than children raised in their birth families, with over half performing at below chance levels even after controlling for verbal ability (Tarullo et al., 2007). Children adopted from institutions after 6 months of age show the greatest deficits in theory of mind (assessed by the Strange Stories task), and theory of mind and executive function difficulties are related to deprivation-specific problems such as ADHD symptoms, indiscriminate friendliness, and quasi-autism (Colvert et al., 2008). It appears that although both theory of mind and executive function may partially mediate the relation between institutional care and deprivation-specific problems, neither fully accounts for the association (Colvert et al., 2008).

Not all of these cognitive outcomes can be attributed to stimulus and social deprivation. Nutritional deficiencies may affect cognitive outcomes as well as neural plasticity during recovery. For example, severity of iron deficiency at adoption is associated with lower IQ in postinstitutionalized children at age 5, while duration of institutional care is not (Doom et al., in press). In addition, children with more severe iron deficiency at adoption or who had spent more than 12 months in an institution before adoption showed the greatest improvements in IQ between 12 months postadoption to 2.5–5 years postadoption (Doom et al., in press). As a result, factors beyond social and physical deprivation should be studied in institutional care in relation to sensitive periods of development and later plasticity in cognitive outcomes.

Emotion

Processing

Although researchers hypothesized that children raised in institutions may have difficulties with facial emotion processing due to lack of experience with consistent caregivers, the BEIP reported no differences between children in institutions and those raised in their biological families between 13 and 30 months of age in responding to peak facial expressions of emotion (Nelson et al., 2006). Differentiating facial expressions, however, is a less complex task than matching facial expressions to situations, something that reflects understanding of both the situations and the meaning of the facial expressions. Here, postinstitutionalized children may be delayed or impaired. A group of postinstitutionalized children compared to family reared children studied around 54 months of age showed difficulty in matching facial expressions to vignettes that reflected situations that would cause children to be happy, fearful, or sad (Fries and Pollak, 2004). These children did not show difficulty matching to angry facial expressions (Fries and Pollak, 2004). The specificity of findings for emotion recognition may be an early risk factor for emotional difficulties if children find it easier to recognize and contextualize angry compared to happy facial expressions. Further neurobiological evidence for altered emotional processing is discussed below.

Emotional difficulties

Although children reared in institutions early in life are often described as having emotional problems, including anxiety, depression and problems regulating emotional behavior, whether or not these problems are particularly associated with institutional care or not and whether they reach clinical levels varies with the child's age, the informant, the instrument used and the comparison group. In the BEIP study they used the Preschool Age Psychiatric Assessment (PAPA) and noted that at 54 months of age, 44.2% of those in the care as usual group were exhibiting clinical levels of internalizing symptoms, while only 22% of those placed in foster care were suffering with significant internalizing symptoms (Zeanah et al., 2009). In contrast, in studies using the Child Behavior Checklist (Achenbach, 1991) or the Rutter Behavioral Scales (Elander and Rutter, 1996), few have reported evidence in childhood that anxiety symptoms are higher in

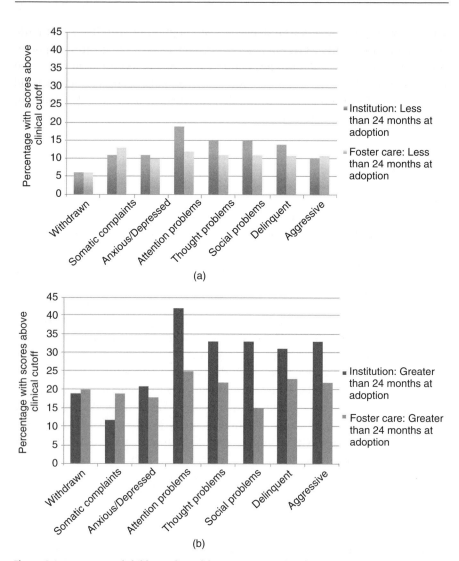

Figure 9.1 Percentage of children adopted from institutional or foster care with CBCL scores of >61 in each domain. (a) Children adopted before 24 months of age. (b) Children adopted after 24 months of age. Regardless of type of care, children adopted later were more likely to express elevated behavior problems. Main effects of institutional care were only noted for attention and social problems. Adapted from Gunnar & van Dulmen, 2007. (See insert for color representation of this figure.)

postinstitutionalized children than in children with other early adverse histories (Figure 9.1; Gunnar and van Dulmen, 2007; Juffer and van Ijzendoorn, 2005). However, when children themselves are interviewed (Wiik et al., 2011) and by age 11 regardless of the informant (Colvert et al., 2008), postinstitutionalized children are more likely to express anxiety disorders and/or preclinical levels of anxiety symptoms than are children from supportive backgrounds or inter-country adopted children arriving from foster care homes. It is not clear whether the PAPA is more sensitive to anxiety in young children or the BEIP children were more anxious.

What does seem clear is that emotional difficulties tend to increase with time since adoption, particularly into adolescence. We do not know why, but there are several possibilities that are not mutually exclusive. First, this could reflect sleeper effects. Thus, neural systems that were impaired early in life begin to produce disorder only with development when the need for those systems to regulate becomes developmentally critical. Second, it may reflect co-morbidities with other problems exhibited by children who experience early deprivation, particularly those that impair school functioning and peer relationships. Parents may be able to scaffold both schoolwork and friendships while the children are young, but with adolescence parental scaffolding gets increasingly removed and deprivation-induced deficits may increasingly affect the child's academic and social standing, which in turn may create the context of significant emotional problems. Finally, in adolescence, issues of identity come to the fore that are very challenging for adopted children, particularly those from racial/ethnic minorities, as are many internationally adopted children. Problems grappling with these identity issues may contribute to emotional burdens that enhance emotional problems with time postadoption.

Behavior

A number of behaviors appear to be characteristic of children and adolescents who have spent a significant duration of time in an institution, with some behaviors becoming less frequent and severe over time and others becoming more frequent and severe. During the time of institutionalization, over 60% of Romanian children experience stereotypies (mean age 22 months), but the frequency of these behaviors decreased significantly over time for the children randomized to the foster care condition, especially with earlier placement and longer duration of foster care in the BEIP (Bos et al., 2010). Remaining stereotypies in the foster care group, but not in the care as usual group, were related to poorer language and cognitive outcomes (Bos et al., 2010). Other behaviors observed at the time of removal from Romanian orphanages include rocking (47%) and self-injurious behavior (Beckett et al., 2002). These behaviors declined in frequency over time, with 18% rocking and 13% self-injuring at 6 years of age. The primary predictor of these unusual behaviors was the duration of time in the institution before adoption (Beckett et al., 2002).

Altered social behaviors have been documented in children experiencing early deprivation, including indiscriminate friendliness and greater likelihood of insecure attachment (Chisholm, 1998), with longer periods in institutional care related to greater indiscriminate friendliness (Bruce et al., 2009). Although indiscriminate friendliness has been interpreted at times as an indication of the lack of an attachment relationship, more recent work now clearly shows that it is not an indication of a disordered attachment (Chisholm, 1998; Zeanah et al., 2002). If not an attachment problem, what is it? Chisholm (1998) argued that it is an adaptive behavior in institutional settings that is not extinguished when children move into more responsive care environments. Others have argued it reflects problems in maintaining appropriate social boundaries (Rutter, 2002), which is consistent with recent evidence that it is not just that postinstitutionalized children are overly friendly. They engage in behaviors, such as touching complete strangers and crawling in their laps, that most family reared children rarely exhibit (Lawler et al., 2014).

Furthermore, although Zeanah and colleagues originally argued that indiscriminate friendliness did not reflect a general impulsivity because it was not associated with aggression (Zeanah et al., 2002), other studies that have examined attention regulation using neuropsychological tasks (Bruce et al., 2009) and attention and hyperactivity problems (Roy et al., 2004) have found significant associations. Thus the current thinking is that it does reflect problems in inhibitory control that results in the failure to appropriately regulate behavior to conform with social boundary expectations.

Brain development

To date there are no published studies of brain development in institutionalized children that have measured development over time. What we have is an emerging literature examining brain structure and function in middle childhood and adolescence of youth who were removed from institutional care when they were infants or young children (average age 2 years). As of yet we cannot say anything about recovery or rebound, although from the behavioral data we know improvement in function has occurred for many children. We can, however, identify systems that years postadoption are structurally and functionally different from what is observed in children who did not spend their early months and years in institutional care. We can also begin to examine effects that are correlated with how long children lived in institutional care.

Both human and animal studies strongly suggest that the prefrontal cortex is directly affected by a harsh early social environment. For example, in neonatal rodents experiencing maternal deprivation, increased rates of cell death in the frontal cortex have been reported (Zhang et al., 2002). Even small but stressful perturbations in the early environment, including brief handling periods multiple times a day, produce structural changes in the pyramidal neurons of the prefrontal cortex (Helmeke et al., 2001). In squirrel monkeys that have experienced intermittent maternal separation, an 8–14% increase in volume of the right ventromedial prefrontal cortex has been observed during adulthood (Lyons et al., 2002). Likewise, maternal deprivation in rhesus monkeys is associated with 10–11% increases in volumes of the dorsal medial prefrontal cortex and dorsal anterior cingulate (Spinelli et al., 2009). Overall, it appears that early social deprivation is linked to specific structural changes in the prefrontal cortex that persist into adulthood.

These findings in animal models have been translated to children experiencing institutional care. Consistent with cognitive delays reported in postinstitutionalized children, decreased prefrontal gray matter volume (Hodel et al., 2015) and alterations in prefrontal white matter (Sheridan et al., 2012) have been documented in formerly institutionalized individuals. Thus, placement out of institutional care and into foster or adoptive homes does not seem to completely ameliorate changes in prefrontal cortex development. In line with findings of poorer cognitive functioning in many formerly institutionalized children, both gray and white matter volumes have been found to be smaller in formerly institutionalized compared to never institutionalized adolescents (Mehta et al., 2009). However, Mehta and colleagues reported no significant differences in hippocampal volume or mid-sagittal area of the corpus callosum after controlling for differences in total brain volume (Mehta et al., 2009). In contrast, examining postinstitutionalized youth from over 25 countries adopted from institutions into US families, our group noted significantly smaller prefrontal cortex volumes regardless of duration of institutional care, and smaller hippocampi that had a dose response association with institutional care duration (Hodel et al., under review). The BEIP also reported smaller cortical gray matter volume for children who had experienced institutional care, but cortical white matter volume was only smaller for the children in the care as usual group (Sheridan et al., 2012). As the group randomized to foster care did not differ from never institutionalized children in cortical white matter volume (Sheridan et al., 2012), it could be that cortical white matter volume in the brain experiences greater plasticity following an improvement in environment but gray matter volume continues to be affected throughout childhood.

Neural connectivity also appears to be altered in individuals who experienced early life institutional care. Adolescents who had experienced early deprivation were found to have a more diffuse pattern of connectivity in the right hemisphere, which is possibly the result of ineffective neural pruning and could be related to ADHD symptoms in this population (Behen et al., 2009). Additionally, alterations in the left uncinate fasciculus, which connects parts of the limbic system to the frontal lobe, appear to be present in children who had previously been institutionalized in Romanian orphanages, which may partially explain cognitive and socioemotional difficulties reported in many studies (Eluvathingal et al., 2006). Further alterations in white matter for children with histories of early deprivation include reduced fractional anisotropy across the frontal, temporal, and parietal lobes (Govindan et al., 2010). This finding included the uncinate and superior longitudinal fasciculi, providing additional evidence that alterations in neural connectivity between frontal and limbic regions may underlie behavioral difficulties. Further, these white matter changes were related to the duration of institutional care and to ADHD symptoms (Govindan et al., 2010), suggesting there are neural underpinnings connecting early experience to later behavior. A recent study reported more diffuse organization of white matter in the prefrontal cortex following institutional care and that this pattern was associated with neurocognitive deficits (Hanson et al., 2013a).

A study of postinstitutionalized children from Romanian orphanages reported decreased bilateral glucose metabolism in several areas, including the infralimbic prefrontal cortex, the orbital frontal gyrus, lateral temporal cortex, the amygdala, the head of the hippocampus, and the brain stem (Chugani et al., 2001). Reduced EEG α-power has been reported in children raised in institutions compared to those raised in their biological families, and this result is partially mediated by cortical white matter volume reductions (Sheridan et al., 2012). As a result, there appears to be both direct and indirect effects of early deprivation on the prefrontal cortex.

Animal studies of stress show that stress produces amygdala plasticity resulting in larger volume and enhanced reactivity to threatening stimuli (reviewed in Tottenham, 2012). Because postinstitutionalized children tend to be anxious and because of the animal work, significant attention has been focused on whether amygdala structure is increased and function is heightened for children with early institutional care histories. Just as some postinstitutionalized children may have difficulties connecting facial expressions with the appropriate eliciting conditions, which may impair responding appropriately to others, some also respond more physiologically to emotional expressions, which may influence behavior in social settings. The results are mixed on structure but consistent so far for function. The mixed results for structure, with some reporting increased volume (Tottenham et al., 2010; Mehta et al., 2009), some decreased volume (e.g, Hanson et al., in press) and some no difference, may be because of both power issues and the challenge of imaging the amygdala. Regardless of whether there is an impact on amygdala volume, the functional studies strongly suggest greater response to threat stimuli. Recent findings in postinstitutionalized children indicate that fearful faces during the Emotional Face Go/Nogo task elicit heightened amygdala responses compared to never institutionalized children (Tottenham et al., 2011). This increased amygdala activity is a mediator of the relationship between early deprivation and decreased eye contact during dyadic interaction, which may be related to socioemotional difficulties in these children (Tottenham et al., 2011). Further, for children with early neglect experiences, about half of whom were adopted from institutional care, threatening information elicited greater activation of the left amygdala and left anterior hippocampus than was noted for children without early neglect experiences (Maheu et al., 2010). Likewise, postinstitutionalized children do not exhibit decreases in ventral PFC activation to fearful faces that are observed in children reared in their birth families (Tottenham et al., 2011). Patterns of reactivity in fearful versus neutral faces in postinstitutionalized children more closely resemble typically developing adults, which may indicate accelerated development of the amygdala and other neural networks responsible for socioemotional processing (Tottenham, 2012). Consistent with neuroimaging results, postinstitutionalized children show a greater number of errors during tasks when negatively valenced faces are present but no differences for positively valenced faces, suggesting difficulty with processing and potentially with attention while negative social stimuli are present (Tottenham et al., 2010). These functional differences are consistent with heightened anxiety discussed earlier as well as with overall atypicalities in social functioning.

Electrophysiology

Electrophysiological measures suggest that early life institutional care alters patterns of neural activity. Several aspects of electrical activity have been examined. First, because internalizing symptoms have been associated with greater EEG activity over right than left frontal regions of the scalp (Davidson, 1998), EEG frontal asymmetry has been examined in institutionalized and postinstitutionalized children. No simple group differences have yet been reported; however, the BEIP group noted that typically developing family reared children showed a greater relative right hemisphere activation from 30 to 42 months, before shifting to the more common mature pattern of greater relative left hemisphere activation (McLaughlin et al.,). This was not observed for all institutionalized children who showed the greater relative right hemisphere activation pattern at older ages, suggesting a delay in maturation. The same delayed pattern of activity has been reported for studies of EEG power. With development, the power spectra observed when the brain is at rest increases (Marshall et al., 2002). For infants sitting quietly, theta rhythms predominate. With development, this shifts to alpha. Several research groups have now shown that when children are in institutional care and soon thereafter, they show a larger percentage of theta rhythms in their resting EEG than children reared in families (Marshall and Fox, 2004; Tarullo et al., 2011). These patterns correlate with attention problems (McLaughlin et al., 2010) and indiscriminate friendliness (Tarullo et al., 2011), both strongly associated with early institutional care as noted above. Importantly, once placed in a supportive home environment, patterns of EEG power show marked development and over time become comparable to those of never institutionalized, family reared children (McLaughlin et al., 2010).

Studies using event-related potentials (ERPs) have also noted differences between children reared in institutions early in life and those reared in family settings. The BEIP group noted that ERPs in responses to faces depicting emotion

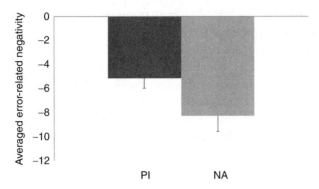

Figure 9.2 Error-related negativity averaged across Flanker and Go-NoGo (counter-balanced) tasks for postinstitutionalized (PI) children and non-adopted (NA) children raised in families comparable to those who adopt children internationally. Bars reflect standard error of the mean. Adapted from Loman et al., 2013.

(i.e, P1, N170, and P400) had smaller amplitudes and longer latencies for care as usual children than for family reared children, with those placed in foster care falling in between, suggesting some recovery (Moulson et al., 2009). Several groups have examined ERPs while children perform tasks that require response inhibition and conflict monitoring (e.g, go/nogo and flanker). The BEIP group reported that children removed from institutional care and placed in foster care showed improved P300 responses compared to the care as usual group but that were still not as good as those of children in the never institutionalized group (McDermott et al., 2013). Likewise, in another study, postinstitutionalized children exhibited smaller attentional responses (N2) and reactions to errors (error-related negativity, ERN) than did never institutionalized, family reared children even after 5 or more years living in enriching family settings (see Figure 9.2; Loman et al., 2013). Thus, the ERP data supports the behavioral findings that early deprivation impairs attention regulation and while improvements may be seen, children frequently continue to struggle with their ability to regulate attention for years following adoption.

HPA activity

The HPA axis serves as a stress-mediating system that prepares the body for physical and psychological challenges. After the stress period has passed, the axis returns to baseline. Evidence from children who have experienced early institutional care indicates that early deprivation has lasting effects on HPA regulation, which in turn is related to subsequent behavior problems. Toddlers living in an institution have demonstrated a flattened diurnal cortisol slope with lower morning and elevated evening cortisol (Carlson and Earls, 1997).

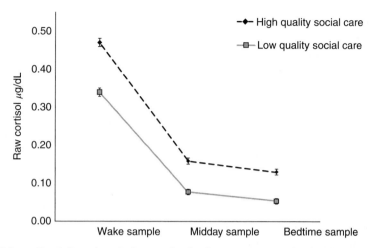

Figure 9.3 Predicted diurnal cortisol across the day for postinstitutionalized children among high- and low-quality social care in institutions. Graphs depict 1 SD above and below the mean of the social care construct as an illustration of high- and low-quality social care. Kalsea J. Koss, Camelia E. Hostinar, Bonny Donzella, Megan R. Gunnar 2014, Figure 2. Reproduced with permission of *Psychoneuroendocrinology*, Elsevier.

Postinstitutionalized children have demonstrated mixed results. One study reported higher cortisol levels over the day for children adopted in the early 2000s from Romania (Gunnar et al., 2001). All the other studies have reported that while some children exhibit a normally steep diurnal cortisol rhythm, other children exhibit a blunted or flattened rhythm either due to lower morning or higher evening levels, or both (Johnson et al., 2011; Kertes et al., 2008). This is also true not only for postinstitutionalized children but also for adults adopted from conditions of deprivation as children (van der Vegt et al., 2009). Notably, a recent longitudinal study of internationally adopted children demonstrated that poorer social care, as opposed to physical care, prior to adoption was related to a more flattened diurnal cortisol slopes that persisted over a 2-year period and mediated behavioral problems reported by parents (see Figure 9.3).

Genetic moderation and epigenetics

Research on single nucleotide polymorphisms has revealed significant moderation of outcomes by genotype. For example, children with the dopamine transporter gene (DAT1) risk allele and who had spent more time in an institution showed the highest levels of ADHD symptoms, and the association strengthened over time (Stevens et al., 2009). Likewise, children with the risk allele of the BDNF gene showed the greatest attention problems when adopted later and fewer attention problems when adopted earlier (Gunnar et al., 2012).

Thus, individual differences in risk and resilience following institutionalization may be partially explained by genetic moderation.

Epigenetic regulation and telomere length have also been studied in relation to institutional care. A study of currently institutionalized children reported greater DNA methylation compared to children raised in their biological families, particularly in regions regulating cellular signaling and the immune response (Naumova et al., 2012). To date, no studies have reported differences in epigenetic regulation years after institutional care, so it is unclear whether there is plasticity in the epigenome following early adversity. DNA telomere length, which is a marker of cellular aging, has also been associated with institutional care. During middle childhood, children with histories of institutional care showed shorter relative telomere length compared to children raised in their biological families (Drury et al., 2012). Notably, in that study girls with longer times in institutional care in infancy and boys with greater times in institutional care including the preschool years had shorter telomeres in middle childhood. Future research is needed to determine whether these genetic alterations are associated with accelerated aging and physical health problems across development.

Evidence for sensitive periods

A large body of evidence suggests the presence of sensitive periods for the development of a number of cognitive, social, and neurobiological domains. The timing of these sensitive periods appears to differ by domain, which is unsurprising considering the varied developmental timing of distinct neural circuits and brain regions. For example, there appears to be a sensitive period for IQ at around 2 years of age, which may reflect the importance of language development in supporting the development of general intelligence (Nelson et al., 2007). Problems with executive functions, attachment, indiscriminate friendliness, and emotional problems may have a different sensitive period. Two studies of Romanian adopted children have suggested that postinstitutionalized children are at heightened risk for problems in these spheres if they are adopted beyond 4 to 6 months of age (Fisher et al., 1997; Kreppner et al., 2007). However, the children in those studies were adopted from conditions of extreme and global deprivation. Children adopted more recently following improvements in institutional care (i.e, adequate physical care, still low social care) appear to have executive function skills comparable to a normative sample when adopted before 9 months of age (e.g, Merz et al., 2013). Broadly, it appears that deprivation very early in life (before 6 months of age) is associated with relatively few lasting impacts compared to infants who experienced more prolonged periods of deprivation. When during infancy long-lasting deficits emerge in different arenas may depend on the timing of maturation of the neural circuits involved in the behavior domain and the severity of the deprivation, with more severe deprivation reducing the age at which full recovery is possible with adoption.

Factors modifying postinstitutional outcomes

Early life social stimulation in the form of sensitive and responsive caregiving may be one of the most important factors influencing subsequent development. As demonstrated by the literature reviewed above, institutional care, which is often characterized by a lack of consistent caregivers, results in a number of social and cognitive deficits. Fortunately, social stimulation and consistent caregiving provided by adults after institutional care are likely the most important factors guiding recovery, which is why placement into an adoptive or foster care home early in life results in more positive outcomes.

The BEIP demonstrated that placing institutionalized children into project-supported foster care dramatically increased the percentage of children who were securely attached to a caregiver (Smyke et al., 2010). Compared to the 18% of securely attached children living in institutions at 42 months, 49% of children placed in foster care and 65% of never institutionalized children showed secure attachment (Smyke et al., 2010). In addition, attachment was shown to mediate between the experiences of institutional care and psychopathology in children randomized to foster care placement in the BEIP study (McGoron et al., 2012). Recent research demonstrates that attachment relationships develop relatively quickly between postinstitutionalized children and caregivers, although children who spent longer periods in an institution took longer to form attachments, and postinstitutionalized children were more likely to have a disorganized attachment pattern than were children reared in their birth families (Carlson et al., 2014). Thus, for most children, institutional care does not appear to disrupt attachment formation long-term after placement into homes with more consistent caregiving, but it may make it difficult for children to form organized and secure attachment relationships.

Researchers are beginning to ask whether and how the quality of parenting postadoption influences the development of postinstitutionalized children and youth. Of course, if children who demonstrate problems have parents who exhibit less positive parenting behaviors, it might be that the problems displayed by the children are affecting parental behavior and not vice versa. This seemed to be the message from an analysis of Romanian children adopted into the United Kingdom. Here the researchers noted that as the children's cognitive functioning improved over time, parents were observed to use more positive parenting behavior (Croft et al., 2001). Nonetheless, most proposed interventions for families with internationally adopted children focus on improving parenting (e.g, Juffer et al., 1997). Parenting interventions developed from research on children in foster care may be useful for promoting the development of attachment between postinstitutionalized children and caregivers. For example, the Attachment and Biobehavioral Catch-up (ABC) intervention has demonstrated effects on stress system regulation and fewer behavior problems for children living in foster care (Dozier et al., 2006; Dozier et al., 2008). An intervention based on the

ABC program is currently being tested with families who have adopted internationally (Dozier, personal communication).

Improving parenting may be important in supporting the postadoption development of internationally adopted children, but it may not address all of the issues in cognitive and social functioning that were noted in this review. For issues with attention problems, inhibitory control, and sensitivity to threat, strategies that help "retrain the brain" to enhance appropriate neural circuits may be needed.

Interventions and evidence for plasticity

While interventions for children experiencing institutional care can provide insights into the elements of deprivation that influence cognitive and social development, the major thrust of these interventions often are to show that it is institutional deprivation and not something inherent about the children that is producing their poor functioning. When this is shown, it encourages countries to change the ways that they are caring for young children who are wards of the state. Certainly, when viewed as an intervention, adoption has massive effects on children's functioning. Indeed, a meta-analysis of adoption studies shows differences in IQ between adopted children and those who stayed in the institution with an effect size of 1.17 (Van IJzendoorn et al., 2005). Improvements in school achievement and attachment security have also been reported at approximately the same effect size as IQ, and adoption produces the best outcomes for children when it occurs before 12 months (Bakermans-Kranenburg et al., 2008). Foster care is a better alternative than institutional care for children without permanent parents, as demonstrated by the BEIP, especially if placement occurs before 24 months (Nelson et al., 2007). However, effect sizes for cognitive outcomes are better for adopted children than for children placed in foster care, whose cognitive outcomes have effect sizes of 0.62 at 42 months and 0.47 at 54 months (Nelson et al., 2007).

While foster care may be better than institutional care, it can only exist if there is a strong infrastructure to support it; thus, intervening to improve the care children receive within institutions and show that it has effects on outcomes are still valuable. Within-institution interventions have included additional tactile, auditory, and visual stimulation by adult caregivers, which have been shown to produce generally positive effects on development.

In the St. Petersburg-USA Orphanage Research project, researchers tried two strategies to improve children's outcomes. One orphanage was provided with trainings for caregivers plus structural changes such as ensuring that individual children are cared for by a few consistent caregivers. Another orphanage was given the caregiver training only. The development of children in these orphanages was compared to that of children in a 'care as usual" orphanage.

In nearly every assessment following the intervention, children in the orphanage with both training and structural changes performed better cognitively and socially than children in the training only or no intervention conditions, suggesting that a combination of educated caregivers and changes that allow for consistent caregiving is best to promote plasticity. As the intervention was largely social in nature, effect sizes were larger in the social domain, including more positive social behaviors for children in the training plus structural changes group. However, cognitive effects were also observed, indicating cross-domain effects are likely for within-institution interventions. Consistent with other institutional interventions, longer exposure to the interventions promoted positive development in typically developing children. In addition, the intervention prevented declines in children with disabilities, and effect sizes were often larger for children with disabilities. This finding suggests that children who are developmentally delayed have the most to gain from improvements in care and demonstrate the most plasticity following early deprivation. This indicates that the treatments provided during the intervention period would need to become a permanent part of institutional care in order to produce lasting positive impacts on children's development.

Nutritional interventions have been implemented in certain institutions in order to prevent the cognitive and socioemotional sequelae of malnutrition and nutrient deficiencies. For example, the SPOON Foundation has worked to improve nutrition and feeding practices in orphanages across the world. Longitudinal research is needed to understand the neurobiological correlates of early nutrition supplementation in institutionalized children.

Within-institution interventions focusing on increasing sensory and social stimulation, as well as improving nutrition, suggest that all three of these components of early deprivation have individual effects on development and should be targeted in future comprehensive interventions. Sadly, in general, gains obtained when institutional conditions are improved often fade when conditions go back to the way they were before the intervention (reviewed in St. Petersburg-USA Orphanage Research Team, 2008). This indicates that for positive gains to become permanent, overall care needs to permanently improve. Indeed, the intervention literature indicates that while adoption is the best intervention for children living in institutions, interventions that include both trained caregivers and structural changes over a prolonged period of time produce the best outcomes for children, especially when implemented early in life while the brain is rapidly developing.

Comparisons with other forms of adversity

Children experiencing other forms of early adversity, including maltreatment and poverty, demonstrate similarities to children who experienced early institutional care. Global cognitive impairments have been noted across experiences for these children (reviewed in Pechtel and Pizzagalli, 2011). Like children who have experienced institutional care, children who have been maltreated have higher rates of internalizing and externalizing problems, including increased rates of ADHD symptoms (Cicchetti and Valentino, 2006). Children adopted from institutional care show the greatest similarities in social behavior to children who have experienced early life neglect. Greater likelihood of insecure attachment and indiscriminate friendliness have been reported for children adopted from Romanian institutions (Chisholm, 1998), which is similar to social patterns observed in children raised by neglectful parents (e.g, Erickson and Egeland, 2002). Children in poverty also show cognitive deficits similar to children with institutional care experiences, such as lower IQ and poorer school achievement (Bradley and Corwyn, 2002). Further, children in poverty have an increased likelihood of psychiatric disturbances (internalizing and externalizing) and social functioning problems, which are observed in postinstitutionalized children (Bradley and Corwyn, 2002).

Likewise, similar patterns of brain development have been reported for children experiencing a variety of different types of adverse care in early development. Thus, reduced brain volume is associated with early institutional care, but this is also true for poverty and maltreatment (Cicchetti and Valentino, 2006; Hanson et al., 2013b). Larger ventricles and reduced hippocampal volume have been observed for maltreated children (Cicchetti and Valentino, 2006), and we have recently noted this for postinstitutionalized children (Hodel et al., under review). One of the reasons why outcomes are not as distinct as we might initially expect for children with these different backgrounds is that they share many similar risks to their development, from prenatal stress and teratogen exposure to neglect of physical and emotional needs to deficits in stimulation. It is difficult to parse out which factors may be contributing to a certain outcome without experimentation (e.g, the BEIP random assignment). In addition, more research following adults who experienced institutionalization as children will provide greater insight into potential development of psychopathology and other socioemotional outcomes in adulthood, which can then be compared to other groups experiencing adversity.

Individual differences and resilience

One theme that cuts across all of these areas is that while some children are negatively affected by adversity, others seem to do much better. The study of resilience in children who have experienced institutionalization closely parallels the literature on maltreated children, citing that supportive relationships and certain characteristics of the child promote resilience against adversity (Cicchetti 2010). Important differences between the groups do exist in terms of resilience as it is unlikely that postinstitutionalized children, who are usually adopted into well-resourced, highly motivated families, experience heightened continued life stress in the same way that maltreated children do. Thus, studies of resilience in postinstitutionalized children may inform studies of maltreated children, particularly if adversity is limited to early in life. Differences between institutionalized children and those experiencing other forms of adversity may help researchers narrow down what outcomes follow each type of adversity as well as the duration and timing of adversity.

Conclusions

Research on the neurobiological correlates of infant institutionalization shows lasting effects of experiences during the first years of life (see Figure 9.4 for a summary). However, studies of children removed from these harsh early environments provide reason for optimism, as there is significant plasticity in cognitive, emotional, and behavioral outcomes following placement in a more enriched environment. Research involving postinstitutionalized children allows researchers to ask questions about the role of a specific time period on

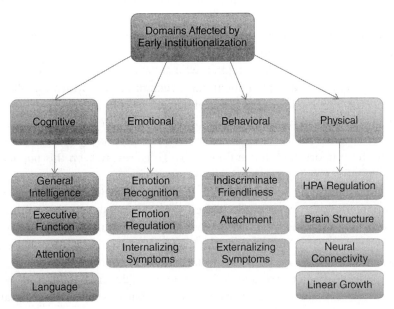

Figure 9.4 Potential effects of early institutional care. These effects are not specific to institutional care, as they may also follow other forms of early adversity. The duration of institutionalization increases the risk of these outcomes. (See insert for color representation of this figure.)

subsequent development, and the timeline of recovery for certain systems can be explored. Importantly, we can also study the factors that promote plasticity and recovery from early life stress. One of the best ways to promote recovery is removal from the depriving environment and placement into a loving family whether through adoption or well-supported foster care. Reuniting the children with their families may also work if the problems that led to institutional placement are addressed. Although there have been some within-institution interventions that have demonstrated success, especially when implemented early in life, further work must be done to improve pre- and postnatal care for children in institutions to ensure the best outcomes possible.

In general, longer periods of deprivation are related to poorer outcomes, and placement into a more enriched environment is best, especially if it occurs early in life. Evidence for sensitive periods differs by the domain studied and the severity of the deprivation. Likewise, certain domains show greater plasticity following adoption or foster care than others. Interventions in this population have demonstrated that improvements in the environment may affect disparate aspects of development. For example, the St. Petersburg study was largely a social intervention, but researchers observed improvements in cognition as well as in social functioning. Findings such as these should influence researchers to study how closely cognitive and social development are related and to probe the potentially shared neural circuitry involved in cognitive and social recovery following deprivation.

Effects of early institutional care are generally consistent with other forms of early adversity. However, unlike other groups of children who experience significant adversity early in life, children who are adopted from institutional care experience a marked and permanent improvement in care, which can allow us more adequately to address questions of plasticity. Work in this population can also allow tests of interventions under optimal conditions of parent participation, before moving the intervention into populations where families may struggle to provide the support the intervention needs. Thus, research on this population may help other groups experiencing early adversity.

Beyond informing scientists about the neurobiological sequelae of early institutionalization, research on children who have experienced institutional care provides valuable information about human nature and development. First, what does early institutional care tell us about human nature? Is institutionalization one extreme on a continuum of social experiences, or is it beyond any experience that a person should have? Research documenting severe delays in functioning in some children would suggest that this is a unique situation for humans, but there are many children who remain resilient in the face of deprivation, which may suggest an extreme end of a continuum that some are able to overcome. Further, should we view alterations in functioning as adaptation to a severely depriving environment, or are these changes maladaptive responses even in the institutional context? One might argue that behaviors such as indiscriminate friendliness may help children gain social interactions that could promote survival in an institution although not necessarily adaptive once in an adoptive family. However, cognitive deficits such as lower IQ do not appear to be adaptive in different contexts, so the argument about the adaptiveness of particular outcomes may be domain-specific. In addition, how long does plasticity occur following removal from institutional care? It likely depends on the timing of the new placement and the severity of deprivation, but this question is important to those interested in neuroplasticity. For example, is the window for plasticity open long enough to allow the adopted child to adapt to their new environment? Ideally, the window would remain open long enough so that children can adapt to their new enriched environment to prevent a mismatch between the child's adaptive skills and their new environment. However, persisting alterations in cognition and behavior suggest that while plasticity may occur for some skills, there may be mismatches between behavior and environment for other capacities. Finally, what factors are essential to human development? The cognitive and social difficulties experienced by children in severely depriving environments suggests that minimum requirements for healthy human development are consistent interactions with sensitive caregivers and a variety of interactions with sensory stimuli. This information is vital for institutional staff as well as any person caring for young children.

Overall, research on children who have experienced early deprivation indicates there are specific cognitive, socioemotional, and neurobiological deficits due to institutional care but also significant opportunities for plasticity following improvements in the environment. Future research in this area should focus on identifying sensitive periods of development for specific domains as well as factors that promote healthy development both within the institution and after placement into an enriched environment. As within-institution interventions and adoption into loving families demonstrate plasticity following deprivation, knowledge gained from research on institutionalized children should continue to inform interventions that promote positive development.

Acknowledgments

The authors are grateful to have support from R01 HD075349-02 (Megan Gunnar, PI), P50MH078105-05 (Megan Gunnar, PI), and T32MH015755 (Dante Cicchetti, PI).

References

Achenbach TM. (1991). *Manual for the Child Behavior Checklist/4–18 and 1991 Profile*. Burlington: University of Vermont, Department of Psychiatry.

Bakermans–Kranenburg MJ, van Ijzendoorn MH, Juffer F. (2008). Earlier is better: A meta–analysis of 70 years of intervention improving cognitive development in institution-alized children. *Monographs Society Research Child Development* 73:279–293.

Beckett C, Bredenkamp D, Castle J, Groothues C, O'Connor TG, Rutter M; English and Romanian Adoptees (ERA) Study Team. (2002). Behavior patterns associated with institutional deprivation: a study of children adopted from Romania. *J Dev Behav Pediatr* 23: 297–303.

Behen ME, Muzik O, Saporta AS, Wilson BJ, Pai D, Hua J, Chugani HT. (2009). Abnormal fronto–striatal connectivity in children with histories of early deprivation: A diffusion tensor imaging study. *Brain Imaging Behavior* 3 292–297.

Bos KJ, Fox N, Zeanah CH, Nelson CA. (2009). Effects of early psychosocial deprivation on the development of memory and executive function. *Frontiers Behavioral Neurosci* 3:16.

Bos KJ, Zeanah CH Jr, Smyke AT, Fox NA, Nelson CA 3rd. Stereotypies in children with a history of early institutional care (2010). *Arch Pediatr Adolesc Med.* 164:406–11.

Bradley R, Corwyn R. (2002). Socioeconomic status and child development. *Annu Rev Psychology* 53:371–399.

Bruce J, Tarullo AR, Gunnar MR. (2009). Disinhibited social behavior among internationally adopted children. *Development Psychpathology* 21:157–171.

Carlson EA, Hostinar CE, Mliner SB, Gunnar MR. (2014). The emergence of attachment fol-lowing early social deprivation. *Development Psychopathology* 26:479–489.

Carlson M, Earls F. (1997). Psychological and neuroendocrinological sequelae of early social deprivation in institutionalized children in Romania. *Annals NY Acad Sci* 807:419–428.

Chisholm K. (1998). A three year follow–up of attachment and indiscriminate friendliness in children adopted from Romanian orphanages. *Child Development* 69:1092–1106.

Choe M, Ortiz–Mantilla S, Makris N, Gregas M, Bacic J, Haehn D, Grant PE. (2012). Regional infant brain development: An MRI–based morphometric analysis in 3 to 13 month olds. *Cerebral Cortex* 23(9):2100–2117. doi: 10.1093/cercor/bhs197.

Chugani HT, Behen ME, Muzik O, Juhasz C, Nagy F, Chugani DC. (2001). Local brain functional activity following early deprivation: A study of post–institutionalized Romanian orphans. *Neuroimage* 14:1290–1301.

Cicchetti D. (2010). Resilience under conditions of extreme stress: a multilevel perspective. *World Psychiatry* 9:145–154.

Cicchetti D, Valentino K. (2006). An ecological–transactional perspective on child maltreatment: failure of the average expectable environment and its influence on child development. In: *Developmental Psychopathology*, Vol. 3. Risk, Disorder, and Adaptation, ed. D. Cicchetti, D.J. Cohen, pp. 129–201. Hoboken, NJ: Wiley.

Colvert E, Rutter M, Kreppner J, Beckett C, Castle J, Groothues, C, et al. (2008). Do theory of mind and executive function deficits underlie the adverse outcomes associated with profound early deprivation? Findings from the English and Romanian Adoptees Study. *J Abnorm Child Psychol* 36:1057–1068.

Croft C, O'Connor TG, Keaveney L, Groothues C, Rutter M. (2001). Longitudinal change in parenting associated with developmental delay and catch–up. *J Child Psychology Psychiatry* 42:649–659.

Croft C, Beckett C, Rutter M, Castle J, Colvert E, Groothues C, et al. (2007). Early adoles-cent outcomes of institutionally–deprived and non–deprived adoptees. II: Language as a protective factor and a vulnerable outcome. *J Child Psychology Psychiatry Allied Disciplines* 48(1):31–44.

Davidson RJ. (1998). Affective style and affective disorders: perspectives from affective neuro-science. *Cogn Emotion* 12:307–330.

Doom JR, Georgieff MK, Gunnar MR. (2015). Institutional care and iron deficiency increase ADHD symptomology and lower IQ 2.5–5 years post–adoption. *Developmental Sci.* 18(3):484–494.

Dozier M, Peloso E, Lindheim O, Gordon MK, Manni M, Sepulveda S, Ackerman J. (2006). Developing evidence–based interventions for foster children: an example of a randomized clinical trial with infants and toddlers. *J Social Issues* 62:767–785.

Dozier M, Peloso E, Lewis E, Laurenceau J, Levine, S. (2008). Effects of an attachment–based intervention on the cortisol production of infants and toddlers in foster care. *Development Psychopathology* 20:845–859.

Drury SS, Theall K, Gleason M, Smyke A, De Vivo I, Wong J, et al. (2012). Telomere length and early severe social deprivation: Linking early adversity and cellular aging. *Mol Psychiatry* 17(7):719–727.

Elander J, Rutter M. (1996). Use and development of the Rutter parents' and teachers' scales. *Intl J Methods Psychiatric Research* 6:63–78.

Eluvathingal TJ, Chugani HT, Behen ME, Juhasz C, Muzik O, Maqbool M, Chugani DC, Makki M. (2006). Abnormal brain connectivity in children after early severe socioemotional deprivation: a diffusion tensor imaging study. *Pediatrics* 117:2093–2100.

Erickson MF, Egeland B. (2002). Child neglect. In: *The APSAC Handbook on Child Maltreatment*, 2nd ed., ed. J.E.B. Myers, L. Berliner, J. Briere, C.T. Hendrix, C. Jenny, and T.A. Reid, pp. 3–20. Thousand Oaks, CA: Sage.

Fisher L, Ames EW, Chisholm K, Savoie L. (1997). Problems reported by parents of Romanian orphans adopted to British Columbia. *Int J Behav Dev* 20:67–82.

Fox NA, Almas AN, Degnan KA, Nelson CA, Zeanah, CH. (2011). The effects of severe psychosocial deprivation and foster care intervention on cognitive development at 8 years of age: findings from the Bucharest Early Intervention Project. *J Child Psychology Psychiatry* 52:919–928.

Fries ABW, Pollak SD. (2004). Emotion understanding in postinstitutionalized Eastern European children. *Development Psychopathology* 16:355–369.

Gao W, Zhu H, Giovanello KS, Smith JK, Shen D, Gilmore JH, Lin W. (2009). Evidence on the emergence of the brain's default network from 2–week–old to 2–year–old healthy pediatric subjects. *PNAS* 106(16):6790–6795. doi:10.1073/pnas.0811221106.

Govindan RM, Behen ME, Helder E, Makki MI, Chugani HT. (2010). Altered water diffusivity in cortical association tracts in children with early deprivation identified with tract–based spatial statistics (TBSS). *Cerebral Cortex* 20:561–569.

Gunnar MR. (2001). Effects of early deprivation: Findings from orphanage–reared infants and children. In: *Handbook of Developmental Cognitive Neuroscience*, ed. C.A. Nelson and M. Luciana, pp. 617–629. Cambridge, MA: MIT Press.

Gunnar MR, Morison SJ, Chisholm K, Schuder M. (2001). Salivary cortisol levels in children adopted from Romanian orphanages. *Development Psychopathology* 13:611–627.

Gunnar MR, van Dulmen MH. (2007). Behavior problems in postinstitutionalized internationally adopted children. *Development Psychopathology* 19(1):129–148.

Gunnar MR, Wenner JA, Thomas KM, Glatt CE, McKenna MC, Clark AG. (2012). The brain–derived neurotrophic factor Val66Met polymorphism moderates early deprivation effects on attention problems. *Development Psychopathology* 24:1215–1223.

Hanson JL, Adluru N, Chung MK, Alexander AL, Davidson RJ, et al. (2013a). Early neglect is associated with alterations in white matter integrity and cognitive functioning. *Child Dev* 84:1566–1578.

Hanson JL, Hair N, Shen DG, Shi F, Gilmore JH, Wolfe BL, Pollak SD. (2013b). Family poverty affects the rate of human infant brain growth. *PLoS One* 8(12):e80954.

Hanson JL, Nacewicz BM, Sutterer MJ, Cayo AA, Schaefer SM, Rudolph KD, Davidson RJ. (in press). Behavioral problems after early life stress: Contributions of the hippocampus and amygdala. *Biological Psychiatry*.

Helmeke C, Ovtscharoff W, Poeggel G, Braun K. (2001). Juvenile emotional experience alters synaptic inputs on pyramidal neurons in the anterior cingulate cortex. *Cerebral Cortex* 11(8):717–727.

Hodel AS, Hunt RH, Cowell RA, Van Den Heuvel SE, Gunnar MR, Thomas KM. (2015). Duration of early adversity and structural brain development in post–institutionalized adolescents 105:112–119.

Hodges J, Tizard B. (1989). Social and family relationships of ex–institutional adolescents. *J Child Psychology Psychiatry Allied Disciplines* 30:77–97.

Hostinar CE, Stellern SA, Schaefer C, Carlson SM, Gunnar MR. (2012). Associations between early life adversity and executive function in children adopted internationally from orphanages. *Proc Natl Acad Sci USA* 109(Suppl 2):17208–12.

Johnson AE, Bruce J, Tarullo AR, Gunnar MR. (2011). Growth delay as an index of allostatic load in young children: Predictions to disinhibited social approach and diurnal cortisol activity. *Development Psychopathology* 23:859–871.

Juffer F, van Ijzendoorn MH. (2005). Behavior problems and mental health referrals of international adoptees: a meta–analysis. *JAMA* 293(20):2501–2515.

Juffer F, Hoksbergen RA, Riksen–Walraven JM, Kohnstamm GA. (1997). Early intervention in adoptive families: supporting maternal sensitive responsiveness, infant–mother attachment, and infant competence. *J Child Psychol Psychiatry* 38(8):1039–1050.

Kertes DA, Gunnar MR, Madsen NJ, Long J. (2008). Early deprivation and home basal cortisol levels: A study of internationally–adopted children. *Development Psychopathology* 20: 473–491.

Kolb B, Mychasiuk R, Muhammad A, Li Y, Frost, DO, Gibb R. (2012). Experience and the developing prefrontal cortex. *Proc Natl Acad Sci USA* 109:17186–93. doi:10.1073/pnas .1121251109.

Kreppner JM, Rutter M, Beckett C, Castle J, Colvert E, Groothues C, Sonuga–Barke EJS. (2007). Normality and impairment following profound early institutional deprivation: a longitudinal follow–up into early adolescence. *Developmental Psychology* 43:931–946.

Kroupina MG, Bauer PJ, Gunnar MR, Johnson DE. (2010). Institutional care as a risk for declarative memory development. In: *Varieties of Early Experience: Implications for the Development of Declarative Memory in Infancy*, ed. P.J. Bauer, pp. 137–159. Advances in Child Development and Behavior 38. London: Elsevier.

Lawler JM, Hostinar CE, Mliner SB, Gunnar MR. (2014). Disinhibited social engagement in postinstitutionalized children: Differentiating normal from atypical behavior. *Development Psychopathology* 26(2):451–464.

Loman MM, Johnson AE, Westerlund A, Pollak SD, Nelson CA, Gunnar MR. (2013). The effect of early deprivation on executive attention in middle childhood. *J Child Psychol Psychiatry* 54(1):37–45.

Lyons DM, Afarian H, Schatzberg AF, Sawyer–Glover A, Moseley ME. (2002). Experience–dependent asymmetric variation in primate prefrontal morphology. *Behavioral Brain Research* 136:51–59.

Maheu FS, Dozier M, Guyer AE, Mandell D, Peloso E, Poeth K, Jenness J, Lau JYF, Ackerman JP, Pine DS, Ernst M. (2010). A preliminary study of medial temporal lobe function in youths with a history of caregiver deprivation and emotional neglect. *Cogn Affect Behav Neurosci* 10:34–49.

Marshall PJ, Fox NA. (2004). A comparison of the electroencephalogram between institution-alized and community children in Romania. *J Cognitive NeuroSci* 16:1327–1338.

Marshall PJ, Bar–Haim Y, Fox NA. (2002). Development of the EEG from 5 months to 4 years of age. *Clinical Neuropsychology* 113:1199–1208.

McCall RB. (2011). Research, practice, and policy perspectives on issues of children without permanent parental care. *Monographs Society Research Child Development* 76(4):223–272.

McDermott JM, Troller–Renfree S, Vanderwert R, Nelson CA, Zeanah CH, Fox NA. (2013). Psychosocial deprivation, executive functions, and the emergence of socio–emotional behavior problems. *Front Hum Neurosci* 7:167.

McGoron L, Gleason MM, Smyke AT, Drury SS, Nelson, CA. 3rd, Gregas MC, Fox NA, Zeanah CH. (2012). Recovering from early deprivation: attachment mediates effects of caregiving on psychopathology. *J Am Acad Child Adolesc Psychiatry* 51(7):683–693.

McLaughlin KA, Fox NA, Zeanah CH, Nelson CA. (2011). Adverse rearing environments and neural development in children: the development of frontal electroencephalogram asymmetry. *Biol Psychiatry* 70:1008–15.

Mehta MA, Golembo NI, Nosarti C, Colvert E, Mota A, Williams SC, Rutter M, Sonuga–Barke EJ. (2009). Amygdala, hippocampal and corpus callosum size following severe early institutional deprivation: the English and Romanian Adoptees study pilot. *J Child Psychology Psychiatry* 50:943–951.

Merz EC, McCall RB, Wright AJ, Luna B. (2013). Inhibitory control and working memory in post–institutionalized children. *J Abnorm Child Psychol* 41(6):879–890.

Moulson MC, Fox NA, Zeanah CH, Nelson CA. (2009). Early adverse experiences and the neurobiology of facial emotion processing. *Developmental Psychology* 45(1):17–30.

Naumova OY, Lee M, Koposov R, Szyf M, Dozier M, Grigorenko EL. (2012). Differential patterns of whole–genome DNA methylation in institutionalized children and children raised by their biological parents. *Development Psychopathology* 24:143–155.

Nelson CA, Parker SW, Guthrie D. (2006). The discrimination of facial expressions by typically developing infants and toddlers and those experiencing early institutional care. *Infant Behavior and Development* 29:210–219.

Nelson CA III,, Zeanah CH, Fox NA, Marshall PJ, Smyke AT, Guthrie D. (2007). Cognitive recovery in socially deprived young children: the Bucharest Early Intervention Project. *Science* 318:1937–1940.

Nishida M, Makris N, Kennedy DN, Vangel M, Fischl B, Krishnamoorthy KS, Grant PE. (2006). Detailed semiautomated MRI based morphometry of the neonatal brain: Preliminary results. *NeuroImage* 32(3):1041–1049. doi:10.1016/j.neuroimage.2006.05.020.

Pechtel P, Pizzagalli DA. (2010). Effects of early life stress on cognitive and affective function: an integrated review of human literature. *Psychopharmacology* 214:55–70.

Pollak SD, Nelson CA, Schlaak MF, Roeber BJ, Wewerka SS, Wiik KL, et al. (2010). Neurodevelopmental effects of early deprivation in postinstitutionalized children. *Child Dev* 81:224–236.

Roy P, Rutter M, Pickles A. (2004). Institutional care: associations between overactivity and lack of selectivity in social relationships. *J Child Psychol Psychiatry* 45(4):866–873.

Rutter M. (2002). Maternal deprivation. In: *Handbook of Parenting*, 2nd ed., ed. M.H. Bornstein, pp. 181–202. Mahwah, NJ: Erlbaum.

Rutter M, Sonuga–Barke EJS, Castle J. (2010). Investigating the impact of early institutional deprivation on development: Background and Research Strategy of the English and Romanian Adoptees (ERA) Study. *Monographs Society Research Child Development* 75(1): 1–20.

Sheridan M, Fox N, Zeanah C, McLaughlin K, Nelson, C. (2012). Variation in neural development as a result of exposure to institutionalization early in childhood. *Proc Natl Acad Sci USA* 109(32):12927–12932.

Smyke AT, Zeanah CH, Fox NA, Nelson CA, Guthrie, D. (2010). Placement in foster care enhances quality of attachment among young institutionalized children. *Child Development* 81:212–223.

Spinelli S, Chefer S, Sumoi SS, Higley JD, Barr CS, Stein E. (2009). Early–life stress induces long–term morphologic changes in primate brain. *Archives General Psychiatry* 66(6):658–665.

St. Petersburg–USA Orphanage Research Team. (2008). The effects of early social–emotional and relationship experience on the development of young orphanage children. *Monographs Society Research Child Development* 73(3):1–298.

Stevens S, Kumsta R, Kreppner J, Brookes K, Rutter M, Sonuga–Barke EJS. (2009). Dopamine transporter gene polymorphism moderates the effects of severe deprivation on ADHD symptoms: Developmental continuities in gene–environment interplay. *Am J Medical Genetics Part B* 150B:753–761.

Tarullo AR, Bruce J, Gunnar MR. (2007). False belief and emotion understanding in post–institutionalized children. *Social Development* 16:57–78.

Tarullo AR, Garvin MC, Gunnar MR. (2011). Atypical EEG power correlates with indiscriminately friendly behavior in internationally adopted children. *Developmental Psychology* 47:417–431.

Tizard B, Joseph A. (1970). Cognitive development of young children in residential care: a study of children aged 24 months. *J Child Psychology Psychiatry Allied Disciplines* 11:177–186.

Tottenham N. (2012). Human amygdala development in the absence of species–expected caregiving. *Development Psychobiology* 54(6):598–611.

Tottenham N, Hare TA, Quinn BT, McCarry TW, Nurse M, Gilhooly T, Casey BJ. (2010). Prolonged institutional rearing is associated with atypically large amygdala volume and difficulties in emotion regulation. *Developmental Sci* 13:46–61.

Tottenham N, Hare TA, Millner A, Gilhooly T, Zevin JD, Casey BJ. (2011). Elevated amygdala response to faces following early deprivation. *Developmental Sci* 14:190–204.

van der Vegt EJ, van der Ende J, Ferdinand RF, Verhulst FC, Tiemeier H. (2009). Early childhood adversities and trajectories of psychiatric problems in adoptees: evidence for long lasting effects. *J Abnormal Child Psychology* 37(2):239–249.

van Ijzendoorn MH, Juffer F. (2006). The Emanuel Miller Memorial Lecture 2006: adoption as intervention. Meta–analytic evidence for massive catch–up and plasticity in physical, socio–emotional, and cognitive development. *J Child Psychology Psychiatry* 47(12):1228–1245.

van Ijzendoorn MH, Juffer F, Poelhuis CW. (2005). Adoption and cognitive development: a meta–analytic comparison of adopted and nonadopted children's IQ and school performance. *Psychological Bulletin* 131:301–316.

van IJzendoorn MH, Luijk MPCM, Juffer F. (2008). IQ of children growing up in children's homes: A meta–analysis on IQ delays in orphanages. *Merrill–Palmer Quarterly* 54(3):341–356.

Walshaw PD, Alloy LB, Sabb FW. (2010). Executive function in pediatric bipolar disorder and attention deficit hyperactivity disorder: in search of distinct phenotypic profiles. *Neuropsychol Rev* 20(1):103–120.

Wiik KL, Loman MM, Van Ryzin MJ, Armstrong JM, Essex MJ, Pollak SD, Gunnar MR. (2011). Behavioral and emotional symptoms of post–institutionalized children in middle childhood. *J Child Psychology Psychiatry* 52(1):56–63.

Windsor J, Benigno JP, Wing CA, Carroll PJ, Koga SF, Nelson CA, Fox NA, Zeanah CH. (2011). Effect of foster care on young children's language learning. *Child Dev* 82:1040–1046.

Windsor J, Moraru A, Nelson CA, Fox NA, Zeanah CH. (2013). Effect of foster care on language learning at eight years: findings from the Bucharest Early Intervention Project. *J Child Language* 40(3):605–627.

Zeanah CH, Smyke AT, Dumitrescu A. (2002). Attachment disturbances in young children. II: Indiscriminate behavior and institutional care. *J Am Academy Child Adolescent Psychiatry* 41:983–989.

Zeanah CH, Egger HL, Smyke AT, Nelson CA, Fox NA, Marshall PJ, et al. (2009). Institutional rearing and psychiatric disorders in romanian preschool children. *Am J Psychiatry* 166(7):777–785.

Zhang L, Levine S, Dent G, Zhan Y, Xing G, Okimoto D, and Smith MA. (2002). Maternal deprivation increases cell death in the infant rat brain. *Developmental Brain Research* 133:1–11.

CHAPTER 10

Impact of infantile massage on brain development

Andrea Guzzetta[1,2,3] and Giovanni Cioni[1,2]

[1] Department of Clinical and Experimental Medicine, Pisa University, Pisa, Italy
[2] Department of Developmental Neuroscience, Stella Maris Scientific Institute, Pisa, Italy
[3] SMILE Lab, Stella Maris Scientific Institute, Pisa, Italy

Introduction

While during intrauterine life the fetus is protected by noxius external stimuli and benefits from positive physiological stimulations such as the continuous and gentle tactile stimulation deriving from the movements inside the womb, birth exposes the fetus to a completely new and potentially stressful environment. This is particularly true in case birth occurs prior to the due date, as in more than 1 in every 19 newborns, when this nonphysiological environment with unfiltered stimuli deprives the infant from the positive stimulations of the womb, potentially resulting in detrimental effects on the development of the immature brain (Saigal and Doyle, 2008). Indeed, it is today well recognized that preterm infants are at higher risk for developmental and cognitive delays, as well as difficulties in the mother–infant relationship across infancy (Feldman and Eidelman, 2006; Vanderveen et al., 2009). Follow-up studies of preterm individuals into the school years consistently found reduced cognitive performance and increased behavioral problems in these children. To minimize the consequences of preterm birth it is of utmost importance to take the highest advantage of enhanced early brain plasticity by devising evidence-based intervention programs centered on the optimization of the infant's environment.

Early intervention programs and infant massage

On these grounds, early intervention programs based on the manipulation of the extra-uterine environment have been used in infants at neurological risk with the aim of optimizing the infant's sensory experience and thus potentially

Environmental Experience and Plasticity of the Developing Brain, First Edition.
Edited by Alessandro Sale.

improving development and functional outcome (Symington and Pinelli, 2006). According to Hadders-Algra (Blauw-Hospers and Hadders-Algra, 2005), early intervention consists of *"multidisciplinary services provided to children from birth to 5 years of age to promote child health and well-being, enhance emerging competencies, minimize developmental delay, remediate existing or emerging disabilities, prevent functional deterioration, and promote adaptive parenting and overall family functioning."* The concept of early intervention thus includes both prevention and rehabilitation and may be interpreted as two different phases of the same process for those children who, at a later age, show a specific neurodevelopmental dysfunction (physical, linguistic, cognitive, educational, behavioral).

Among the early intervention programs, infant massage and interventions based on the provision of skin-to-skin contact have demonstrated important positive effects. Infant massage is based on tactile, vestibular, auditory, visual, and kinesthetic stimulations, used alone or in various multisensory combinations, in order to make up for the impoverishment of the various stimuli that preterm infants would otherwise experience in the intrauterine environment or with postnatal mothering care (Montagu, 1978). Massage therapy was introduced in the neonatal intensive care unit (NICU) primarily with the aim of improving weight gain, in particular in low birth-weight subjects during their hospital admission and, as a consequence, to obtain an earlier hospital discharge (Field, 2002).

The term "massage" refers to any form of tactile skin stimulation performed by human hands. There are differences in technique, for example, in the pressure applied and the sequences in which each body part is massaged. The type of massage used in NICU is gentle, slow stroking and involves all parts of the body. In the model proposed by Tiffany Field (Scafidi and Field, 1996), preterm infants receive 15-minute massage three times a day for 10 days, and each stimulation session consists of three standardized 5-minute phases (Figure 10.1). Tactile stimulation is given during the first and third phases, while kinesthetic stimuli are applied during the middle phase. Massage therapy begins with the infant in a prone position followed by a middle supine phase and a final prone one. Gentle stroking is carried out with warm hands following a well-defined and sequenced methodology. Gentle, "minimal" touch is another technique applied by nurses who place their hands on the infants gently as they sleep. The hands should not move or stroke the skin and are removed after 15 or 20 minutes. Another kind of approach called "positive touch" has been proposed by Bond (Bond, 2002). This method is primarily practiced by parents and involves various types of infant touch interaction including handling, holding, kangaroo care (or skin-to-skin contact care), and massage.

Several studies using infant massage have shown positive effects on weight gain, behavioral reactions, postnatal complications, and hospital discharge (Wheeden et al., 1993; Scafidi and Field, 1997). Hormonal changes, in particular decreased blood cortisol, have also been reported in massaged preterm infants

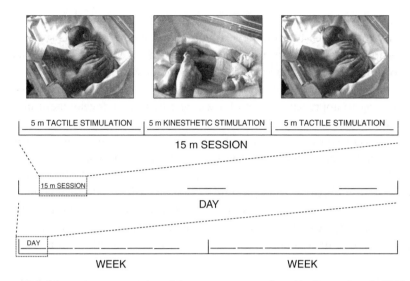

Figure 10.1 Schematic representation of the massage protocol used in Guzzetta et al., 2009, based on the one proposed by Tiffany Field. The protocol consists of 2 weeks of intervention with 1-day pause, with three 15-minute sessions per day. Each session is composed of two 5-minute tactile stimulations and one 5-minute kinesthetic stimulation.

(Schanberg and Field, 1987; Acolet et al., 1993). In a recent Cochrane Review by Vickers et al. (2004), it was reported that massage intervention improved daily weight gain and reduced the length of hospital stay, although there were methodological concerns about the blindness of the observers on this outcome. There was also some evidence that massage intervention has a slight positive effect on postnatal complications and weight at 4–6 months. It is of interest that the effects of these interventions on brain development have been dramatically less explored in the scientific literature, probably also due to the challenges correlated with the implementation of early instrumental evaluations on such vulnerable populations.

Infant massage as a model of environmental enrichment

In Chapter 1, the model of environmental enrichment as a noninvasive paradigm for plasticity enhancement was extensively reviewed and discussed. For several reasons, infant massage has been considered as a valid model of environmental enrichment in humans. Indeed, it represents a well-known and widely used approach in NICUs, and since data in rodents show that pups reared in an enriched environment receive in their first days of life a greater amount of tactile stimulation, through maternal licking, grooming, and physical contact, it can be hypothesized that tactile stimulation represents a crucial component in early environmental enrichment. Also, preterm infants can be considered to some extent exposed to an impoverished environment, where sensory stimulations and human contacts are reduced or disturbed. Massage has an effect in both counteracting the stress-inducing stimuli of the NICU (bright light, constant noise, and so on) and providing an additional amount of tactile stimulation, thus constituting an approach capable of assisting growth and development in these selected newborns.

In a recent study in preterm infants we have reported a significant effect of massage on the maturation of visual function, in line with the findings of a parallel protocol in a mouse model (Guzzetta et al., 2009). We found a larger latency shortening of the most prominent peak of flash visual evoked potentials, N300, between pre- and postmassage assessments in massaged babies, relative to a control group, associated with an increase of behavioral visual acuity persisting beyond 3 months of post-term age (Figure 10.2). The effects of massage on

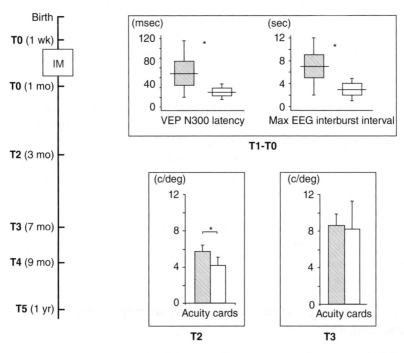

Figure 10.2 Schematic representation of the results from Guzzetta et al., 2009. On the left side the time of intervention and the time of assessments are indicated. In the insets, main results are shown. T1-T0: Difference between premassage and postmassage assessment of VEP N300 latency and maximum EEG interburst interval. Boxes indicate median (black horizontal line), interquartile values, and range. Massaged infants show larger differences between T1 and T0, which are statistically significant from those in controls. T2 and T3: Behavioral visual acuity measured in cycles per degree (c/deg) by means of the Vital-Durand Acuity Cards at 3 and 7 months corrected age. Bars indicate mean values and SEM. Visual acuity in massaged infants is significantly higher than in controls at 3 months, but the difference is no longer present at 7 months.

visual acuity development were evident at 3 months of age – that is, more than 2 months after the end of the massage protocol – but were no longer present at 7 months of age. This might be related to a greater sensitivity of the earliest phases of visual acuity development, characterized by the most rapid maturation of the visual cortex and visual acuity, or to the endogenous factors modulated by massage for the rather short period of the intervention.

In the same study, we also found an increase in IGF-1 blood levels in the subgroup of preterm infants receiving massage as opposed to controls. The same finding had been previously reported in preterm infants undergoing massage therapy (Field et al., 2008) and was considered as one of the underlying mechanisms for massage-related weight gain (Field et al., 2011). It is reasonable that IGF-1 could also play a role as a mediator of the effects of therapeutic massage on visual development in infants, as in rats. This could occur through an acceleration of the maturation of the intracortical inhibitory circuits that shape the receptive fields of the visual cortex (Sillito, 1975; Ciucci et al., 2007). Recently, the presence of lower plasma levels of IGF-1 and IGF-1 binding protein in premature subjects has been correlated with an increased incidence of retinopathy of prematurity (ROP) (Hellstrom et al., 2003; Lofqvist et al., 2007). Thus, therapeutic massage, causing an increase in plasma IGF-1 and to a lesser extent IGF binding protein-3, could have a clinical application in preterm infants, especially between 30 and 35 weeks of postmenstrual age when typically ROP is induced (Hellstrom et al., 2003).

The effects of infant massage do not seem to be limited to the visual system. A visual analysis of electroencephalography (EEG) showed a much larger degree of shortening of the interburst intervals during quiet sleep between pre- and postmassage assessments in massaged babies, relative to a comparison group, suggesting a more global effect of massage on brain electrical activity. In a further study, we found a significant difference in spectral power during active sleep between preterm newborns who underwent massage therapy and those who did not. In particular, the variation of global EEG power before and after intervention was significantly different between the two groups for the slow frequencies (0.5 to 4 Hz), owing to a reduction of delta power in control infants relative to the massaged ones (Guzzetta et al., 2011). This difference was especially observed in the perirolandic regions. More recently, acceleration of brain maturation as measured with different parameters of EEG complexity was also reported in healthy preterm infants undergoing skin-to-skin contact, a different kind of neurodevelopmental intervention (Scher et al., 2009; Kaffashi et al., 2013). Furthermore, an increase in the EEG power in the frontal polar region at higher frequencies (10–48 Hz) was reported in a large group of 134 preterm infants undergoing a neurodevelopmental intervention that included touch (Welch et al., 2014). The intervention consisted of sessions designed to achieve mutual calm and promote communication of affect between infants and their mothers throughout the NICU stay. Effects were significant in both quiet and active sleep, regardless of gender, singleton-twin status, gestational age (26–30 or 30–35 weeks), or birth weight (<1500 or >1500 g).

The effects of infant massage on brain electrical activity have also been tested directly during the administration of the intervention (Rudnicki et al., 2012). Rudnicki et al. found that massage therapy can benefit infants born preterm by stimulating electrical activity in the brain, therefore promoting brain maturation. In a study with 35 infants born preterm with gestational ages ranging from 28 to 37 weeks, massage significantly increased the amplitude of amplitude-integrated electroencephalography (aEEG) and also affected dominant frequency delta waves.

Taken together, all these electrophysiological findings support the assumption that infant massage, or other interventions based on human touch, have the potential to modify brain electrical activity in preterm newborns, a key element being the ability to maintain high-power EEG activity, and in particular slow wave activity during sleep. Indeed, the reduction of slow wave power seems to be a typical effect of extra-uterine life in preterm born infants, as shown by the consistent reports of lower delta power in preterm infants at term age compared with term newborns (i.e., at a comparable postconceptional age) (Scher et al., 1994a, 1994b; Scher et al., 1997), and by the observation that in preterm infants EEG spectral power tends to decrease from birth to term age (Bell et al., 1991; Okumura et al., 2003). Also, preterm infants born at different gestational ages have undistinguishable EEG power at similar postnatal age, suggesting that energy reduction is related to postnatal age (and thus to the duration of extra-uterine life) rather than gestational age (Batuev et al., 2008).

The relatively low spectral power in preterm infants at term has been interpreted as the effect of a functional alteration in brain development related to the untimely exposure to the extra-uterine environment (Scher et al., 1994a, 1994b). More specifically, it has been proposed that the extra-uterine environment is inadequate to support the maturation of the thalamocortical network, resulting in an impoverishment of neuronal aggregates in this network, with the consequence of the reduction of the oscillatory potentials. It is of interest that a direct link has been already demonstrated in adults between exploratory behavior, cortical expression of brain-derived neurotrophic factor, and spectral power of slow wave activity, supporting the notion that sleep EEG is heavily influenced by the richness of preceding wakefulness (Faraguna et al., 2008). This effect on sleep does not seem to involve its induction (Underdown et al., 2006; Yates et al., 2014) nor its overall duration, which was reported to be, on the contrary, reduced (Dieter et al., 2003). Rather, it might affect the quality of sleep and with it the duration of the wakefulness following it (Yates et al., 2014).

The effect of massage seems to have a topographic distribution. In our study, the increase of local absolute power of delta and beta band activity was indeed limited to the central regions, which seem to be therefore a target region for early neurodevelopmental intervention. Regional patterns of sleep EEG modification after local activation of brain regions during wakefulness have been reported both in the animal model and in humans (Kattler et al., 1994; Vyazovskiy et al., 2006). In preterm infants, some reports show reduced white matter development in several frontal lobe projections compared with healthy term infants imaged at the same postmenstrual age (Rose et al., 2008). Interestingly, Als et al. (2004) studied a group of preterm infants enrolled in a neurodevelopmental intervention (NIDCAP) trial, reporting higher relative anisotropy in frontal white matter and increased coherence between frontal and occipital brain regions. Altogether these findings may suggest that in preterm infants the maturation of the connectivity of the central regions is sensitive to the exposition to extra-uterine environment and can be effectively modulated by early intervention.

Summary and conclusions

The evidence of the effects of infant massage on brain development is still very scanty. What is fascinating, however, is the hypothesis that the effects observed in massaged infants, both at an electrophysiological and structural level, are directly related to the postnatal enrichment represented by the multisensorial stimulation, mediated by an action on synaptic activity similar to that observed in enriched animals. On these grounds, it is safe to suggest that in low-risk preterm infants massage therapy favors a process of maturation of brain electrical activity similar to that observed (in utero) in term infants, probably through an attenuation of the discrepancies between the extra- and the intrauterine environments. It is not clear whether other types of intervention might have the same effects, and to some extent it is very likely that all those interventions that are based on early intersubjectivity and meaningful human interaction will produce similar positive results. We are still walking the first steps of a long path of knowledge, but the chances are high that it will lead us to a fuller understanding of the deep mechanisms of early neurodevelopment in both typical conditions and that we will proficiently use this knowledge for early intervention in adverse conditions.

References

Acolet D, Modi N, Giannakoulopoulos X, Bond C, Weg W, Clow A, Glover V. (1993). Changes in plasma cortisol and catecholamine concentrations in response to massage in preterm infants. *Arch Dis Child* 68(1 Spec No):29–31.

Als H, Duffy FH, McAnulty GB, Rivkin MJ, Vajapeyam S, Mulkern RV, et al. (2004). Early experience alters brain function and structure. *Pediatrics* 113(4):846–857.

Batuev AS, Iovleva NN, Koshchavtsev AG. (2008). Comparative analysis of the EEG in babies in the first month of life with gestation periods of 30–42 weeks. *Neurosci Behav Physiol* 38(6):621–626.

Bell AH, McClure BG, McCullagh PJ, McClelland RJ. (1991). Variation in power spectral analysis of the EEG with gestational age. *J Clin Neurophysiol* 8(3):312–319.

Blauw-Hospers CH, Hadders-Algra M. (2005). A systematic review of the effects of early intervention on motor development. *Dev Med Child Neurol* 47(6):421–432.

Bond C. (2002). Positive Touch and massage in the neonatal unit: a British approach. *Semin Neonatol* 7(6):477–486.

Ciucci F, Putignano E, Baroncelli L, Landi S, Berardi N, Maffei L. (2007). Insulin-like growth factor 1 (IGF-1) mediates the effects of enriched environment (EE) on visual cortical development. *PLoS One* 2(5):e475.

Dieter JN, Field T, Hernandez-Reif M, Emory EK, Redzepi M. (2003). Stable preterm infants gain more weight and sleep less after five days of massage therapy. *J Pediatr Psychol* 28(6):403–411.

Faraguna U, Vyazovskiy VV, Nelson AB, Tononi G, Cirelli C. (2008). A causal role for brain-derived neurotrophic factor in the homeostatic regulation of sleep. *J Neurosci* 28(15):4088–4095.

Feldman R, Eidelman AI. (2006). Neonatal state organization, neuromaturation, mother-infant interaction, and cognitive development in small-for-gestational-age premature infants. *Pediatrics* 118(3):e869–878.

Field T. (2002). Massage therapy. *Med Clin North Am* 86(1):163–171.

Field T, Diego M, Hernandez-Reif M, Dieter JN, Kumar AM, Schanberg S, Kuhn C. (2008). Insulin and insulin-like growth factor-1 increased in preterm neonates following massage therapy. *J Dev Behav Pediatr* 29(6):463–466.

Field T, Diego M, Hernandez-Reif M. (2011). Potential underlying mechanisms for greater weight gain in massaged preterm infants. *Infant Behav Dev* 34(3):383–389.

Guzzetta A, Baldini S, Bancale A, Baroncelli L, Ciucci F, Ghirri P, Putignano E, Sale A, Viegi A, Berardi N, Boldrini A, Cioni G, Maffei L. (2009). Massage accelerates brain development and the maturation of visual function. *J Neurosci* 29(18):6042–6051.

Guzzetta A, D'Acunto MG, Carotenuto M, Berardi N, Bancale A, Biagioni E, Boldrini A, Ghirri P, Maffei L, Cioni G. (2011). The effects of preterm infant massage on brain electrical activity. *Dev Med Child Neurol* 53 Suppl 4:46–51.

Hellstrom A, Engstrom E, Hard AL, et al. (2003). Postnatal serum insulin-like growth factor I deficiency is associated with retinopathy of prematurity and other complications of premature birth. *Pediatrics* 112(5):1016–1020.

Kaffashi F, Scher MS, Ludington-Hoe SM, Loparo KA. (2013). An analysis of the kangaroo care intervention using neonatal EEG complexity: a preliminary study. *Clin Neurophysiol* 124(2):238–246.

Kattler H, Dijk DJ, Borbely AA. (1994). Effect of unilateral somatosensory stimulation prior to sleep on the sleep EEG in humans. *J Sleep Res* 3(3):159–164.

Lofqvist C, Chen J, Connor KM, et al. (2007). IGFBP3 suppresses retinopathy through suppression of oxygen-induced vessel loss and promotion of vascular regrowth. *Proc Natl Acad Sci U S A* 104(25):10589–10594.

Montagu A. (1978). *Touching : The Human Significance of the Skin*. New York: Harper & Row.

Okumura A, Kubota T, Toyota N, et al. (2003). Amplitude spectral analysis of maturational changes of delta waves in preterm infants. *Brain Dev* 25(6):406–410.

Rose SE, Hatzigeorgiou X, Strudwick MW, Durbridge G, Davies PS, Colditz PB. (2008). Altered white matter diffusion anisotropy in normal and preterm infants at term-equivalent age. *Magn Reson Med* 60(4):761–767.

Rudnicki J, Boberski M, Butrymowicz E, et al. (2012). Recording of amplitude-integrated electroencephalography, oxygen saturation, pulse rate, and cerebral blood flow during massage of premature infants. *Am J Perinatol* 29(7):561–566.

Saigal S, Doyle LW. (2008). An overview of mortality and sequelae of preterm birth from infancy to adulthood. *Lancet* 371(9608):261–269.

Scafidi F, Field T. (1996). Massage therapy improves behavior in neonates born to HIV-positive mothers. *J Pediatr Psychol* 21(6):889–897.

Scafidi F, Field T. (1997). Brief report: HIV-exposed newborns show inferior orienting and abnormal reflexes on the Brazelton Scale. *J Pediatr Psychol* 22(1):105–112.

Schanberg SM, Field TM. (1987). Sensory deprivation stress and supplemental stimulation in the rat pup and preterm human neonate. *Child Dev* 58(6):1431–1447.

Scher MS, Sun M, Steppe DA, Banks DL, Guthrie RD, Sclabassi RJ. (1994a). Comparisons of EEG sleep state-specific spectral values between healthy full-term and preterm infants at comparable postconceptional ages. *Sleep* 17(1):47–51.

Scher MS, Sun M, Steppe DA, Guthrie RD, Sclabassi RJ. (1994b). Comparisons of EEG spectral and correlation measures between healthy term and preterm infants. *Pediatr Neurol* 10(2):104–108.

Scher MS, Steppe DA, Sclabassi RJ, Banks DL. (1997). Regional differences in spectral EEG measures between healthy term and preterm infants. *Pediatr Neurol* 17(3):218–223.

Scher MS, Ludington-Hoe S, Kaffashi F, Johnson MW, Holditch-Davis D, Loparo KA. (2009). Neurophysiologic assessment of brain maturation after an 8-week trial of skin-to-skin contact on preterm infants. *Clin Neurophysiol* 120(10):1812–1818.

Sillito AM. (1975). The contribution of inhibitory mechanisms to the receptive field properties of neurones in the striate cortex of the cat. *J Physiol* 250(2):305–329.

Symington A, Pinelli J. (2006). Developmental care for promoting development and preventing morbidity in preterm infants. *Cochrane Database Syst Rev* (2):CD001814.

Underdown A, Barlow J, Chung V, Stewart-Brown S. (2006). Massage intervention for promoting mental and physical health in infants aged under six months. *Cochrane Database Syst Rev* (4):CD005038.

Vanderveen JA, Bassler D, Robertson CM, Kirpalani H. (2009). Early interventions involving parents to improve neurodevelopmental outcomes of premature infants: a meta-analysis. *J Perinatol* 29(5):343–351.

Vickers A, Ohlsson A, Lacy JB, Horsley A. (2004). Massage for promoting growth and development of preterm and/or low birth-weight infants. *Cochrane Database Syst Rev* (2):CD000390.

Vyazovskiy VV, Ruijgrok G, Deboer T, Tobler I. (2006). Running wheel accessibility affects the regional electroencephalogram during sleep in mice. *Cereb Cortex* 16(3):328–336.

Welch MG, Myers MM, Grieve PG, et al. (2014). Electroencephalographic activity of preterm infants is increased by Family Nurture Intervention: a randomized controlled trial in the NICU. *Clin Neurophysiol* 125(4):675–684.

Wheeden A, Scafidi FA, Field T, Ironson G, Valdeon C, Bandstra E. (1993). Massage effects on cocaine-exposed preterm neonates. *J Dev Behav Pediatr* 14(5):318–322.

Yates CC, Mitchell AJ, Booth MY, Williams DK, Lowe LM, Whit Hall R. (2014). The effects of massage therapy to induce sleep in infants born preterm. *Pediatr Phys Ther* 26(4):405–410.

Index

Environmental Experience and Plasticity of the Developing Brain, First Edition.
Edited by Alessandro Sale.
© 2016 John Wiley & Sons, Inc. Published 2016 by John Wiley & Sons, Inc.